Making Decisions

EVIDENCE AND INFORMATION

CANADA HEALTH ACTION: BUILDING ON THE LEGACY
PAPERS COMMISSIONED BY THE NATIONAL FORUM ON HEALTH

Making Decisions

EVIDENCE AND INFORMATION

ÉDITIONS
MULTIMONDES

FORUM NATIONAL
SUR LA SANTÉ

NATIONAL FORUM
ON HEALTH

Canadian Cataloguing in Publication Data

Main entry under title:

Canada Health Action: Building on the Legacy

Issued also in French under title: La santé au Canada: un héritage à faire fructifier
To be complete in 5 v.
Includes bibliographical references.
Contents: v. 1 Childen and Youth – v. 2. Adults and Seniors – v. 3. Settings
and Issues – v. 4. Health Care Systems in Canada and Elsewhere – v. 5 Evidence
and Information.
ISBN 2-921146-62-2 (set)
ISBN 2-921146-53-3 (v. 5)

1. Public health – Canada. 2. Medicine, Preventive – Canada. 3. Children – Health
and hygiene – Canada. 4. Adulthood – Health and hygiene – Canada. 5. Aged –
Health and hygiene – Canada. I. National Forum on Health (Canada).

RA449.C28 1998   362.1'0971   C97-941659-0

Linguistic Revision: Traduction Tandem
Proofreading: Traduction Tandem and Robert Paré
Cover Design: Gérard Beaudry
Graphics: Emmanuel Gagnon

Volume 5: Evidence and Information
ISBN 2-921146-53-3   Cat. No.: H21-126/6-5-1997E
Legal Deposit– Bibliothèque nationale du Québec, 1998
Legal Deposit – National Library of Canada, 1998
© Her Majesty the Queen in Right of Canada, 1998

The series The National Forum on Health can be ordered at this address:
Éditions MultiMondes
930, rue Pouliot
Sainte-Foy (Québec)
G1V 3N9 CANADA
Telephone: (418) 651-3885; toll free in North America: 1 800 840-3029
Fax: (418) 651 6822; toll free in North America: 1 888 303-5931
E-mail: multimondes@multim.com
Internet: http://www.multim.com

Published by Éditions MultiMondes in co-operation with the National Forum on Health, Health
Canada, and Canadian Government Publishing, Public Works and Government Services Canada.

In this publication the masculine form is used solely for ease of readability.

FOREWORD

In October 1994, the Prime Minister of Canada, The Right Honourable Jean Chrétien, launched the National Forum on Health to involve and inform Canadians and to advise the federal government on innovative ways to improve the health system and the health of Canada's people. The Forum was set up as an advisory body with the Prime Minister as Chair, the federal Minister of Health as Vice Chair, and 24 volunteer members who contributed a wide range of knowledge founded on involvement in the health system as professionals, consumers and volunteers.

To fulfil their mandate, the Forum focused on long-term and systemic issues. They saw their task as formulating advice appropriate to the development of national policies, and divided the work into four key areas – Values, Striking a Balance, Determinants of Health, and Evidence-Based Decision Making.

The complete report of the National Forum on Health consists of two volumes:

Canada Health Action: Building on the Legacy
The Final Report of the National Forum on Health
and
Canada Health Action: Building on the Legacy
Synthesis Reports and Issues Papers

Copies available from: Publications Distribution Centre, Health Canada Communications, PL. 090124C, Brooke Claxton Building, Tunney's Pasture, Ottawa, Ontario K1A 0K9. Telephone: (613) 954-5995. Fax: (613) 941-5366. *(Aussi disponible en français.)*

The Forum based its recommendations on 42 research papers written by the most eminent specialists in the field. The papers are brought together in a five-volume series:

VOLUME 1 – CHILDREN AND YOUTH
VOLUME 2 – ADULTS AND SENIORS
VOLUME 3 – SETTINGS AND ISSUES
VOLUME 4 – HEALTH CARE SYSTEMS IN CANADA AND ELSEWHERE
VOLUME 5 – EVIDENCE AND INFORMATION

Individual volumes or the complete series can be ordered from: Editions MultiMondes, 930, rue Pouliot, Sainte-Foy (Québec) G1V 3N9. Telephone: 1 800 840-3029. Fax: 1 888 303-5931. *(Aussi disponible en français.)*

Values

The Values working group sought to understand the values and principles that Canadians hold about health and health care, so that the system continues to reflect and respond to these values. To explore Canadian core values that are connected to the health care system and to understand the implications for decision making, the group conducted some original public opinion research, using scenarios or short stories which addressed many of the issues being investigated by the other working groups of the Forum. The scenarios were tested in focus groups. Quantitative research supplemented the focus groups making the findings more generalizable. The group also contributed to a review of public opinion research on health and social policy. Finally, a review of Canadian and international experience with ethics bodies was commissioned to identify the contribution that such groups can make to continuing the discusssion of values in decision making.

Striking a Balance

The Striking a Balance working group considered how to allocate society's limited resources to best protect, restore and promote the health of Canadians. Attention was given to the balance of resources within the health sector and other sectors of the economy. The group commissioned a series of papers to assist in their deliberations. They conducted a thorough review of international trends in health expenditures, use of resources, and outcomes. They paid considerable attention to public and private financing issues, health system oganization and federal-provicial transfers. The group produced a separate discussion paper on public and private financing, and a position paper on the Canada Health and Social Transfer.

Determinants of Health

The Determinants of Health working group sought to answer the question: In these times of economic and social hardship, what actions must be taken to allow Canadians to continue to enjoy a long life and, if possible, to increase their health status? The group consulted specialists to assist in identifying appropriate actions on the non-medical determinants of health. Specialists were asked to prepare papers on issues of concern to the health of the population related to the macro-economic environment, the contexts in which people live (i.e. families, schools, work and communities), as well as on issues of concern to people's health at different life stages. Each paper presents a review of the literature, examples of success stories or failures, and relevant policy implications.

Evidence-Based Decision Making

The working group on Evidence-Based Decision Making considered how individually practioners and policy makers can have access to, and utilize the best available evidence in making decisions. The group held two workshops with leading authorities to discuss how health information can be used to support and encourage a culture of evicence-based decision making, and to consider what information Canadians need to be better health care consumers and how to get that information to them. The group commissioned papers to: examine the meaning and concepts of evidence and evidence-based decision making as well as cases that illustrate opportunities for improvement; identify the health information infrastructure needed to support evidence-based decision making; examine tools which support more effective health care decision making; and identify strategies for assisting and increasing the role of Canadians in decision making in health and health care.

Members

William R.C. Blundell, B.A.Sc. (Ont.)	Margaret McDonald, R.N. (NWT)
Richard Cashin, LL.B. (Nfld.)	Eric M. Maldoff, LL.B. (Que.)
André-Pierre Contandriopoulos, Ph.D. (Que.)	Louise Nadeau, Ph.D. (Que.)
Randy Dickinson (N.B.)	Tom W. Noseworthy, M.D. (Alta.)
Madeleine Dion Stout, M.A. (Ont.)	Shanthi Radcliffe, M.A. (Ont.)
Robert G. Evans, Ph.D. (B.C.)	Marc Renaud, Ph.D. (Que.)
Karen Gainer, LL.B. (Alta.)	Judith A. Ritchie, Ph.D. (N.S.)
Debbie L. Good, C.A. (PEI)	Noralou P. Roos, Ph.D. (Man.)
Nuala Kenny, M.D. (N.S.)	Duncan Sinclair, Ph.D. (Ont.)
Richard Lessard, M.D. (Que.)	Lynn Smith, LL.B., Q.C. (B.C.)
Steven Lewis (Sask.)	Mamoru Watanabe, M.D. (Alta.)
Gerry M. Lougheed Jr. (Ont.)	Roberta Way-Clark, M.A. (N.S.)

Secretary and Deputy Minister, Health Canada

Michèle S. Jean

Secretariat Staff

Executive Director
Marie E. Fortier

Joyce Adubofuor

Lori Alma

Rachel Bénard

Kathy Bunka

Barbara Campbell

Marlene Campeau

Carmen Connolly

Lise Corbett

John Dossetor

Kayla Estrin

Rhonda Ferderber

Annie Gauvin

Patricia Giesler

Sylvie Guilbault

Janice Hopkins

Lucie Lacombe

Johanne LeBel

Elizabeth Lynam

Krista Locke

John Marriott

Maryse Pesant

Marcel Saulnier

Liliane Sauvé

Linda St-Amour

Judith St-Pierre

Nancy Swainson

Catherine Swift

Josée Villeneuve

Tim Weir

Lynn Westaff

We extend our sincere thanks to all those who participated in the various production stages of this series of publications.

TABLE OF CONTENTS – VOLUME 5

EVIDENCE

THE ISSUES OF VALUES

Evidence

Factors That Influence
Evidence-Based Decision Making

JOAN E. TRANMER

Principal Investigator, Kingston General Hospital

SUSAN SQUIRES

Project Coordinator, Queen's Health Policy

KEVIN BRAZIL

Queen's Health Policy

JACQUELYN GERLACH

Kingston General Hospital

JOHN JOHNSON

Hotel Dieu Hospital

DIANNE MUISINER

Kingston, Frontenac and Lennox & Addington Health Unit

BILL SWAN

Queen's Health Policy

RUTH WILSON

Faculty of Medicine, Queen's University

SUMMARY

Purpose

This study had a twofold purpose: to identify the influence of various factors on how evidence was used in practice and policy decision making within the Canadian health care system, and to recommend strategies to strengthen the influence of these positive factors and lessen the influence of these negative factors for evidence-based decision making.

Methods

Case studies were used to explore the nature of evidence-based decision making with 12 selected health care issues (primary cases) across four broad realms: clinical practice, pharmaceutical practice, health care delivery, and health care management. Evidence included information obtained from scientific evaluation (e.g., experimental and nonexperimental studies), expert opinion (e.g., consensus statements, published commission reports), and historical or experiential perspectives.

Successful cases were selected following one or more of these criteria:
— *availability of highly accessible and compelling evidence;*
— *a predominant pattern of outcomes presumed to be reflective of evidence adoption; and*
— *the relevance of the case to a broad spectrum of health care providers or consumers.*

Opportunities for improvement were selected based on one or more of the following criteria:
— *availability of highly accessible and compelling evidence;*
— *a highly varied or poor pattern of outcomes presumed to be reflective of poor evidence adoption;*
— *a predominant pattern of outcomes presumed to be reflective of questionable evidence adoption; and*
— *the relevance of the case to a broad spectrum of health care providers or consumers.*

A balance of successes and opportunities for improvement was sought. However, it was recognized that characteristics of both were evident in each primary case.

The 12 primary cases were:

Primary cases

Realm	Health issue – Primary cases
Clinical practice	Routine electronic fetal surveillance and use of cesarean section
	*Selection of cases for carotid endarterectomy
	Selection of BPH cases for prostatectomy
	*Implementation of the Ottawa Ankle Rules
Pharmaceutical practice	Promoting appropriate medication use by elderly persons
	*Appropriate timing of thrombolysis in acute myocardial infarction
Health care delivery	Implementation of second-dose measles vaccine program
	Implementation of addiction treatment programs for Aboriginal people
	*Implementation of breast-screening programs
	Implementation of acupuncture programs
Health care management	Hospital closures
	Labour substitution in acute care nursing

* Identified as potential successes.

A multistage, key informant, sampling strategy identified specific sites for each issue. Sites were identified by direct measures of outcomes (operative rates, program implementation), qualitative measures (expert opinion), and geographical representation. Sampling ensured that the extremes of presumed evidence adoption were assessed.

Data were collected by survey either by questionnaire or by detailed telephone interviews. These data collection tools addressed specific factors related to evidence adoption as defined in the literature: quality of the evidence, dissemination strategies, and environmental influences (administrative, economic, political, community, educational, and personal).

Findings

Within each realm and within each primary case a range of influential factors was identified.

Influential factors

Primary case	Range of adoption	Identified influential factors	
		Barriers	Enablers
Clinical			
1. Routine electronic fetal surveillance and use of cesarean section	Varied	• Negative caregiver attitude • Limited knowledge (nursing) • Litigation • Technological (information) environment • One decision maker • Complex decision rules	• Quality of evidence • Dissemination (consensus guidelines, database) • Quality assurance monitoring • Positive caregiver attitude • Consumer influence
2. Selection of cases for carotid endarterectomy	Good for selected criteria	• Dissemination • One decision maker • Economic disincentive	• Quality of evidence • Positive caregiver attitude
3. Selection of BPH cases for prostatectomy	Varied	• Negative caregiver attitude toward patient involvement in decision making • Questionable cost-effectiveness • Economic disincentive • Pharmaceutical industry	• Quality of evidence • Dissemination • Quality assurance monitoring • Multidisciplinary programs
4. Implementation of the Ottawa Ankle Rules	Good—except in geographically isolated areas	• Dissemination (poor to remote areas) • Liability • Physician attitude	• Quality of evidence • Dissemination (guidelines, tools) • Ease of implementation

Influential factors (cont.)

	Primary case	Range of adoption	Identified influential factors	
			Barriers	Enablers
Pharmaceutical				
5.	Promoting appropriate medication use by elderly persons	Varied	• Quality of evidence poor for program effectiveness • Lack of financial support • Poor applicability of guidelines • Lack of organized approach to the issue	• Quality of evidence sound for description of problem • Expert opinion • Local initiatives
6.	Appropriate timing of thrombolysis therapy in acute myocardial infarction	Good	• Negative caregiver attitude • Lack of nursing expertise	• Quality of evidence • Dissemination (consensus guidelines, Canadian Association of Emergency Physicians – CAEP) • Multidisciplinary approaches • No economic disincentive
Health care delivery				
7.	Implementation of second-dose measles vaccine program	Good	• Poor link between evidence and local planning and implementation of programs	• Quality of evidence • National goal • Dissemination (consensus conference)

Influential factors (cont.)

	Primary case	Range of adoption	Identified influential factors	
			Barriers	Enablers
Pharmaceutical (cont.)				
8.	Implementation of addiction treatment programs for Aboriginal people	Varied	• Poor link between scientific and historical evidence • Poor sharing of information	• Quality of experiential/historical evidence • Culture • Opinion leaders • Planned programs
9.	Implementation of breast-screening programs	Good	• Lag of scientific evidence • Varied regulatory powers • Physician attitude • Poor coordination of different programs	• Quality of evidence • Dissemination (consensus conference) • Multidisciplinary implementation
10.	Implementation of acupuncture programs	Varied	• Varied quality of evidence • Difficult to determine effectiveness in current system • Economic costs • Professional boundaries	• Quality of evidence sound for documentation of problem • Consumer demand • Culture

Influential factors (cont.)

Primary case	Range of adoption	Identified influential factors	
		Barriers	Enablers
Health management			
11. Hospital closures	Varied	• Poor quality of evidence concerning planning and implementation • Complex decisions • Political • Consumer pressure • Multiple stakeholders	• Quality of experiential/historical evidence • Culture • Opinion leaders • Planned programs
12. Labour substitution in acute care nursing	Varied	• Poor quality of evidence • Complex decision • Poor accessibility to evidence • Multiple stakeholders • Questionable effectiveness	• Philosophy of care • Qualitative, descriptive evidence

Conclusions

- *Between cases within each realm, common enabling factors and barriers exist. However, the degree to which these common factors enhance or obstruct evidence adoption varies. As well, each case has its own unique set of influential factors and barriers.*
- *Adoption of evidence into* clinical *decision making is facilitated by: quality evidence, organized approach to dissemination (consensus guidelines, planned educational initiatives), interdisciplinary approach to implementation, quality assurance monitoring of outcomes, positive caregiver attitude, cost-effectiveness (personal and organizational), and consumer support.*
- *Barriers to the adoption of evidence into* clinical *decision making are: poor dissemination, nonsupportive caregiver attitude, sole decision-making responsibility (e.g., physician), perceived economic disincentive, fear of litigation, technological (informational) environment, lack of resources, and complexity of decision.*
- *Adoption of evidence into* administrative *decision making is facilitated by: quality of informational evidence, expert opinion, perceived national (provincial) support and commitment, planned group or program approach, consumer demand, cultural environment, and supportive policy directions.*
- *Barriers to the adoption of evidence into* administrative *decision making are: poor quality of evidence, questionable cost-effectiveness of decisions, stakeholder boundaries, lack of resources (education, time, and financial), and complexity of decision.*

Recommendations

Evidence-based decision making or problem solving is complex within the health care system.

Decision making is influenced by the quality of the evidence, dissemination of the evidence, and the environment in which the decision making and incorporation of the evidence is taking place. The incorporation of evidence into decision making is an active process. Best practices do not spontaneously occur. Strategies need to be developed to ensure that high-quality evidence is produced, disseminated, synthesized, and incorporated into decisions. Outcomes of successful (or nonsuccessful adoption) need to be regularly monitored and evaluated. Within the Canadian health care system, this is both a professional and public responsibility. However, a significant, collaborative effort is required to develop, coordinate, and support strategies.

The following recommendations are submitted for consideration as potential strategic directions for professional and public policy. These recommendations suggest directions to facilitate the identified enablers for successful evidence adoption: quality evidence, effective dissemination, and supportive environment.

- *The nature of evidence is varied. The definition of evidence-based decision making within the Canadian health care system should be clearly articulated and address the different sources of facts and knowledge, the process through which these facts and knowledge are assessed (efficacy, effectiveness, appropriateness, affordability filters), and the process for incorporating evidence into decision making (e.g., implementation strategies).*

- *Encourage granting bodies to continue to support research activities that generate the development of quality evidence for both clinical and administrative decision makers.*

- *Professional organizations should continue to develop clinical guidelines and consensus approaches to high-risk, high-volume health care issues. These guidelines must reflect high-quality evidence and be widely disseminated to all appropriate caregivers.*

- *Provincial and national health ministries should collaborate with the professional organizations to develop, where appropriate, bodies or systems that collate, review, interpret, disseminate, and monitor health care evidence. This would facilitate the incorporation of clinical and nonclinical evidence into accessible and comprehensive databases and increase the availability, timeliness, comprehensiveness, and accessibility of informational data to decision makers (e.g., practitioners, hospitals, programs).*

- *Public programs should be developed to encourage consumers to be more knowledgeable of the evidence and actively involved in decision making regarding its adoption or nonadoption.*

- *Encourage granting bodies to support further research on complex health care decisions. Studies need to: describe the nature and influence of influential factors in complex administrative and clinical decisions, determine effective methods for collation and synthesis of evidence in relation to individual/ community experiences, and determine effective implementation and evaluation strategies.*

- *Economic resources and reimbursement should facilitate and support the adoption of evidence. As forms of health care payments are reviewed, the incorporation of the best available evidence into practice seems to be facilitated when fees for service are not a significant component of the decision-making process.*

- *At all levels (national, provincial, hospital, community, professional) the incorporation of evidence into practice and administrative decisions must be a planned process that formally integrates all significant stakeholders. Decision making is rarely confined to one discipline or one site; thus decision makers and resources to support the adoption of the evidence should be consolidated where possible. Decisions should be evaluated through quality assurance monitoring of defined outcomes. Quality assurance programs need to collect and evaluate information in relation to appropriate peers and programs. Outcomes need to be congruent with expected norms (e.g., utilization rates, national trends, accepted values).*

- *Professional organizations need to develop strategies that ensure professional standards reflect consistent adoption of the best available evidence. Where appropriate, provincial and national ministries need to be reassured, either through reporting or surveillance, that standards are being achieved.*
- *The role of the consumer in adopting practice changes in relation to evidence adoption is underdeveloped. Encourage professional organizations and provincial ministries to collaborate on the development of strategies to ensure consumers are knowledgeable of health evidence and are actively involved in review and synthesis of the evidence into their community.*

TABLE OF CONTENTS

LIST OF FIGURES

LIST OF TABLES

What is evidence?

> *The rules of evidence control the presentation of facts before the court. Their purpose is to facilitate the introduction of all logically relevant facts without sacrificing any fundamental policy of the law which may be of more importance than the ascertainment of the truth... Laws of evidence regulate 1) what matters are or are not admissible before the courts, and 2) the method by which admissible facts are placed before it.*
>
> J. Sopinka and S. Lederman,
> *The Law of Evidence in Civil Cases* (1974)

What are the rules of evidence that control presentation and introduction of logically relevant facts to the health care system? What evidence is admissible and how is this evidence assessed, presented, and utilized?

SECTION I – PROJECT REPORT

WHAT FACTORS INFLUENCE EVIDENCE-BASED DECISION MAKING WITHIN THE CANADIAN HEALTH CARE SYSTEM?

Background

The value of evidence as a basis for decision making within health care is well established. However, despite extensive research exploring the determinants of evidence utilization, the incorporation of evidence remains inconsistent (Brook 1993; Kelly and Toepp 1992).

This research identifies factors influencing implementation of evidence-based decision making.

Factors Influencing Evidence Adoption

The factors influencing the adoption of evidence into practice and policy by health care decision makers have been studied extensively, particularly by those in management and the clinical sciences.

Both medicine and nursing have explored determinants of evidence use in clinical decision making (Funk, Tornquist, and Champagne 1995; Grimshaw and Russell 1993; Mittman, Tonesk, and Jacobsen 1992). Research has clearly demonstrated that a range of factors frequently prevents the adoption of evidence into practice, despite clear benefits of evidence-based practice to both patient and practitioner. For example, clinical guideline development has provided some of the most robust evidence that research-based information is not readily adopted into practice (Kelly and Toepp 1992). While clinical guidelines have been carefully designed to promote research transfer, they have had limited impact on medical practice (Grimshaw and Russell 1995; Lomas 1993). Promotion of nursing research utilization has proven equally difficult (Luckenbill 1989; Funk et al. 1991, 1995). Although some differences exist between factors influencing the adoption of evidence within health care professions, several common determinants of evidence use have been identified. These include individual practitioner characteristics; the practitioner community; patients (and their families); organizational administrative structures and processes; economic, social, and regulatory environments within which the organization or practitioner exist (Funk, Tornquist, and Champagne 1995; Lomas 1993; Funk et al. 1991); and the quality, relevance, and presentation of the information (VanAmringe and Shannon 1992).

In general, administrative decision making has been explored as a barrier or enabler to clinical practice change. However, the extensive literature addressing the determinants of evidence use in administrative decision making has demonstrated that many factors apparent at the clinical level are equally relevant at the administrative and policy-making levels. Factors that have demonstrated association to adoption of evidence at the administrative level include the context within which the case arises and must be managed (similar to the environment described in clinical research), the quality and timing of the evaluation process, and the personal/professional characteristics of the decision makers at various levels (Alkin, Daillak, and White 1979; Lester and Wilds 1990).

Studies in both the clinical and administrative arena have generally evaluated single or narrowly focused research transfer strategies. The fact that the extensive research generated has not translated into more successful strategies for promoting evidence-based practice suggests that a more comprehensive approach is required (Mittman, Tonesk, and Jacobsen 1992; Lomas 1993; Fitch 1992).

Evidence adoption by administrative and clinical decision makers is complex. Decision makers base decisions on a diverse range of evidence or information. Evidence is obtained from experimental and nonexperimental research, informational sources (cost analysis, prevalence studies, utilization data, needs assessments, program evaluations, surveys, research literature, commissioned reports, comparative analyses), and historical or experiential perspectives. Decision makers often find that evidence is difficult to interpret, reflective of conflicting expert opinions, not relevant or specific enough to the practice or policy being questioned, and not timely enough for operational needs. Moreover, many personal and organizational factors influence decision makers' capability to change practice: values and beliefs, economical imperatives, regulatory bodies, organizational and professional boundaries, geographical location, and educational background. Decision makers need evidence that is presented in a manner that not only includes relevant information but also addresses the implications of incorporating the evidence into decisions.

Lomas (1993) has synthesized most of the research on evidence use into a coordinated implementation model, that defines those factors that influence evidence-based practice. Lomas suggests that evidence utilization depends on multiple interacting factors (figure 1).

These multiple positive and negative influences are likely to be portrayed in examples or stories of where the best available evidence influenced decision making within the health care system. This study explored the process of adopting evidence into decision making in selected cases across four realms: clinical practice, pharmaceutical care, health care delivery, and health care management.

Nature of Evidence

Evidence was defined as information based on historical or scientific evaluation of a practice that was accessible to decision makers in the Canadian health care system. The types of evidence considered include:
- experimental (randomized clinical trials, metanalysis, and analytic studies);
- nonexperimental (quasi-experimental, observational);
- expert opinion (consensus, commission reports) (consensus statements were considered only if based on published literature and a consensus process); and
- historical or experiential.

Nature of Evidence Adoption

A continuum exists for evidence adoption, ranging at the extremes from the complete adoption of best available evidence to nonadoption of the evidence. Successful implementation of evidence-based decisions usually results in the more appropriate use of resources and no increase in risk or reduction in patient health status, or in a clear improvement in quality of care or services. Nonsuccessful adoption of evidence usually results in inappropriate change (e.g., no change) in practice or in a consistent pattern of change in light of insufficient evidence to support the specific change. Within these two extremes there is a middle range of evidence adoption. Evidence is either partially or slowly adopted.

Figure 1

Coordinated implementation model

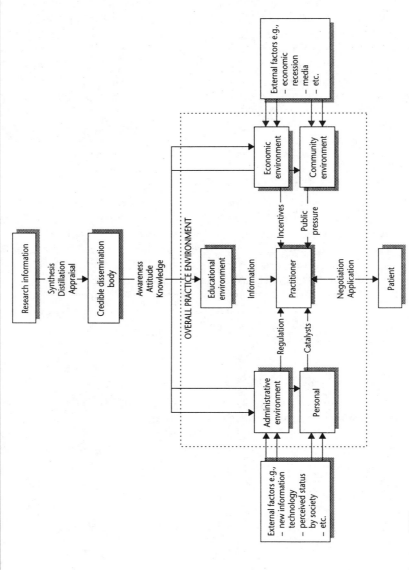

Source: J. Lomas, 1993.

Methods

Case Study Design

A case study approach was used to explore the impact of influential factors, as identified in the Lomas model, on utilization of evidence in decision making in the Canadian health care system. The complex interaction of influential factors in the adoption of evidence can best be studied by methods where context and nonlinear interaction patterns can be more readily evaluated, such as in a case study.[1]

The program-effects case study type was used for this investigation (Yin 1994). In accordance with this type, an embedded, multiple case replication design and multiple methods of data collection were used. Multiple case design involves identification and analysis of replication case studies to produce more compelling evidence regarding the relationship between the variables of interest. Embedded case study design involves the examination of natural subunits (e.g., sites, individual programs) within each case to allow more accurate and in-depth description of each case as a whole.

The primary cases investigated comprised health care issues for which sound evidence was available to support decision making. Embedded cases within each primary case comprised examples (sites or programs) of utilization within the Canadian health care system.

Primary Case Selection

Two types of cases were the basis for the evaluation of factors contributing to evidence-based decision making in the Canadian health care system: those where primary outcomes suggested adoption of the best available evidence and those where primary outcomes suggested poor or nonadoption of the best available evidence. A balance of successes and opportunities for improvement were sought. However, it was recognized that characteristics of both were evident with each primary case.

Primary cases were selected from four targeted realms: clinical practice, pharmaceuticals, health care delivery, and health care management. Within each realm, cases were determined on the basis of the following criteria: evidence characteristics including quality, accessibility, and stability of evidence across time; degree of evidence adoption across Canada; and relevance to a broad spectrum of consumers/providers and potential for significant effectiveness gains or cost savings without compromising quality of care. Preliminary assessments of evidence adoption across Canada were based on published utilization rates, studies evaluating evidence adoption, and expert opinion.

---

1. General Accounting Office, Case Study Evaluations, 1990 (abstract).

In addition, the feasibility of studying each case was evaluated. Feasibility was determined by: the ability to adequately assess the adoption of evidence at each site, the ease of identifying sites and participants for interview and questionnaire within each site, and the likelihood of documentation of planning and outcomes of practice change. In most cases, compliance with these criteria was estimated based on available written evidence and expert opinion.

Success Identification

Successes were selected on the basis of case-specific successful outcomes, assuming this was due to a predominant pattern of evidence adoption. Therefore, prerequisites included: availability of highly accessible and compelling evidence over a period of at least one year, a predominant pattern of outcomes presumed to be reflective of evidence adoption, and relevance of case to a broad spectrum of consumers/providers. Low degrees of practice variation, where evidence was available, research findings or expert opinion indicating practice consistent with evidence were used to determine success. In some case, some aspects of evidence had been widely adopted while other aspects had not.

Opportunities for Improvement

Opportunities for improvement were selected on the basis of case-specific negative outcomes, assuming this was due to a predominant pattern of failure to adopt sound evidence or to adopt evidence of uncertain validity. Therefore, prerequisites included: availability of highly accessible and compelling evidence over a period of a least one year, a highly varied or poor pattern of outcomes presumed to be reflective of poor adoption of evidence, a pattern of outcomes presumed to be reflective of adoption of questionable evidence, and evidence that the case was relevant to a broad spectrum of consumers/providers. High degrees of practice variation, when evidence was available, research findings or expert opinion indicating inconsistent practice with evidence (or consistent with questionable evidence) were used to determine opportunity for improvement status.

Cases selected for study are listed in table 1.

Embedded Case Selection

Several sites or examples within each were identified for study. A program-effects approach to case study required that the identification of selected sites represented a range of evidence use outcome within each primary case. That is, examples of highly successful adoption as well as of less successful adoption were identified.

Table 1

Primary cases

Realm	Health issue – Primary cases
Clinical practice	Routine electronic fetal surveillance and use of cesarean section
	*Selection of cases for carotid endarterectomy
	Selection of BPH cases for prostatectomy
	*Implementation of the Ottawa Ankle Rules
Pharmaceutical practice	Promoting appropriate medication use by elderly persons
	*Appropriate timing of thrombolysis in acute myocardial infarction
Health care delivery	Implementation of second-dose measles vaccine program
	Implementation of addiction treatment programs for Aboriginal people
	*Implementation of breast-screening programs
	Implementation of acupuncture programs
Health care management	Hospital closures
	Labour substitution in acute care nursing

* Identified as potential successes.

The process of identifying sites for inclusion depended on the availability of quantitative or qualitative date that could be used to determine evidence adoption.

Direct Measures of Outcome

Direct measures of outcome included utilization rates where these were available for the appropriate population and implementation of program under study. Rates were available for cesarean section, carotid endarterectomy, and prostatectomy. Evidence of program implementation was available for second-dose measles vaccine, acupuncture, medication use, and addiction treatment for Aboriginal people.

Qualitative Measures of Outcome

In some cases, quantitative measures of outcome were not readily available. Here, consultation with experts in the field and appropriate organizations (health ministries, professional bodies) was used. As well, this approach was used to validate site selection based on quantitative data.

Geographical Representation

To ensure appropriate representation across Canada, when qualitative and quantitative measures were relatively equal, cases were selected based on geographical location.

Multistage Key Informant Sampling

Initially, first-stage key informants for each of the 12 primary cases were identified and contacted by telephone. These individuals (key informants) were experts or opinion leaders in their respective fields. Each key informant was asked to identify potential embedded sites for inclusion in this study.

After the embedded sites had been identified, one second-stage key informant per site was identified. The identification of the second-stage key informant was made either by a first-stage key informant or by virtue of the second-stage key informant's position (e.g., for prostatectomy primary case, the second-stage key informant was the head of urology). The second-stage key informant was then sent a fax to inform him about this study and to ask for the key informant's participation in the study and cooperation in identifying three to 10 other individuals in his site who would be appropriate for inclusion in the survey. A follow-up telephone call was made to obtain the second-stage key informant's consent and, as well, to add to the survey sampling frame the names of the third- (and final) stage key informants. All second- and third-stage key informants were included in the final survey database (sampling frame).

Measures

Multiple sources of data were used to identify the factors that influenced evidence-based decision making in the 12 primary cases: quantitative survey data, qualitative interview data, and case-specific documentation.

Questionnaire

The survey questionnaire was used to determine the frequency and degree of impact of specific factors on adoption of evidence in the 12 primary cases. Utilization of evidence in decision making has been widely studied within and outside the health care system. Multiple factors have been identified in individual research studies, literature reviews, and dissemination theory. The questionnaire was used to describe the known or hypothesized influential factors.

Interview

While the list of factors known and hypothesized to have an impact on decision making in health care is extensive, the use of quantitative studies in the past may have limited the range of factors identified. Moreover, evidence-based decision making is a complex process, with factors interacting to determine the ultimate outcome. In-depth interviews were combined with the questionnaire to obtain more information than could be acquired by questionnaire alone.

Questionnaire Design

Design of the questionnaire followed accepted survey design procedures. Constructs were based on the literature addressing dissemination theory and its testing. The constructs defined on the basis of the literature included:
- Credibility of information:
  stability – consistency of evidence across studies and time;
  quality – rigour of the methodologies used to generate the evidence; and
  quantity – the number of replication or related studies and the representativeness of the populations studied.
- Dissemination:
  what – which information was disseminated and synthesized;
  how – what methods of presentation and distribution were used; and
  who – credentials of the organizations/persons who have disseminated the information.
- Environment:
  administrative – organizational culture, structure, policy, and practice patterns;
  economic – status of local, provincial, and national economy;
  community – community culture, political structure and behaviour;
  educational – teaching status of health care organizations and structure of continuing education programs within the organization; and
  person/profession – beliefs and attitudes of individual decision maker.

A pilot test of the questionnaire was completed. Ten individuals from a range of settings were asked to respond to the questionnaire. Pilot test results and a final revision of the instrument were completed before distribution.

Expert Panel Review

A panel composed of expert decision makers from academic, community, hospital, district health council, provincial ministry and health unit settings participated in the interpretation of findings. This interpretative session was facilitated by a health economist. Participants reviewed the findings, discussed their significance, interpreted their relevance and relationship with evidence-based decision making and recommended strategic direction for the facilitation of evidence-based decision making. Their feedback was incorporated into the final conclusions and recommendations.

Findings Reported across Clinical and Administrative Realms

Sample

Three hundred and thirty informants were identified through the key informant sampling process. Overall, 51 percent (114/225) of identified informants completed and returned the questionnaire and 69 percent (90/130) informants participated in interviews. Within the clinical realms (clinical and pharmaceutical issues), 51 percent (51/101) completed the questionnaire and 57 percent (36/63) participated in interviews. Within the administrative realms (health care delivery and management), 51 percent (63/124) completed the questionnaire and 81 percent (54/67) participated in interviews (figure 2).

Figure 2

Response rates for questionnaire and interview by issue

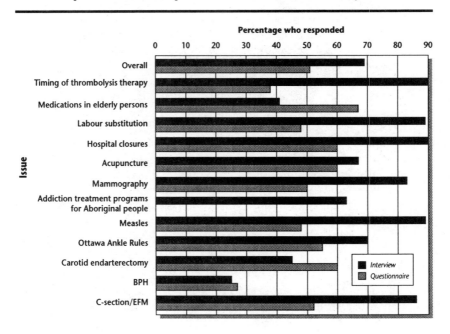

The sample consisted of relatively equal numbers of females and males, distributed predominantly between 35 and 55 years of age. Most had attended university and obtained postgraduate degrees: master's (22 percent), professional (41 percent), and doctorate (9 percent) (figure 3).

Figure 3

Age

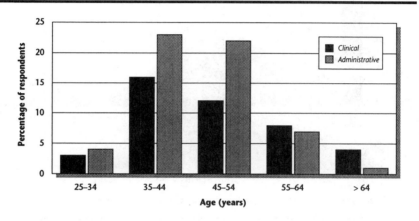

Age (years)

Approximately half the informants worked within a clinical setting, the most common being a hospital. Others worked within provincial programs, professional organizations, and community settings. Half the work settings were associated with a university and most were located in urban centres.

Within the clinical and pharmaceutical realms, the primary health care role was practitioner (physician and nurse) and, within the administrative realms, the primary health care role was administrator (manager, administrator, policymaker). Other reported roles included researcher, educator, and consultant (figure 4).

Range of Adoption of Evidence

Adoption of the best available evidence varied (figure 5). Within all realms, the majority of respondents indicated that evidence was partially adopted. Approximately half the respondents indicated that practice was not consistent with the best available evidence. Generally, practice was changing to become more consistent with the best available evidence (figure 6). However, a substantial number of decision makers, especially those within the clinical realms, did not perceive this to be the direction. The degree of adoption of evidence was based on the informants' opinion. However, review of utilization data, published literature, and expert reports substantiated their opinion in most cases.

Figure 4

Primary health care role

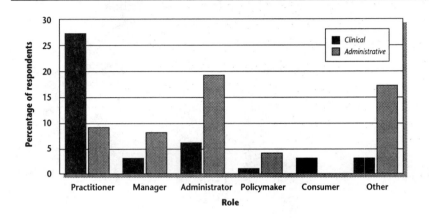

Figure 5

Practice is consistent with the best available evidence

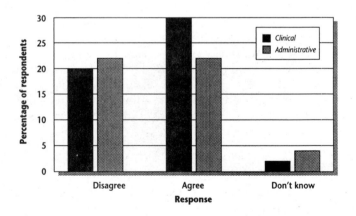

Quality of the Evidence

The stability, credibility, and quantity of best available evidence for each issue was explored (figures 7 and 8). Clinical and administrative research evidence demonstrated inconsistency over time. While the evidence was not perceived to be stable, that which was available was perceived to be credible. Respondents in both realms expressed concern about the quality, timeliness, appropriateness, and applicability of the evidence. Only half

Figure 6

Practice is changing to become more consistent with the evidence

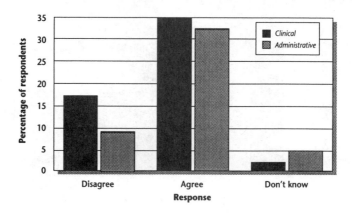

Figure 7

The evidence is stable

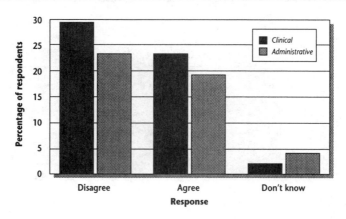

the clinicians and administrators felt the evidence was compelling and comprehensive. Commission reports, expert opinion and informational databases were common sources of administrative evidence. Published research, when available, was used in both realms as a primary source of evidence.

Sixty percent of informants believed that the evidence regarding effectiveness for the stated issues was convincing (figure 9). However, within the clinical realms, more respondents raised concern about the effectiveness and cost-effectiveness of the suggested practice change if the best available evidence was adopted. This was not the case with respondents in the

Figure 8

The evidence is credible

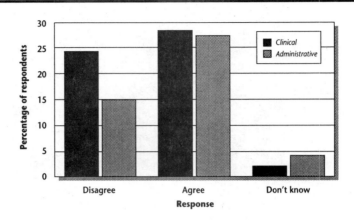

Figure 9

Evidence indicates effectiveness

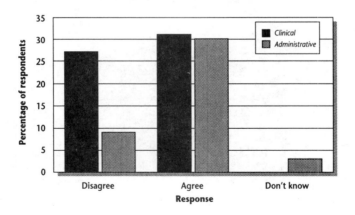

administrative realms. Cost-effectiveness is rarely a focus for clinical research but is often the focus of administrative studies. This may account for the perception that evidence for clinical issues did not consistently demonstrate cost-effectiveness (figure 10).

The quality of evidence for clinical issues is often perceived to be stronger evidence, as research designs are more experimental and controlled. Clinicians, in comparison to administrators, were more critical of the stability, credibility, and effectiveness of this evidence. Evidence used for administrative decision

Figure 10

Evidence indicates cost-effectiveness

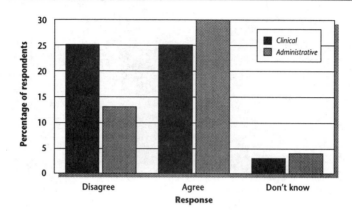

making is not as controlled; yet, administrators perceived the available evidence as credible, cost effective, and effective. This perception of high-quality evidence may be reflective of the wider scope and nature of evidence used to make complex, administrative decisions. Administrative evidence tends to reflect the most current status of issues (e.g., hospital closures, labour substitution), whereas clinical evidence is not as grounded in current practice. Interventions are used in trials and being tested in a controlled experimental manner, thus limiting assessment of the impact of other influential factors, such as the economic, political, and personnel environment, on decisions. However, all clinicians acknowledged the importance and significance of well-controlled experimental research (e.g., clinical trials) to generate the best-quality evidence.

Dissemination

The content and method of dissemination strategies was explored. Reports and publications regarding evidence related to the identified issues were available in most work settings. Research was reported clearly and readably. The most successful dissemination strategies included consensus reports, clinical guidelines, national conferences, and planned workshops. Research was not consistently disseminated to remote geographical areas (e.g., Ottawa Ankle Rules). Response was mixed when informants were asked whether local research was used to validate or adopt information about identified issues. Similarly, information was not consistently disseminated to the consumer, suggesting that dissemination ends with the practitioner or decision maker and that collection, collation, and interpretation of evidence for local initiatives is not shared with the community. Overall, dissemination to health care providers was perceived to be relatively positive (figures 11 and 12).

Figure 11

Dissemination to health care providers is good

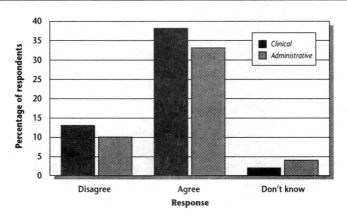

Figure 12

Dissemination to consumers is good

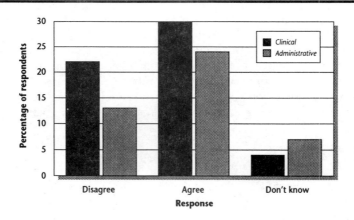

Environmental Factors

Administrative

The influence of administrative factors including the organizational structure, culture, beliefs, policies, and practice was explored. Organizational processes and structures had substantial influence. Most respondents believed that the administrative environment facilitated the adoption of evidence. Evidence was more consistently adopted in clinical settings that used a systematic approach (e.g., interdisciplinary task forces) and maintained this approach for evaluation (quality assurance monitoring). A broad-based program approach facilitated evidence adoption within the clinical realms (e.g., provincial breast screening, second-dose measles vaccine campaign). Singular attempts at evidence adoption did not have the same national effect (e.g., programs for medication misuse in elderly persons). Regulations or polices related to issues prevented changes suggested by the best available evidence but this did not seem to be a major influential factor (e.g., facility regulations for breast screening). Most respondents perceived that evidence would not be adopted in organizational environments that were in conflict with the direction of the suggested practice changes (e.g., electronic fetal surveillance).

Economic Conditions

Economic conditions explored the influence of the local, provincial, or national economy on evidence adoption. Generally, respondents felt that there were adequate facilities or resources within their community to support the suggested practice. However, those respondents in administrative realms believed that economic conditions strongly influenced evidence adoption within their community (e.g., hospital closures, labour substitution). The economic conditions initiated the examination of administrative issues and set the parameters in which the evidence could be examined and adopted. Within the clinical realms, most felt economic conditions did not influence evidence adoption. This is consistent with the finding that clinical cost-effectiveness evidence is perceived to be poor. Practitioners tend to focus on individual well-being in comparison to societal or organizational well-being. Overall, economic conditions were not perceived to be a barrier (figures 13 and 14).

Political Factors

Political factors considered the influence of key persons or organizations. Opinion leaders, experts, and organizations were influential in evidence adoption across all realms. Endorsement by professional organizations was a substantial influential factor for clinical evidence adoption. Expert and consensus opinion validated the evidence. If experts perceive that the evidence is poor, clinicians and administrators are not likely to consider its adoption. However, professional and expert support does not guarantee evidence adoption (e.g., fetal electronic surveillance). Political factors had an influence at local, provincial, and national levels (figure 15).

Liability

Concerns were expressed with regards to liability. These concerns varied within issues (e.g., thrombolysis, electronic fetal surveillance) and across issues.

Figure 13

Economic conditions influence evidence adoption

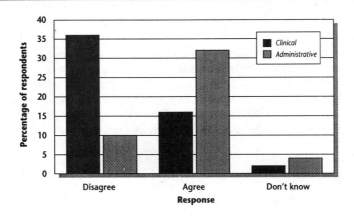

Figure 14

Economic conditions are a barrier to evidence adoption

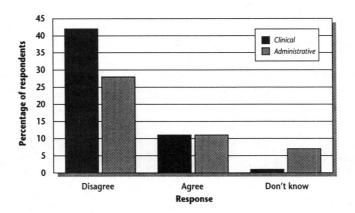

Liability was more of a concern within the clinical realms. Concern about litigation strongly inhibited evidence adoption. Liability concerns were more apparent if practitioners thought they, as individuals, were more at risk for litigation. Some suggested that legal actions need to consider more the contribution of the practice setting (e.g., hospital organization) as well as the individual (e.g., the physician) for determination of fault (or no fault) (figure 16).

Figure 15

Political factors influence evidence adoption

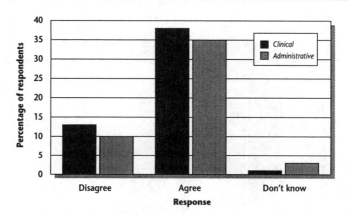

Figure 16

Liability concerns influence evidence adoption

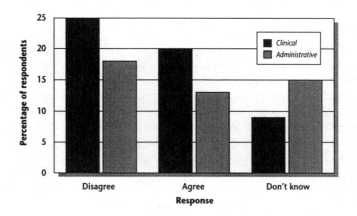

Consumer Influence

Across the realms, decision makers believed that the public did not strongly influence evidence adoption. In some cases, consumer influence was very strong. Consumers initiated the drive to change practice (e.g., regulation of acupuncture) and ensured that the practice was appropriate for their community (e.g., addiction treatment programs). However, for most issues this was not the case. In some cases, consumer (or patient) involvement was a negative influence (e.g., implementation of the Ottawa Ankle Rules). Consumers were not aware of the evidence and the implications of evidence adoption for their health (figure 17).

Figure 17

Consumer pressure influences evidence adoption

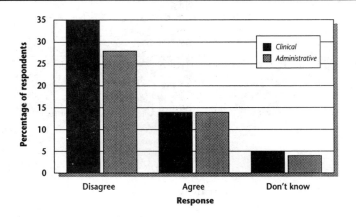

Personal/Professional Factors

The influence of personal/professional beliefs, and attitude toward evidence adoption was explored. Overall, personal attitude strongly influenced evidence adoption. Most decision makers supported basing practice on evidence, regularly attended conferences, regularly reviewed research reports, were comfortable interpreting findings, influenced how evidence-based practice was carried out in their community and were aware of the most current research related to their issue. However, 72 percent of all respondents felt that knowledge gained from experience was more important to decision making than the incorporation of the best available evidence. The actual incorporation of evidence seemed to be filtered through one's personal/ professional attitude toward its use and personal/professional experience. There did not appear to be any criteria on which personal/professional experiential evidence was weighed or utilized: it was a personal decision (figures 18 and 19).

Figure 18

Personal/professional attitude influences evidence adoption

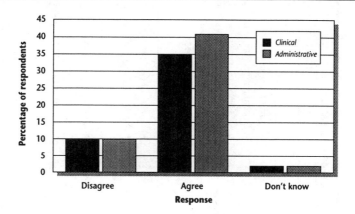

Figure 19

Knowledge gained from experience is less important than other forms of evidence to decision making

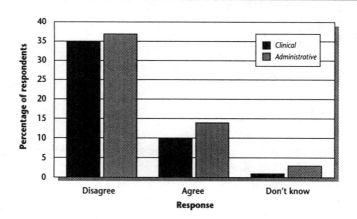

Summary of Findings

Within each realm and primary case, a range of influential factors was identified (table 2).

Table 2

Influential factors

	Primary case	Range of adoption	Identified influential factors	
			Barriers	Enablers
Clinical				
1.	Routine electronic fetal surveillance and use of cesarean section	Varied	• Negative caregiver attitude • Limited knowledge (nursing) • Litigation • Technological (information) environment • One decision maker • Complex decision rules	• Quality of evidence • Dissemination (consensus guidelines, database) • Quality assurance monitoring • Positive caregiver attitude • Consumer influence
2.	Selection of cases for carotid endarterectomy	Good for selected criteria	• Dissemination • One decision maker • Economic disincentive	• Quality of evidence • Positive caregiver attitude
3.	Selection of BPH cases for prostatectomy	Varied	• Negative caregiver attitude toward patient involvement in decision making • Questionable cost-effectiveness • Economic disincentive • Pharmaceutical industry	• Quality of evidence • Dissemination • Quality assurance monitoring • Multidisciplinary programs
4.	Implementation of the Ottawa Ankle Rules	Good—except in geographically isolated areas	• Dissemination (poor to remote areas) • Liability • Physician attitude	• Quality of evidence • Dissemination (guidelines, tools) • Ease of implementation

Influential factors (cont.)

Primary case	Range of adoption	Identified influential factors	
		Barriers	Enablers
Pharmaceutical			
5. Promoting appropriate medication use by elderly persons	Varied	• Quality of evidence poor for program effectiveness • Lack of financial support • Poor applicability of guidelines • Lack of organized approach to the issue	• Quality of evidence sound for description of problem • Expert opinion • Local initiatives
6. Appropriate timing of thrombolysis therapy in acute myocardial infarction	Good	• Negative caregiver attitude • Lack of nursing expertise	• Quality of evidence • Dissemination (consensus guidelines, Canadian Association of Emergency Physicians – CAEP) • Multidisciplinary approaches • No economic disincentive
Health care delivery			
7. Implementation of second-dose measles vaccine program	Good	• Poor link between evidence and local planning and implementation of programs	• Quality of evidence • National goal • Dissemination (consensus conference)

Influential factors (cont.)

Primary case	Range of adoption	Identified influential factors	
		Barriers	Enablers
Pharmaceutical (cont.)			
8. Implementation of addiction treatment programs for Aboriginal people	Varied	• Poor link between scientific and historical evidence • Poor sharing of information	• Quality of experiential/historical evidence • Culture • Opinion leaders • Planned programs
9. Implementation of breast-screening programs	Good	• Lag of scientific evidence • Varied regulatory powers • Physician attitude • Poor coordination of different programs	• Quality of evidence • Dissemination (consensus conference) • Multidisciplinary implementation
10. Implementation of acupuncture programs	Varied	• Varied quality of evidence • Difficult to determine effectiveness in current system • Economic costs • Professional boundaries	• Quality of evidence sound for documentation of problem • Consumer demand • Culture

Influential factors (cont.)

Primary case	Range of adoption	Identified influential factors	
		Barriers	Enablers
Health management			
11. Hospital closures	Varied	• Poor quality of evidence concerning planning and implementation • Complex decisions • Political • Consumer pressure • Multiple stakeholders	• Quality of experiential/historical evidence • Culture • Opinion leaders • Planned programs
12. Labour substitution in acute care nursing	Varied	• Poor quality of evidence • Complex decision • Poor accessibility to evidence • Multiple stakeholders • Questionable effectiveness	• Philosophy of care • Qualitative, descriptive evidence

Conclusions

- Between cases within each realm, common enabling factors and barriers exist. However, the degree to which these common factors enhance or obstruct evidence adoption varies. As well, each case has its own unique set of influential factors and barriers.
- Adoption of evidence into *clinical* decision making is facilitated by: quality evidence, organized approach to dissemination (consensus guidelines, planned educational initiatives), interdisciplinary approach to implementation, quality assurance monitoring of outcomes, positive caregiver attitude, cost-effectiveness (personal and organizational), and consumer support.
- Barriers to the adoption of evidence into *clinical* decision making are: poor dissemination, nonsupportive caregiver attitude, singular responsibility and accountability for decision making, perceived economic disincentive, fear of litigation, technological (informational) environment, lack of resources, and complexity of decision.
- Adoption of evidence into *administrative* decision making is facilitated by: quality of informational evidence, expert opinion, perceived national (provincial) support and commitment, planned group or program approach, consumer demand, cultural environment, and supportive policy directions.
- Barriers to the adoption of evidence into *administrative* decision making are: poor quality of evidence, questionable cost-effectiveness of decisions, stakeholder boundaries, lack of resources (education, time, and financial), and complexity of decision.

Recommendations

Evidence-based decision making or problem solving is complex within the health care system.

Decision making is influenced by the quality of the evidence, dissemination of the evidence, and the environment in which the decision making is taking place. The incorporation of evidence into decisions is an active process. It does not occur spontaneously. Strategies need to be developed which ensure that high-quality evidence is produced, disseminated, synthesized, and incorporated into decisions. Outcomes of successful (or non-successful) adoption need to be regularly monitored and evaluated. Within the Canadian health care system, this is both a professional and public responsibility. However, a significant, collaborative effort is required to develop, coordinate, and support strategies.

The following recommendations are submitted for consideration as potential strategic directions for professional and public policy. These recommendations suggest directions to facilitate the identified enabling factors for successful evidence adoption: quality evidence, effective dissemination, and supportive environment.

The quality of evidence available for health care decision makers is varied. Within the clinical realms, the quality of the evidence is perceived as scientifically sound, generalizable and credible. Concern was raised about the lag of scientific evidence, expense of randomized trials, and the focus of research evidence on popular themes. Within the administrative realms, the quality of evidence was perceived as less credible when compared to usual scientific research indicators. However, decision makers acknowledged the richness and value of evidence gained from information reports, opinion leaders, colleagues, databases, and personal experience.

- The nature of evidence is varied. The definition of evidence-based decision making within the Canadian health care system should be clearly articulated and address the different sources of facts and knowledge, the process through which these facts and knowledge are assessed (efficacy, effectiveness, appropriateness, affordability filters), and the process for incorporating evidence into decision making (e.g., implementation strategies).
- Encourage granting bodies to continue to support research that generates the development of quality evidence for both clinical and administrative decision makers.

Dissemination of evidence varied across realms. Within clinical realms, dissemination was most effective if evidence was reviewed and synthesized into *national* clinical guidelines or consensus reports. Endorsement by professional experts and organizations was essential. Within administrative realms, dissemination was most effective if reports and facts were synthesized at a national or provincial level and policy directions established. Dissemination is effective when the knowledge level of both the decision maker and consumer are enhanced. The evidence message must consider multilevel professionals and the consumer.

- Professional organizations should continue to develop clinical guidelines and consensus approaches to high-risk, high-volume health care issues. These guidelines must be widely distributed and disseminated to all appropriate caregivers.
- Provincial and national health ministries should collaborate with the professional organizations to develop, where appropriate, bodies or systems that collate, review, interpret, disseminate, and monitor health care evidence. This would facilitate the incorporation of clinical and non-clinical evidence into accessible and comprehensive databases and increase the availability, comprehensiveness, and accessibility of informational data to decision makers (e.g., practitioners, hospitals, programs).
- Public programs should be developed to encourage consumers to be more knowledgeable of the evidence and actively involved in decision making regarding its adoption or nonadoption.

Environmental factors (administrative, economical, community, political, personal/professional, consumer, cultural) strongly influence the adoption of evidence.

Environmental factors contribute to the complexity of the decision-making process. The number and nature of influential factors involved in the decision-making process influences the direction and degree of adoption. Environmental factors are either significant facilitators or barriers. If evidence facilitates the process and is not in contradiction to important factors, evidence is easily adopted (e.g., Ottawa Ankle Rules, carotid endarterectomy), but if evidence is perceived to complicate and is in conflict with important factors, practice is not readily changed (e.g., fetal monitoring).

- Encourage granting bodies to support further research on complex health care decisions. Studies need to describe the nature and influence of influential factors in complex administrative and clinical decisions, determine effective methods for collation and synthesis of evidence in relation to individual/community experiences, and determine effective implementation and evaluation strategies.

Economic conditions were a strong driving force for the initiation of examination of the evidence (e.g., hospital closures). Economic conditions within the clinical realm at times were a barrier if the evidence-based change was perceived to be an economic disincentive (e.g., appropriate use of prostatectomy). Economic influence needs to be neutralized where possible.

- As forms of health care payments are reviewed, the incorporation of the best available evidence into practice seems to be facilitated when fees for service are not a significant component of the decision-making process. Economic resources and reimbursement should facilitate and support the adoption of evidence.

Incorporation of evidence is facilitated by interdisciplinary approaches within clinical settings and programs (provincial or national). These approaches ensure a broad-based, organized approach to assessment and implementation of the evidence. Furthermore, continuation of these approaches through quality assurance monitoring ensures that presumed outcomes are achieved.

- At all levels (national, provincial, hospital, community, professional) the incorporation of evidence into practice and administrative decisions must be a planned process that formally includes significant stakeholders. Decision making is rarely confined to one discipline or one site; thus decision makers and resources to support the adoption of the evidence should be consolidated where possible. Decisions should be evaluated through quality assurance monitoring of defined outcomes. Quality assurance programs need to collect and evaluate information in relation to appropriately approved standards and outcomes. Outcomes need to be congruent with expected norms (e.g., utilization rates, national trends, accepted values).

Personal and professional beliefs strongly influence evidence sought, interpretation of evidence, and incorporation of evidence into practice. Clearly, personal and professional judgment influences the decision-making process. However, if evidence is compelling and professional endorsement of suggested evidence adoption exists, providers of publicly financed services should be obliged to adopt the evidence into their practices.

There is a continuum of responsibility and accountability for evidence adoption: sole private practices to national programs. Along this continuum, evaluation of practice in relation to the best available evidence and accountability for practice in relation to professional or public standards are required. The boundary between professional and public responsibility and accountability is unclear.

- Professional organizations need to develop strategies that ensure professional standards reflect consistent adoption of the best available evidence. Where appropriate, provincial and national ministries need to be reassured, either through regular reporting or surveillance, that standards are being achieved.

The role of the consumer in relation to evidence-based decision making is underdeveloped. Many professionals believe that the consumer exerts little influence on the adoption of evidence into practice. However, in specific examples, the consumer exerted a very strong influence on the development, assessment, and synthesis of the available evidence (e.g., acupuncture, addiction treatment programs, fetal monitoring). We need to recognize the importance of the consumer and provide appropriate education and opportunities to share in the development of, and responsibility for, health care decisions.

- Encourage professional organizations and provincial ministries to collaborate on the development of strategies to ensure consumers are knowledgeable of health evidence and are actively involved in review and synthesis of the evidence into their community.

Summary

To ensure more comprehensive health care, the Health Action Lobby (HEAL) proposes a decision-making framework in which policy demands, originating from consumers, providers, political consideration or science, are subject to a decision-making process of three sequential policy filters: efficacy and effectiveness (health research), appropriateness (policy advisory), and affordability (government). These policy filters assist decision makers in assessments of benefits and risks by developing strategies for careful revision of the evidence, ensuring input from health professionals and consumers and interpretation in relation to societal values by the government (Health Action Lobby 1994). Adoption of evidence into practice is rarely sequential. Many factors are interacting simultaneously to influence the degree and direction of evidence adoption. If the HEAL framework was further developed and refined to incorporate the important components of evidence-based decision making (evidence, dissemination, influential factors), a comprehensive framework could be created. A comprehensive framework for further research and development of evidence-based decision making is required.

Evidence-based decision making is complex. Across the health care system there are enablers and barriers to decision making. A system that recognizes these important influential factors and establishes process and structures to support the adoption of evidence will better ensure comprehensive, effective health care.

SECTION I – BIBLIOGRAPHY

ALKIN, M., R. DAILLAK, and P. WHITE. 1979. Toward a theory of evaluation utilization. In *Using Evaluations: Does Evaluation Make a Difference?*, (Anonymous) Beverly Hills (CA): Sage Publications.

BROOK, R. 1993. Using scientific information to improve quality of health care. *Annals of the New York Academy of Science* 703: 74–85.

FITCH, M. 1992. Fostering research growth in a nursing department. *Canadian Journal of Nursing Administration* 5(1): 11–27.

FUNK, S., E. TORNQUIST, and M. CHAMPAGNE. 1995. Barriers and facilitators of research utilization. *Nursing Clinics of North America* 30: 395–407.

FUNK, S., M. CHAMPAGNE, E. TORNQUIST, and R. WIESE. 1995. Administrator's views on barriers to research utilization. *Applied Nursing Research* 8: 44–49.

FUNK, S., M. CHAMPAGNE, R. WIESE, and E. TORNQUIST. 1991. Barriers to using research findings in practice: The clinician's perspective. *Applied Nursing Research* 4: 90–95.

GRIMSHAW, J., and I. RUSSELL. 1993. Effect of clinical guidelines on medical practice: A systematic review of rigorous evaluations. *The Lancet.* 342: 1217–1322.

HEALTH ACTION LOBBY. 1994. *Getting to the Core of Comprehensiveness: A Discussion Paper by the Health Action Lobby.* Published in cooperation with the Canadian Hospital Association, the Canadian Long-Term Care Association, the Canadian Medical Association, the Canadian Nurses Association, the Canadian Psychological Association, the Canadian Public Health Association, and the Consumers Association of Canada.

KELLY, J., and M. TOEPP. 1992. Practice parameters: Development, evaluation, dissemination, and implementation. *Quality Review Bulletin* 18(12): 405–409.

LESTER, J., and L. WILDS. 1990. The utilization of public policy analysis: A conceptual framework. *Evaluation and Program Planning* 13: 313–319.

LOMAS, J. 1993. Retailing research: Increasing the role of evidence in clinical services for childbirth. *The Millbank Quarterly* 71: 439–475.

LUCKENBILL, B. 1989. Organizational integrative mechanisms and adoption of innovations by nurses. *Nursing Research* 38: 105–110.

MITTMAN, B., X. TONESK, and P. JACOBSEN. 1992. Implementing clinical practice guidelines: Social influence strategies and practitioner behaviour change. *Quality Review Bulletin* 18(12): 413–422.

VANAMRINGE, M., and T. SHANNON. 1992. Awareness, assimilation, and adoption: The challenge of effective dissemination and the first ACHPR-sponsored guidelines. *Quality Review Bulletin* 18(12): 397–404.

YIN, R. 1994. *Case Study Research: Design and Methods.* Thousand Oaks (CA): Sage Publications.

SECTION II – PRIMARY CASE SYNOPSES

Clinical Practice Case Synopses

Routine Electronic Fetal Surveillance and Use of Cesarean Section

The use of routine electronic fetal surveillance and rates of cesarean section vary within Canada. The best available evidence suggests there is no improvement in neonatal outcome with electronic fetal monitoring and, in fact, maternal outcome may be adversely affected (Neilson 1994). The best available evidence recommends that appropriate use of cesarean section delivery is associated with the following practices: trial of labour for breech (under specific conditions) and previous uterine scar, accurate diagnosis of dystocia, and accurate determination of fetal distress (Canadian Medical Association 1986).

Stable evidence strongly indicates a change toward lower usage of electronic fetal monitoring and cesarean section, but practice across Canada is inconsistent, suggesting that the available evidence has had little influence on decision making (Helewa 1995). The focus of this case was to identify the influence of various factors on how evidence was used in practice decisions regarding routine electronic monitoring and cesarean sections.

Classification

This case was identified as an opportunity for improvement because incorporation of the best available evidence was inconsistent and there was potential for gain in both efficiency and effectiveness.

Sample

Twelve sites with high and low cesarean section (C/S) rates were identified from the Health Canada Reports (1994). Four sites (two with the highest rates and two with the lowest rates) were chosen for interview. Interviews were not obtained from the two sites with high rates: one refused to participate and the other did not return initial contact calls. Two sites (six participants) were surveyed by interview. Questionnaire response rate was 53 percent (21/40).

Findings

Quality of the evidence – The evidence was perceived as credible, stable, and convincing by half the respondents (figure 20). However, some individuals reported that study findings, specifically those related to electronic fetal monitoring (EFM) were difficult to interpret and contradictory. There was no reported use of the Cochrane Collaboration Pregnancy and Childbirth Database. As one expert reported: "The evidence regarding appropriate use of electronic fetal surveillance is compelling, yet clinicians choose to question methods and results because the findings are not congruent with their beliefs."

Figure 20

The best available evidence is credible

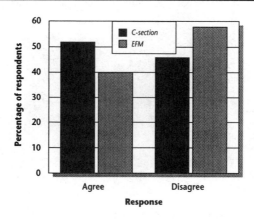

Degree of adoption – As expected, EFM practice varied, with the range for its use being continuous, intermittent, on admission only, as needed, or for specific conditions (epidural, oxytocin stimulation).

Usage of C/S was more consistent. Most sites conducted trials of labour with breech presentations and previous uterine scar. The most common indication for primary cesarean section was failure to progress. Most were aware of the Canadian consensus guidelines regarding C/S but found them difficult to implement as diagnosis of dystocia and fetal distress was complex (figure 21).

Attempts to manage C/S use better were more consistently reported. Most decision makers (60 percent) felt that EFM practice was not changing to become more consistent with best available evidence (figure 22).

Dissemination – Evidence related to electronic fetal surveillance and cesarean section was disseminated through consensus guidelines, organized regional perinatal educational programs, local research initiatives, and published reports. An extensive database of randomized clinical trials, the Cochrane Childbirth and Pregnancy Collaboration, is available but many clinicians did not use this resource (figure 23).

Administrative support – The hospital administrative environment was a substantial influential factor (figure 24). Hospitals' culture, beliefs, policy, and programs facilitated the incorporation of evidence into practice. For example, to monitor effectiveness, some sites implemented quality assurance programs.

Figure 21

Practice in my community is consistent
with the best available evidence

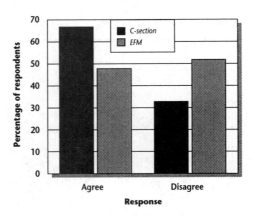

Figure 22

Practice in my community is changing to become more consistent
with the best available evidence

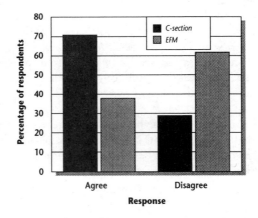

One clinician reported: "Along with the CMDP [College of Physicians, Dentists and Pharmacists] and the local obstetrical review committee, we are doing an awareness campaign to promote decreased use of EFM. We have established a interdisciplinary committee that looks at the rate and type of interventions."

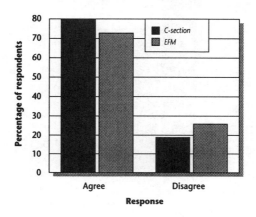

Figure 23

Dissemination to health care providers is good

Figure 24

Administrative factors have a positive influence on evidence adoption

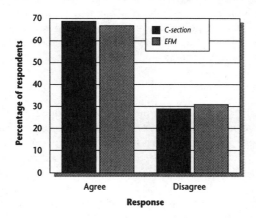

Administrative support was necessary for the adoption of evidence for both C/S and EFM.

Caregiver attitude – Caregiver attitude was a substantial influential factor and was diverse. In interview sites with high cesarean section rates, caregivers did not want to share their experience. Caregivers in interview sites with low rates and questionnaire respondents readily shared their diverse philosophy and attitudes regarding the incorporation of evidence into practice (figure 25).

Figure 25

Personal factors influence evidence adoption

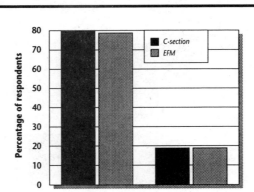

One physician reported:

C/S decisions come from personal experience and attitude of trying to de-medicalize the birthing process, [from] personal and colleagues' experience. Rarely does evidence play a role in decision making as this is not a university centre. Nurses are not trained to read the strips. The interpretation is done by the physician. A policy is available on when to use EFM but we use personal experience and knowledge more. Initial decision making about EFM comes from the nurse and then it is ordered by the physician.

One nurse manager reported:

My knowledge of research is limited. My knowledge comes from experience not just the evidence. Nursing personnel rely on the information brought to them by the residents. EFM is used quite extensively within the hospital, but I do not believe we overuse it. Evidence is used to develop and implement protocols on interpretation of fetal monitoring strips. The hospital wants EFM to be used. There is some preoccupation with litigation. Often EFM is used to protect staff from legal suits and is used as a basis for proving the fetus is not in distress. EFM is well known by consumers. They could go into a court of law and state they did not receive EFM, whereas their roommate did. Research is useful as it keeps you informed—however, it is not well distributed. Nurses rely heavily on hearsay from those deemed to be experts (i.e., residents). As we are in the process of merger, research is not an important issue—other priorities are more important. Researchers say EFM should not be used all the time, yet EFM is a very useful tool. It would be very difficult to give it up.

Liability – Liability was voiced by some as a large concern. In this case, this concern was a barrier to the adoption of the best available evidence. Electronic fetal monitoring was used more readily as caregivers perceived continuous information, available from a continuous recording, was better evidence and, therefore, reduced liability (figure 26).

Figure 26

Liability concerns influence evidence adoption

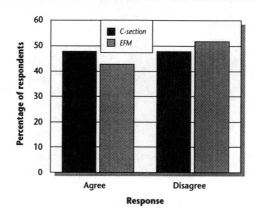

Consumer influence – Interestingly, most decision makers did not perceive that public pressure influenced evidence adoption. However, in those sites where there was strong consumer and cultural influence, practice reflected this influence (figure 27). For example, in a Quebec site with a low C/S rate, a physician reported that consumers were insisting on less EFM and C/Ss, based on information obtained from a popular book by H. Vadeboncœur, *Une autre césarienne? Non merci.*

Conclusions

Decision making regarding EFM and C/S is complex, a high-stake outcome (birth) with many substantial influential factors involved in the decision-making process: personal attitude, litigation, availability of information (e.g., continuous record versus intermittent), consumer influence, education (e.g., nursing knowledge about interpretation of fetal monitoring strips), and hierarchical health care team structure. These influential factors are either strong barriers or enablers to the adoption of evidence. The culture of the practice environment seems to be the filter through which these factors become enablers or barriers. An environment that reflects an interventionist approach to childbirth, is fearful of litigation, is not program based nor open to consumer input is more likely not to adopt the evidence.

Figure 27

Public pressure influences evidence adoption

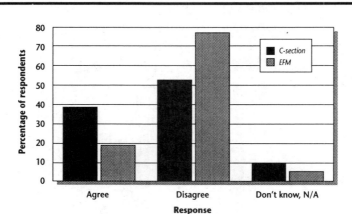

The evidence is stable, convincing, and available for dissemination (database, published reports, consensus guidelines) but its impact remains varied. There are many unanswered questions:

- Why are the C/S rates the lowest where there is no clear adoption of the evidence?
- Are culture and attitude the most influential factors in this case?
- Why are the rates higher where there is easy access to regional perinatal educational expertise?

This case demonstrated the importance of opinion leaders (attitude) and environment. Initiatives to demedicalize childbirth resulted in low C/S rates despite barriers to evidence adoption.

Selection of Cases for Carotid Endarterectomy

Evidence clearly demonstrates that carotid endarterectomy is beneficial for selected patient groups, particularly those with high-grade stenosis (Gentleman and Parson 1994; Matchar and Goldstein 1992). Diagnosis and medical treatment of those patients at risk for ischemic stroke and asymptomatic disease has proven problematic in evaluating the appropriate use of carotid endarterectomy. Consensus guidelines suggest that several additional groups of patients, where there are not definitive findings, may be appropriate for this procedure (Moore and Barnett 1995). Early diagnosis and treatment (surgical) determine the effectiveness of this procedure on patient outcome.

The focus of this case was to identify the influence of various factors on how evidence was used in practice decisions regarding the selection of cases for carotid endarterectomy.

Classification

This case was classified as a successful adoption of evidence. Utilization rates between the early 1980s and the present reflect the incorporation of the best available evidence.

Sample

Six sites were identified from the examination of the Health Canada Reports (1994). Four sites were identified for interview: two with the highest rate and two with the lowest rate. The two sites with the highest rates did not consent to participate in the interview process. An alternate hospital site within close geographical proximity was approached. This site also refused. Interview response rate was 25 percent (2/8) and questionnaire response rate was 60 percent (3/5).

Findings

Degree of adoption – The degree of adoption was difficult to determine from the responses. It was presumed, from the utilization rates, that the evidence was adopted partially to completely.

Quality of evidence – Generally, practitioners felt that the evidence was sound and clear for symptomatic patients with 70 percent stenosis. Evidence was less clear regarding asymptomatic diagnosis, intraoperative shunting versus nonshunting, patch closure or not, timing after incomplete stroke, use of carotid endarterectomy in combination with aneurysm repairs, and optimal preoperative cardiovascular assessment. Evidence of the effectiveness was compelling, but evidence of cost-effectiveness was not.

Dissemination – Evidence was presented well but not distributed, as one clinician reported, in a "digestible fashion." Practitioners were responsible for reviewing, critiquing, and interpreting the studies for implications related to practice. Many practitioners stated they did not have the time or resources to do this and felt that high-quality evidence, such as was available with this case, needed to be easier to interpret and read. One clinician reported that "CME does not work—doctors go to talks but do not change practice and patients are not referred appropriately."

Liability – Liability concerns were present but did not seem to be a driving force.

Administrative support – The administrative environment seemed to have little influence on the adoption of this evidence into practice. However, in those sites with quality assurance programs, evidence was used as a benchmark to monitor surgical rates and effectiveness.

There were no written policies: decision making was practitioner driven. Evaluation and monitoring of community surgeons (even though there were not many) were more difficult if they were not associated with major referral centres.

Attitude – All clinicians interviewed strongly supported the use of evidence in practice and often attended professional conferences.

Conclusions

Credible, stable, quality evidence was available for one aspect of this case, specifically, the selection of patients with greater than 70 percent stenosis for surgery. The interpretation of evidence with other patient groups and with diagnosis or assessment of stenosis was more difficult.

Evidence has not been incorporated into clear guidelines. Dissemination to relevant stakeholders in the community and nonteaching hospitals is varied.

Practice was sole-practitioner driven. If the practitioner was not within a teaching hospital and with quality assurance programs, there were few checks and balances in the decision-making process. As evident through those sites which declined to participate, some physicians were reluctant to discuss the rationale for their practice decisions.

Selection of BPH Cases for Prostatectomy

Benign prostate hyperplasia (BPH) is a benign neoplasm with a high prevalence rate that increases progressively with age. Four conditions are associated with the disease process of BPH: anatomic prostatic hyperplasia, the presence of symptoms commonly referred to as prostatism, the urodynamic presence of obstruction, and the response of the bladder muscle to obstruction. The etiology of the disease is poorly understood. Outcome data regarding the natural history and treatment of BPH are lacking and, because of these uncertainties, there is substantial geographic variation in BPH treatment patterns.

The best available evidence has been incorporated into guideline recommendations (McConnell and Barry 1994). The goals of the guidelines are to identify the most appropriate and effective diagnostic methods for detecting BPH and assessment of its severity, and select the most appropriate treatment approach. Since BPH is rarely life threatening, many patients choose a regime of watchful waiting rather than more active treatments. Guidelines detail the relative benefits and harms associated with invasive and noninvasive treatment methods. Laser prostatectomy and thermal therapy are emerging modalities for which the evidence of effectiveness is not well established.

Ultimately, the decision to proceed with a prostatectomy should be a shared decision between the patient and physician. Decision tools (interactive videos) have facilitated the decision-making process and are used in many, but not all, programs. The use of video to help make decisions is associated with increased selection of watchful waiting rather than surgery (Kaspar and Mulley 1992; Wagner and Barrett 1995).

The focus of this case was to identify the influence of factors on how evidence was used in practice decisions regarding the selection of BPH cases for prostatectomy.

Classification

This case was classified as an opportunity for improvement as there was a wide range of prostatectomy rates across Canada suggesting that clinicians and patients are using different decision criteria (Gentleman and Parson 1994).

Sample

Nine sites for study were identified from the examination of Health Canada Reports (1994). Four sites (two with the highest rate and two with the lowest rate) were approached for interview. Two of the identified interview hospital sites with high surgical rates refused to participate as they did not want to provide information about what influenced their decisions to perform surgery or not. Questionnaire response rate was 27 percent (3/11), and interview response rate was 25 percent (2/8). The sample for this case was small but those clinicians who were interviewed provided some interesting responses to the posed questions.

Findings

Degree of adoption – The degree of adoption of the evidence was difficult to determine due to the poor survey response rate. Based on utilization rates and interview comments, it was presumed that evidence adoption was varied.

Quality of evidence – The quality of evidence was perceived as good. There were many randomized trials with reliable long-term data. The clinical practice guidelines were based on a review of the evidence by a panel of experts and the American Public Health Service, in conjunction with the Department of Health.

Some aspects of the evidence were not found useful enough to support clinical practice (i.e., scoresheet), suggesting that physicians may disregard these and recommend surgery for the patient. Cost-effectiveness of watchful waiting was questioned: "If surgery is not being done, then extra testing and drug prescriptions are involved which may be just as costly as surgical intervention. These costs are not tracked."

Dissemination – Detailed comprehensive guidelines are available. Some clinicians reported that multiple guidelines are available and some of the information is confusing and conflicting. One clinician reported: "All guidelines need to be individualized for the patient. One person's discomfort may be another person's agony."

Administrative support— Administrative support was a positive influential factor. Quality assurance monitoring in a hospital with a low rate ensured a process was in place to implement and monitor practice change. "In our hospital, all patients see the video as part of the divisional program for this condition. The practice is monitored through the quality assurance program, an elaborate system that measures disease outcome and patient satisfaction."

Economic conditions— High surgical rates may be related to the potential reduction in physician's income. There was an economic disincentive to perform less surgery. However, one physician researcher reported that many drug studies are currently targeting urologists for participation in trials. Most of these studies have honorariums attached with them.

Personal attitude – Physician attitude toward patient involvement in decision making influences use of decision-making tools. One physician reported:

> The video may not be useful as the patient comes away more confused than clear. The more intelligent patient will ask more questions and pursue more options. The medical community wants to offer the patient more input, and this is the modern trend now. I don't necessarily agree. A five-minute video does not make a patient competent. Some patients want the doctor to make the decision.

Conclusions

The quality of evidence was perceived as sound, scientific, and applicable to the general population.

Dissemination of evidence was widespread through the use of guidelines and professional associations.

Individual practice patterns remain varied. This may be related to economic disincentive (loss of income with surgery) and more time required with medical management.

Individual practitioners' beliefs regarding patient involvement in care decisions influence the degree that patient decision-making aids are used.

Administrative programs that included an interdisciplinary approach, application of accepted guidelines, and a quality assurance component facilitated patient involvement in decision making.

Implementation of the Ottawa Ankle Rules

Evidence suggests that nonradiographic assessment methods can determine ankle fracture in selected cases. Single and multisite trials have demonstrated 93 to 100 percent sensitivity for the Ottawa Ankle Rules (OAR) with a substantial reduction in radiological determination and associated costs (Lucchesi and Jackson 1995; Pigman and Klug 1994). Since its recent introduction in 1992, adoption of the OAR seems fairly well spread (Stiell and Greenberg 1992; Stiell and McKnight 1994). The rules have been widely published and disseminated in a variety of forms (pocket cards, video) and appear easy to implement in emergency room settings.

The focus of this study was to identify the influence of various factors on how evidence was used in decision making regarding the implementation of the OAR in emergency room departments.

Classification

This case was classified as a success because there appears to be widespread adoption of the best available evidence into clinical practice resulting in more appropriate use of resources.

Sample

Fourteen emergency departments in community hospitals or larger teaching hospitals across Canada were approached to participate. Three sites were identified for interviewing and five sites were surveyed by questionnaire. Many sites (six) declined to be involved; some were not familiar with the rules. Questionnaire response rate was 55 percent (11/20) and interview response rate was 70 percent (7/10).

Findings

Degree of adoption – Fifty-five percent of the clinicians reported that practice was not consistent with the best available evidence. The Ottawa Ankle Rules were either partially or completely adopted. However, in most centres, practice was changing to become more consistent with the evidence (figure 28).

Quality of the evidence – Clinicians familiar with the guidelines felt the available evidence was scientifically sound, stable, and applicable to the general population. The overall conclusion was that use of the OAR was a safe and effective practice (figure 29).

Dissemination – Dissemination of the OAR varied. In a smaller, northern community hospital, emergency physicians and nurse administrators were not familiar with the rules and unable to answer the questions related to evidence adoption regarding implementation. But these practitioners provided some useful feedback regarding how evidence was assessed and obtained within their isolated geographical site: "Clinical practice guidelines are not filtering down. I finished my education three years ago, and my practice is based pretty much on what I was taught then. I think guidelines based on good evidence are important but they need to be accessible and easy to read. Unfortunately, I cannot access the journals each week to determine what is the best evidence for my practice."

Figure 28

Practice is consistent with the best available evidence

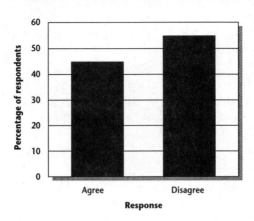

Figure 29

Evidence is credible

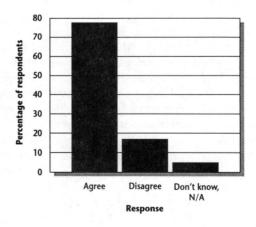

Although no one had presented the OAR guidelines to them, they felt their practice was fairly consistent with recommended practice.

Clinicians familiar with the guidelines felt that the evidence was well published in appropriate journals (figure 30). Findings were incorporated into easy to read "cards." Decision-making tools and educational programs were available for staff and patients.

Figure 30

Dissemination of evidence to health care providers is good

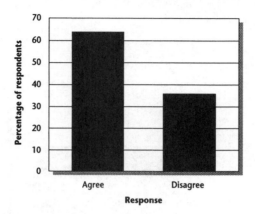

Administrative support – Administrative support was perceived as a substantial influential factor. Administrative support facilitated orientation of nursing staff and the establishment of policies to support practice changes (figure 31).

Figure 31

Administrative factors have a positive influence on evidence adoption

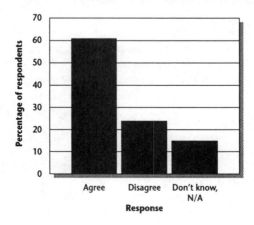

Liability – Concern about liability and patient attitude potentially influenced the application of the OAR by some physicians (figure 32).

One physician reported: "The CMPA newsletter stated that one of the areas of highest liability in the emergency department is because doctors are not X raying limbs enough—so we do more X rays."

Figure 32

Liability concerns influence evidence adoption

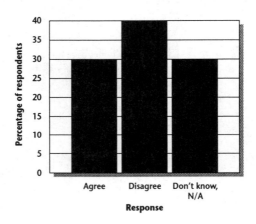

Physician attitude– Sites reported that implementation of the rules was difficult as there were isolated incidents where patients required an X ray. As a result, some physicians did not believe the rules could replace an X ray. Feedback or evaluation data were not regularly received.

One physician reported: "It almost seems that, for physicians to accept guidelines, they need to develop them on their own which is not really feasible. We did not create a hospital policy but we are now involved in an evaluation process and this information will be useful."

Generally, it was felt that professional attitude toward evidence adoption influenced decision making. If emergency department physicians were supportive of the evidence, practice changes occurred readily (figure 33).

Conclusions

Quality evidence is available and incorporated into easy-to-read guidelines with clear decision rules.

Guidelines were disseminated in published journals and through professional organizations, such as the Canadian Association of Emergency Physicians (CAEP).

Figure 33
Personal factors influence evidence adoption

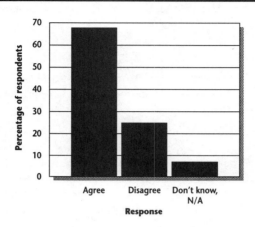

Guidelines provided simple direction for individual practitioner care; hospital policies were not created.

Guidelines were not consistently disseminated to more geographically remote areas.

Evidence was easily incorporated into nursing or physician practice in emergency room settings. Decision making was not complex.

Individual practitioners are influenced by perceived consumer need for more information (e.g., X ray) and fear of liability (e.g., missing something).

Pharmaceutical Case Synopses

Promoting Appropriate Medication Use by Elderly Persons

The best available evidence suggests that inappropriate use of medications by elderly persons is a common occurrence in Canada, resulting in substantial preventable health care costs (Canadian Medical Association 1993; Coambs and Jensen 1996). Several factors contribute to improper use of medications, including, but not limited to, multiple prescription, drug packaging, poor assessment of patient capability, inadequate patient teaching, and poor prescription tracking (Canadian Medical Association 1993; Davidson and Molloy 1994). More appropriate use of medication is possible with careful prescribing, medication monitoring, and patient education (Tamblyn and McLeod 1994). Health ministries, pharmacists, physicians, and consumers can contribute to improved medication use (Pharmaceutical Inquiry of Ontario 1990).

Some provinces have initiated programs such as provincial information systems, others have not. The focus of this case was to identify the influence of various factors on how evidence was used in the planning and implementation of initiatives to reduce inappropriate use of medications by elderly persons.

Classification

This case was classified as an opportunity for improvement because it is a high-cost, high-volume occurrence for which there are potential gains in effectiveness and efficiency.

Sample

Eight provincial sites were identified for participation. Sites had either implemented programs to address medication use in elderly persons or were in the process of addressing the issue. Questionnaire response rate was 67 percent (8/12), and interview response rate was 41 percent (7/17).

Findings

Quality of the evidence – The evidence was convincing for identifying the problem, specifically, that prescription drug use increases with age and that the hazards of drug use are most evident in older patients and are associated with hospital admissions.

Evidence was less convincing on the effectiveness of programs to address the problem. Programs surveyed included consumer-oriented help lines, screening of persons at high risk for drug dependence, and a community-based pharmaceutical care model (a pharmacy consultation service) for elderly persons.

Institution-based studies demonstrate that pharmacists can influence prescribing, resulting in fewer inappropriate medication choices, fewer drug reactions, and fewer adverse drug effects. Few effectiveness and cost-effectiveness evaluations of community-based programs exist.

One pharmacist reported: "We have a lot of anecdotal evidence of effectiveness. We get 2,300 calls per year and, if 10 admissions to hospital were prevented, the cost of the line would be covered."

Dissemination – Annual reports facilitated communication within the pharmacy profession. Reports need to be more readily available to other stakeholders (physicians, consumers). Access to a locus of pharmacy experts and current drug information programs were perceived as necessary supports for community medication information (e.g., line) operations.

There was no organized or program approach to dissemination of the information.

Economic conditions – There was a perceived lack of funding to assess effectiveness of intervention programs. Most of the research literature in this area is descriptive, and few centres or programs are objectively and scientifically evaluated.

Conclusions

Clearly, inappropriate medication use in elderly persons has been identified by ministries and experts as an important health care issue. That misuse is associated with increased costs to the health care system (increased hospital admissions). However, the evidence on the type of interventions needed to address the issue is less convincing. There is little evidence of effectiveness of provincial initiatives and interventions.

Most initiatives to address this issue are spearheaded by expert individuals and local interest.

While guidelines have been developed for physicians and pharmacists, these seem to have little impact on prescription practices and, ultimately, on consumer compliance or noncompliance (intentional or nonintentional) with medication therapy.

It is perceived that a more organized approach that incorporates expert opinion and available evidence from pharmacists, physicians and consumers would facilitate the generation of quality evidence on which to base practice change.

Appropriate Timing of Thrombolysis Therapy in Acute Myocardial Infarction

Evidence suggests that the timing of thrombolytic therapy for the management of acute myocardial infarction (AMI) is essential to successful patient outcome (Cairns and Armstrong 1994; Franzosi and Maggioni 1994; Van de Werf and Topol 1995).

Recommendations for ensuring early thrombolytic therapy for acute myocardial infarction require streamlining of current practices and enhanced cooperation among health care professionals to expedite care. Early recognition of AMI symptoms by the public and health care professional, early access to emergency medical services, and early action by emergency care providers in administering thrombolytic therapy (within 30 minutes of patients' arrival in department) is recommended (Cairns and Armstrong 1994; Weston and Penny 1994).

Classification

This issue was classified as a success as several reports suggest that use of thrombolytic therapy is widespread and extends to rural and northern areas in Canada (Hindle and Norheim 1995; Hutten-Czapski 1993; Pachos and Normand 1994).

Sample

Key informants were identified at nine community and teaching hospitals. Four interviews were arranged with emergency (ER) or cardiology department heads. Questionnaire response rate was 67 percent (8/12) and interview response rate was 41 percent (7/17).

Findings

Degree of adoption – Emergency physicians reported that patients with cardiac symptoms are triaged immediately (some in the ambulance), diagnostic tests completed (ECG) and medication administered within 30 to 35 minutes. Choice of medication depends on location of the myocardial infarction, duration of symptoms (i.e., more than six hours) and patient history. Some centres administered the medication in emergency or after immediate transfer of patient directly to a coronary care unit (CCU).

All centres interviewed reported that they monitored the "door to needle" time with the goal being administration of thrombolysis within 30 minutes of admission.

Quality of the evidence – Physicians reported that the evidence was convincing in that there were:
- a number of large, scientifically sound, clinical trials; and
- trial outcome results were consistent—early thrombolysis treatment results in less morbidity and mortality.

As one physician reported: "There is overwhelming, indisputable evidence, that is stable across time, reproducible, scientifically sound criteria, applicable to any setting, worldwide."

Dissemination – The Canadian consensus guidelines were useful in that they provided specific recommendations in terms of indications, contra-indications, and adjunct medications. Experts synthesized the findings from the clinical trials. Generally, the guidelines were reviewed by cardiologists and emergency physicians and were used as guidelines for hospital policy development: "Based on the guidelines we made the following changes: (1) nursing staff performed ECGs—not a technician, (2) the ECG was shown immediately to a physician and not filed on rack, and (3) a practice policy was developed and disseminated by the Nurse Manager."

The Canadian Association of Emergency Physicians (CAEP) developed and delivered a series of workshops in at least 18 different cities across Canada. The workshop was designed to teach ER physicians how to recognize and manage acute myocardial infarction with thrombolysis therapy. This was an effective dissemination method.

Administrative support – The formation of hospital committees ensured that the appropriate organizational supports were available for the practice change. Interdisciplinary committees planned for and ensured orientation of hospital staff. Quality assurance programs involving regular chart reviews which focused on timing of drug administration ensured that practice was changing.

Some centres reported that, with recent hospital restructuring, inexperienced nurses are reassigned into the ER. Educated and qualified nursing staff members are essential to the early recognition of cardiac symptoms and appropriate triage and facilitation of therapy.

Personal/professional attitude – Some reported that some ER physicians are intimidated by complications associated with thrombolytic therapy and are concerned about liability.

Conclusions

This case demonstrated successful adoption of evidence.

Scientifically sound evidence was available and disseminated in an organized manner (consensus conference, CAEP presentations).

These rules were relatively easy to implement within hospital settings that provided the necessary education and resources. No attitudinal barriers existed. Care was perceived to be more efficient and effective with the suggested changes.

Health Care Delivery Case Synopses

Implementation of Second-Dose Measles Vaccine

Measles continues to be a public health problem in developed and developing countries, despite the availability of an effective vaccine (Orenstein and Markowitz 1994). Full control of the disease has not been achieved, in part due to primary and secondary vaccine failure. In Canada, in 1988, measles immunization coverage of one year was reported as 85 percent, using a single dose of measles vaccine with mandatory school entry vaccination. The measles incidence rate dropped from 9.4 per 100,000 (1987) to 2.4 per 100,000 (1988). Despite the introduction of routine vaccination programs, epidemics have occurred in highly immunized populations (Atkinson and Orenstein 1995).

Single-dose vaccine coverage will not achieve the measles eradication goal set because of the difficulties in obtaining 95 percent coverage in infancy and the primary-dose vaccine failure. A second-dose measles vaccination program is recommended to achieve this goal (Ontario Ministry of Health 1995; Tulchinsky and Ginsberg 1993).

In 1992, the Measles Consensus Conference recommended a national goal of measles elimination by the year 2005. To achieve this goal, each province examined its practice and implemented the following policy changes (table 3).

Table 3

Measles programs in Canada – updated March 1996

Province/territory	Routine second dose
British Columbia	Yes
Alberta	Yes
Saskatchewan	Yes
Manitoba	Yes
Ontario	Yes
Quebec	Yes
Nova Scotia	Possible – FY 96/97
New Brunswick	No
Prince Edward Island	Yes
Newfoundland	Possible – January 1997
Yukon	Yes
Northwest Territories	Yes

Source: KFLA Health Unit, Kingston, Ontario.

The focus of this case was to identify the influence of various factors on decision making regarding the implementation of provincial second-dose measles vaccine programs.

Classification

This case was classified as a success, for there was widespread adoption of evidence.

Sample

All provinces were surveyed. Informants in New Brunswick, the Northwest Territories, Nova Scotia, and Ontario were interviewed. Questionnaire response rate was 48 percent (20/42) and interview response rate was 89 percent (8/9).

Findings

Degree of adoption – As expected, practice was consistent with the best available evidence and provincial programs were implementing a second-dose measles vaccine program. While some provinces were in the planning and implementation stages, all reported that practice was changing or actually was consistent with the national direction (figure 34).

Figure 34

Practice in my community is consistent with the best available evidence

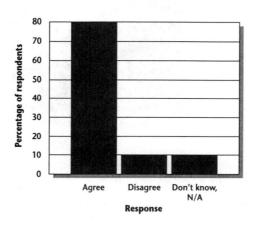

Quality of evidence – Epidemiological evidence from other countries, especially those that had implemented second-dose measles vaccine programs, was very convincing (figure 35). Yet, comments were made that the evidence was not applicable to local situations: "We only have a few scattered outbreaks, suggesting that our single dose is effective."

Evidence for cost-effectiveness was limited in some provinces. In the Northwest Territories, cost-effectiveness of second-dose measles vaccine was easily documented, as most illnesses require a medi-vac to fly the ill person to a southern hospital, and outbreaks were occurring every six to seven years. Conversely, in Nova Scotia, there were not significant treatment costs and only sporadic cases were reported.

Dissemination – The Canadian Consensus Conference, held in August 1995 in conjunction with the Laboratory Centre for Disease Control (LCDC), was effective in building a consensus approach to the problem. Access to international experts who had previous experience with measles campaigns was facilitated. The conference created a momentum or, as one interviewee stated, "a bandwagon." Evidence regarding program content and implementation was disseminated in a variety of ways, for example, through newsletters or communiqués (physicians) (figure 36).

Figure 35

The best available evidence is credible

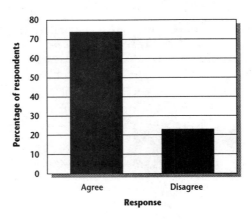

Figure 36

Dissemination to health care providers is good

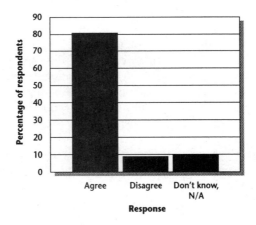

Political support – The national political environment and direction was a key influence. There was a domino effect within the provinces in that they did not want to be perceived as not following the national trend (figure 37).

Administrative support – There was little evidence available for planning and implementation of the policy regarding second-dose schedules. Other factors, such as community, clinician responsibilities, other competing

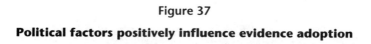

Figure 37

Political factors positively influence evidence adoption

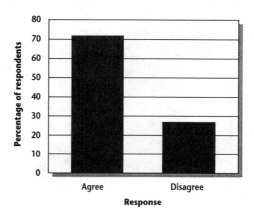

immunization programs (Hepatitis B), other public health priorities, and funding were deemed important considerations.

Personal/professional attitude – Concern was raised about the flow between policy and evidence (figure 38). One administrator reported:

> Policy makers depend on the ability of national or provincial groups to steer them in the desired direction. Sometimes the groups do not translate the information to a relevant level for the province. The flow of evidence is slow and may not be readily available for policy decisions. Another issue is that one cannot be certain that the evidence is unbiased—researchers are only part of the picture. I have two messages:
>
> 1. Evidence is only part of the picture. Researchers are painting an evidence picture; when they make recommendations, they must consider the policy implications and the context in which decisions are made.
>
> 2. Research should not drive policy; policy should drive research. There is a need to do active research to drive policy agendas not create them (or conflicts). Second-dose measles vaccine created a policy dilemma in the country. The evidence did this. The momentum for initiating changes was not driven by the policymakers and, as a result, they had to make an agenda item that was not necessarily their priority.

Conclusions

Best available evidence was perceived as essential to policy decisions but decision makers also considered the economical, political, and geographical implications of the evidence.

Figure 38

Personal factors influence evidence adoption

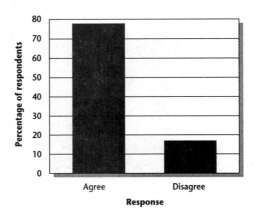

Strong epidemiological evidence was nationally disseminated and discussed (consensus conference). Development of a national policy direction ensured that all provinces addressed the evidence as best they could, taking into account their economic conditions, geography, and program priorities. Concern was raised about the local community implications, but this was raised as an organizational concern and did not influence program implementation. A strong political influence facilitated adoption of the best available evidence.

Implementation of Addiction Treatment Programs for Aboriginal People

Aboriginal health services are based on strong religious and cultural belief systems (Avery 1991; Zubek 1994). Harmony of body, mind, and spirit are the cornerstones of the system. Health practices focus on maintaining or restoring harmony. The evidence to support Aboriginal practice is largely historical and anecdotal in nature, yet these health practices have been successfully employed in many Aboriginal-based programs, including treatment of addictions. While their efficacy is well accepted within Aboriginal communities, this is not necessarily the case within the non-Aboriginal communities where there is more reliance on scientific evidence. As the different types of practices are adopted within the various programs, concessions to traditional Western medicine evidence and strong Aboriginal beliefs and historical evidence are made (Drew 1992; Lechky 1991; Woodard and Edourd 1992).

The focus of this case was to explore the influence of factors on how evidence was used in the development of treatment programs for addictions within the Aboriginal population.

Classification

This case was classified neither as an opportunity for improvement nor a success, for the nature of the case study was to explore the influence of the various factors on evidence adoption within programs.

Sample

Eight treatment centres were approached by phone and by fax. Of those contacted, three agreed to participate (two with interviews and one with a survey questionnaire). We were unable to connect with representatives from four sites, and one site refused. Interview response rate was 63 percent (5/8).

Findings

Nature of the evidence – Evidence was available from two sources: program or site reports, and experiential or historical evidence from within the Aboriginal community. As one administrator reported:

> Evidence is usually not expert opinion nor someone with a professional degree. We are not a culture that likes to write everything down but the evidence that I have read (and believe) shows that Aboriginal needs are based in culture, spirit and need to be really strongly holistic. I am convinced of this evidence when I see clients 'turn around' because they truly own the information they receive and they have really bought into it. You can see their life turn around and that comes from the spiritual and cultural aspect: from the heart, not from the head.

Range of adoption – Adoption of any evidence was strongly centred in a holistic approach, with a strong cultural, spiritual, and family component. The Aboriginal community made it easier to adopt change because of their spiritual and cultural depth. "There are some barriers to the implementation of what we feel is the best evidence: justification to funding bodies, but we do have a strong political board that takes the political heat so that the service providers can do their job. As an administrator, I need to walk in both worlds; to justify our work to funders and deal with the Aboriginal program needs. I have these skills."

One advisor reported:

> I feel there is no strong evidence about the effectiveness of Native addiction treatment centres. The priority of centres is very low, and our connection with the government levels is different with the restructuring.

We have a provincial, not a federal contact person. Most times I feel that we are in a reactionary phase and use more informational data. We cannot control the issues that demand our attention. In order to work with the evidence, we need to have a sense of control and stability. Research evidence is generally useful for informational purposes but, within my organization, I need to make it relevant to the situation.

Aboriginal centres are very different than other addiction centres. Evidence provides caregivers with ideas but, because they speak different dialects and each community is unique, many different factors were taken into consideration when addiction programs were planned.

Dissemination – Evidence (information) was shared between centres in a verbal way through informal networks. At times, administrators reported a sense of isolation and verbalized a desire to share resources and information more.

Reports were readily available from the National Native Alcohol and Drug Abuse Program (NADAP) of Health Canada and organized associations (e.g., Aboriginal Nurses Association, National Addiction Awareness). Reports provided the general structure of programs and direction for the communities to implement within their culture and community.

Conclusions

Awareness of, or reliance on, documented evidence was not a substantial influential factor.

There was an extremely strong base of historical and cultural evidence—a potential wealth of information. Scientific research did not easily translate into applied programs for this issue.

Programs seem to be driven by provincial/federal directions but actual services were based on community need and input and, thus, were sensitive to important cultural, religious, and family values.

There was a sense of isolation with persons in management positions. They felt that evidence and information could be more effectively shared.

Implementation of Breast-Screening Programs

Breast cancer is the most common malignancy and is the leading cause of death in Canadian women (Miller, Baines, and Wall 1992). The epidemiology of breast cancer involves several factors that may be useful in deciding who to recommend for breast cancer screening. The most important factor is age: the evidence consistently reports that mammography screening every two to three years reduces breast cancer mortality in women aged 50 to 69. The evidence on reducing mortality in younger women is not convincing (Shapiro 1994).

Classification

The case was classified as a success, as provinces have either initiated mammography programs for women 50 and older or are in the process of planning them.

Sample

All provinces and territories were invited to participate. Four were interviewed, the remaining provinces were surveyed by questionnaire. Questionnaire response rate was 50 percent (14/28) and interview response rate was 83 percent (5/6). Participants included administrators, researchers, clinicians, and managers.

Findings

Degree of adoption – Breast-screening programs are available and, for the most part, are based on the best available evidence. Partial adoption usually reflected that the program was not successful in screening all women above the age of 50 years (figure 39).

Figure 39

**Practice in my community is consistent
with the best available evidence**

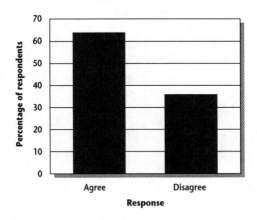

Quality of the evidence – The quality of evidence was perceived as good: scientific, international and national sources, generally applicable to selected populations and stable across time (figure 40). Evidence regarding the effectiveness of breast-self examination was less convincing. Best available evidence was strong enough to support policy direction for women age 50 and over.

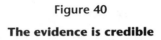

Figure 40

The evidence is credible

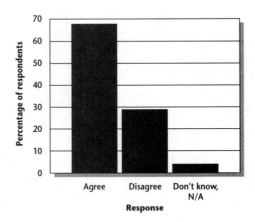

Concern was raised about the lag of scientific evidence, especially in light of better-quality mammography. Perhaps different results would be obtained now (i.e., in the 40 to 49 age group) with better diagnostic equipment and screening.

Screening was perceived as cost effective if the protocols were implemented as provincial programs and recruitment were active in the targeted age group.

Dissemination – Evidence was readily accessible and widely published and distributed (figure 41). Evidence was incorporated quickly and efficiently at the national level; thus all provinces looked at the issue within their ministries.

A national consensus conference on breast screening confirmed policies and directions for practice. Provinces were directed to consider the development of programs for screening women over 50 years, with no upper age limit, every two years. There was no policy direction established for high-risk screening.

Administrative support – Administrative support was essential to the development of programs. One province, in the proposal stage of planning a program, developed an interdisciplinary committee consisting of radiologists, nurses, physicians, breast cancer survivors, and policymakers to examine the evidence and determine direction (figure 42).

There was less available evidence on how to plan and implement programs. For example, one site reported three screening providers: a population health–based screen test only available in urban and some rural centres (through a mobile van), individual radiologists who provided mammography through

Figure 41

Dissemination to health care providers is good

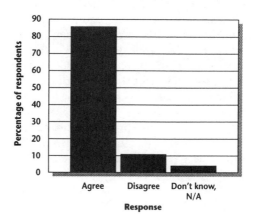

Figure 42

**Administrative factors have a positive influence
on evidence adoption**

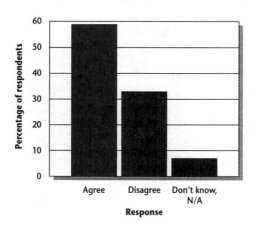

private clinics (limited number), and hospital-based programs. Currently a policy council is trying to organize all providers under one provincial-based program, with active recruitment of women aged 50 to 69 years. The recruitment strategy, evaluation, and quality assurance component of the programs will be based on recommendations from a detailed special task force report. Evidence was key in the development of this strategy.

Implementation of screening programs was influenced by the availability of mammography facilities. In Ontario, a program advisory committee of experts in policy and medical fields provided policy direction for improvement of facilities but believed that the government regulations remained weak. Regulations focused on equipment standards and not on the overall monitoring and regulation of facilities.

Consumer influence – Most participants felt that the consumer was becoming more involved in the implementation of breast-screening programs. However, at least 30 percent thought that there was little consumer influence, either due to lack of opportunities or to lack of knowledge and awareness of issues (figure 43).

Personal/professional attitude – Physician attitude toward screening had an impact on the recruitment of women for screening. Some physicians felt that they could adequately screen for breast cancer (figure 44).

Most providers supported research activities and detailed collection of data. Surveillance data and creation of a national database were perceived as essential for program development and evaluation.

Figure 43

Public pressure influences evidence adoption

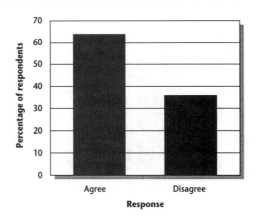

Conclusions

Scientifically sound evidence was accessible and available.

National and provincial commitments to the adoption of evidence facilitated its incorporation into policy. A provincial programmatic approach to evidence adoption seemed the most effective for this case.

Stakeholders (consumer and professional) influenced the adoption of evidence at the local level.

Figure 44
Personal factors influence evidence adoption

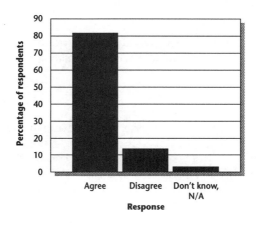

Implementation of Acupuncture Programs

There is a solid scientific base of objective research that acknowledges acupuncture as a form of treatment that stimulates known neuroendocrine elements of human physiology (Han 1982; Lewith and Kenyon 1984). This can have a wide-ranging influence on human function and, in particular, on pain management. Most of the Western medical literature on acupuncture discusses placebo effect, release of endorphins, "gate" theories, and release of serotonin (Millman 1977; Eisenberg et al. 1993). As with many prescription medications, the exact nature in which acupuncture works cannot be fully explained. It has been demonstrated that there is a specific body of knowledge related to acupuncture and that development of this knowledge has led to the development of professional bodies of acupuncturists.

Across Canada, the training of acupuncturists from within their own professional community or other health professionals is diverse. A distinction is commonly made between individuals who are comprehensively trained in acupuncture and use Chinese medicine principles as the basis of their diagnosis and treatment (comprehensively trained) and those who use acupuncture (either Chinese or Western) as an adjunctive therapy within an existing scope of practice of another health care professional (focused trained). Three provinces—Alberta, Quebec, and British Columbia—have legislated and regulated acupuncture as a profession. Other provinces are considering various submissions from professional organizations.

The focus of this case was to identify the various influential factors on how evidence was used in decisions regarding the planning and implementation of acupuncture services within provinces.

Classification

This case was classified as an opportunity for improvement because provincial adoption of acupuncture as an alternate pain management therapy across Canada is diverse.

Sample

Acupuncture professional organizations, ministries of health, and other health professions were approached for inclusion in the study. Six interview and three questionnaire sites were identified. Questionnaire response rate was 60 percent (3/5) and interview response rate was 63 percent (5/11). Participants were administrators involved with policy decisions.

Findings

Quality of evidence – Sources of evidence were perceived as varied and included scientific studies, anecdotal evidence, and historical documents. Evidence consistently concluded that acupuncture is a safe, effective, pain relief measure with minimal side effects.

Effectiveness was perceived to be strongly demonstrated by the historical evidence. Acupuncture has been used therapeutically for over 5,000 years. The effectiveness of the evidence was difficult to determine within the current system, as acupuncturists tended to receive those cases where everything else has failed. To determine the effectiveness in comparison with more traditional care, it was felt that acupuncture care needs to be integrated as a component of the health care system. This would more likely happen as regulation for controls on education and practice standards were established and recognized.

Economic conditions – Economics influenced the adoption of acupuncture services, as most services are not reimbursed in provincially funded programs. Currently, the patient pays for the services unless they are provided within a publicly funded centre. Some private health insurance plans cover acupuncture expenses.

Consumer/culture – Consumer and cultural support strongly influenced the development of acupuncture programs within specific provinces. In Quebec, the consumer played the largest role in the drive to regulate acupuncture. This was probably related to the French cultural influence, as most acupuncture schools are Francophone. Most Anglophone therapists in Quebec are of Oriental origin. Likewise in British Columbia, the cultural influence was significant as a large proportion of the Asian population wished to use acupuncture as a form of therapy.

Political conditions/professional attitude – Evidence was available on the effectiveness of acupuncture as an alternate form of therapy, but evidence carried little weight when there was not a receptive political climate. Informants reported conflict with the medical associations during the discussions regarding establishment of acupuncture programs. Acupuncturists felt that physicians were reluctant to give up aspects of care to acupuncture therapy.

As one advisor stated: "We don't seem to subject medical practice to the same scrutiny to determine whether their procedures should be replaced with less costly nonmedical ones—perhaps we should."

Conclusions

Evidence was used to support the decision to regulate acupuncture, but it was not fundamental. All sources of evidence—commission reports, scientific studies, practice in other communities, and opinion evidence—was reviewed and submitted to form the basis of advisory reports. This generated the necessary background information for the development of professional requirements, practice scope, educational requirements, and governance. The incorporation of the evidence was facilitated by local practitioners, community participants, leaders, consultants, and experts. These factors facilitated the development of a regulated profession and programs within each province, but they were not the driving force to the initial decision to pursue regulation. Culture and consumer influence were the driving forces.

Strong coordinated efforts were required by those provinces that regulated the profession. Continuing effort will be required to further incorporate acupuncture as a truly integrated health service.

Heath Care Management Case Synopses

Hospital Closures

Within the organizational sector of the health care system, many changes are occurring. Restructuring and reform are taking place at federal, provincial, regional, and local levels. The goal is to restructure the system so that it becomes more efficient and cost effective and, ultimately, results in smaller overall expenditures for health care services (Angus 1991; Angus and Turbayne 1995). It is within this context of reorganization and restructuring that hospital closures have taken place. The decision to close a hospital is complex. There are many factors—culture, religion, physical plant, available services, board allegiances, professional unions, etc.—that influence this decision-making process. It is difficult to determine the nature and effect of the best available evidence on such complex decisions as hospital closures.

The purpose of this case study was to determine the influence of various factors on how evidence was used in the decisions to close hospitals.

Classification

Not all provinces are explicitly pursuing hospital closures as a method of cost containment. However, some have implemented partial closures and amalgamations. This case was classified as an opportunity for improvement because of the overall resistance to these decisions, the varied pattern of implementation, and the influence of political conditions and stakeholders on decision making.

Sample

Hospital sites were chosen because they had either closed or were in the process of deciding to close a hospital. Geographical representation across Canada was achieved. Interviews were conducted at three sites. Questionnaire response rate was 60 percent (12/20), and interview response rate was 90 percent (9/10). Participants included administrators involved with policy decisions and consumers (hospital board members).

Findings

Degree of adoption – Participants were relatively split in their opinion regarding the degree of adoption of the evidence for hospital closures. For the most part, administrators felt that decisions were made within their community with the most available evidence and information.

Only 25 percent of the respondents felt that the decision to close a hospital was consistent with the available evidence. The others either disagreed or were not sure. This was reflective of the complex nature of the evidence about hospital restructuring.

Quality of evidence/dissemination – Evidence regarding hospital closure was available in national, provincial, and hospital reports. In addition, evidence included provincial utilization data, hospital medical record data, professional organization reports, and consultant reports. Reports and evidence were shared between hospital administrators. Little research literature was available on the effectiveness of hospital closure strategies.

Political/economical conditions – The economical and political climate were substantial driving forces to the examination of the evidence regarding hospital closures. The economic conditions drove the decision making; the administrative environment facilitated or was a barrier to the adoption of change.

The factors influencing hospital closure decision making were complex. One site reported:

The decision to close two facilities was based on expert opinion and evidence gained from consultant reports, examination of existing data, engineering and architectural reports, surveys of community opinion and projections of patient volume. Open forums with presentations from stakeholders (physicians, nurses, community, politicians) were held. Information from these presentations was merged with an inventory of facts. There were no studies that directly influenced this decision.

Literature regarding program clustering and effective use of resources was examined. The most important source of information was an inventory of facts. Some of the data was poor and not useful (i.e., HMRI) and may have been presented in a biased manner—especially when positions were at stake. The evidence suggested that this site was overbedded, services were fragmented and more services could be shifted to the community.

We didn't have any good evidence but there was dialogue and consensus with the community and the providers. The consumer perspective was a strong influence as there were many stakeholders: OMA, Catholic Church, labour unions and professionals. The fear of change was a real barrier.

Commitment, including a provincial financial commitment was an important support.

An independent group to guide the process (i.e., District Health Council) examined the evidence in an unbiased manner. We started out with a focus on acute care hospital change and ended up with a total system reconfiguration.

Decisions were made on the best available information but planners were frustrated when information was either not available or was dated. The impression was that evidence related to hospital closures is soft, sociological and political in nature. Planners are focused on being agents of change and feel that they do not have the time to evaluate the nature of the evidence as it relates to proposed changes.

Another site reported:

We formed a corporation that governs eight facilities, three hospital-based schools of nursing, regional ambulance service and a central laundry. The new structure was not voluntarily sought by the institutions, and the conclusive evidence to support the wisdom of regional approaches does not yet exist—yet the strength and traditions of the eight facilities, the positive working relationships between the health care system and the Department of Health, and the province's characteristic resilience in the face of adversity gave the corporation confidence that health care delivery would be improved.

Personal/professional factors – Public opinion and personal beliefs and attitude strongly influenced evidence adoption. Community and interdisciplinary input influenced the direction of hospital closures. The economic conditions initiated the decision making; the personal influence of the community shaped the incorporation of the best available evidence.

Conclusions

There was no scientific evidence to support hospital closures, yet there was detailed information available on which to base decisions (databases, descriptive studies, expert opinion, commission reports).

All changes were economically driven.

Changes were based on opinion, consensus, effective management of change process, underlying principles or beliefs, and multiple community stakeholders. These strong societal forces shaped the incorporation of the evidence.

Labour Substitution in Acute Care Nursing

Health care reform takes many shapes in many provinces, but it is universally driven by the need to control costs while maintaining and, perhaps, enhancing the quality of health care. The polices associated with health care reform have had a significant impact on health human resource planning, specifically in nursing as hospitals downsize or close (Carr-Hill et al. 1995; International Council of Nurses 1993).

The decision to substitute registered nurses with either licensed practical nurses, nonregulated multiskilled assistants, or no one at all is influenced by potential stakeholders and interest groups, with varying degrees of power, including but not limited to hospital associations, nurses' associations, unions, medical associations, and professional bodies. The lack of integrated health (nursing) human resource planning has allowed hospitals, the major employers of nurses, to estimate nursing requirements and to add, subtract, and transfer resources in a somewhat ad hoc manner. Nurses do influence these decisions but the difficulty for nurses is that, while planning to ensure the right provider is in the right place and the role of the nurse in the system is clarified, it may mean fewer nurses in the future.

Therefore, this case focused on the influence of various factors on evidence adoption with respect to policy decisions regarding the planning and implementation of labour substitution within acute care nursing.

Classification

This issue was classified as an opportunity for improvement because the decision making demonstrated widespread implementation based on uncertain evidence.

Sample

Key informants were drawn from experts in health human resources, appropriate professional organizations (Canadian Nurses Association, provincial nurses' associations), and individuals involved in integrated health human resource development. Three hospital sites and all provincial nursing organizations were surveyed. Questionnaire response rate was 48 percent (14/28) and interview response rate was 89 percent (17/19).

Findings

Degree of adoption – Nursing substitution varied across Canada. At the sites interviewed, each had implemented different policies for nurse staffing: no labour substitution, substitution of registered nurses (RN) with registered practical nurses (RPN), or substitution of RNs with unskilled workers.

Decision makers felt that decisions were not reflective of the best available evidence because the evidence was of poor quality and did not provide direction.

Quality of the evidence – There was a lack of experimental evidence to support the direction of labour substitution but strong historical and expert evidence existed. Descriptive studies suggested that hospital length of stay, patient satisfaction, and morbidity decreased with an increased RN-to-patient ratio. It was difficult to interpret qualitative studies. Findings from these studies provided important evidence for nursing care as they addressed many of the factors involved in caring for complex patients (i.e., decision making, caring, communication, reporting, assessment). Studies regarding labour substitutions often did not address many important variables, including but not limited to staff ratios of RN:RPN, patient acuity and mix, available support services, staff nurse education level, and different models of care. Studies were often single site, limiting the ability to generalize the findings.

Overall, concern was raised about the nature and quality of evidence used. One administrator reported: "Change is often based on workload statistics, medical diagnosis, patient days—measures not reflective of nursing work."

Dissemination – Many administrators reported that with all the changes going on within their organizations, they had little time to search research literature. Most relied on expert opinion, anecdotal evidence, and their own individual preference or philosophy of care. Some sites were implementing changes based on consultant reports, usually from the United States.

Political environment – Administrative support, economic conditions, political influence, and professional beliefs strongly influenced the adoption of the available evidence.

Union representatives raised concern:

Many administrators are implementing labour substitution based on information from consultants from the United States. They are using information from a different health care system. I don't believe they are promoting the research that has been done. They are trying to sell this— nurses need to have more time to do what nurses do. They are substituting with less trained, less educated workers and we have the same number of staff and more acute patients. We are doing the same, if not more work, but with less knowledgeable staff.

Middle nurse managers and union representatives felt that staffing decisions were made with little input from front-line workers, which they believed was the "best available evidence."

All administrators reported that fiscal restraint was the driving force that influenced their decision to reassess and change nurse staffing ratios.

Some nurse administrators clearly stated that, although the evidence was weak, planning should be consistent with conceptual frameworks or principles commonly reported in the literature.

One nurse manager reported:

Planning should not be based on the best bandwagon but should reflect principles such as:

— matching competence of individual's skill and education with care requirements;

— cost-effectiveness;

— flexibility;

— patient centered;

— continuity of care; and

— coordination of care, and above all quality care.

Unfortunately, staffing is a budget issue. We need to do things differently or better with existing or less resources.

Conclusions

Quality and utility of scientific evidence was perceived as poor.

Financial resources were the driving force to examine nurse substitution, but individuals' experience and professional beliefs strongly influenced the direction of the substitution.

There was a desperate need to conduct research related to nurse resource planning and to evaluate the cost-effectiveness and effectiveness.

Personal and professional attitudes and beliefs influenced the interpretation of the evidence.

Consumer pressure was not perceived to be an influential factor.

Joan E. Tranmer, *RN, M.Sc., Ph.D. (candidate), is the director of nursing research at Kingston General Hospital, and holds a joint appointment as an assistant professor at the School of Nursing, Queen's University. She has worked extensively in the perinatal field as a practitioner, administrator, and researcher. Currently her research interests are focused on patients' symptom experiences, and decision making within clinical and administrative realms.*

Acknowledgments

The research team acknowledges the important contribution of all informants who participated in the study, the Kingston General Hospital Nursing Research Unit for facility support, and interviewers C. Laroque, F. Mawani, S. McFarlane, and J. Monahan for their detailed interviewing and reporting.

Expert Panel

C. Bolton, Queen's Health Policy
D. Brindle, Ontario Ministry of Health
J. Dorland, Queen's Health Policy
D. Farquhar, Faculty of Medicine, Queen's University
P. Glynn, Kingston General Hospital
J. Hoey, Kingston, Frontenac and Lennox & Addington Health Unit
D. Hunter, Health Information Partnership of Eastern Ontario
J. McBride, Kingston General Hospital
B. McIver, Kingston, Frontenac and Lennox & Addington District Health Council
B. Smith, Faculty of Medicine, Queen's University
D. Walker, Faculty of Medicine, Queen's University
H. Walker, Queen's Health Policy

SECTION II – BIBLIOGRAPHY

ANGUS, D. E. 1991. *Review of Significant Health Care Commissions and Task Forces in Canada Since 1983–84.* The Canadian Medical Association, the Canadian Nurses Association, and the Canadian Hospital Association. Ottawa.

ANGUS, D. E., and E. TURBAYNE. 1995. Path to the future: A synopsis of health and health care issues (abstract). Part of the National Nursing Competency Project. Canadian Nurses Association. Ottawa.

ATKINSON, W., and W. ORENSTEIN. 1992. The resurgence of measles in the United States, 1989–1990. *Annual Review of Medicine* 43: 451–463.

AVERY, C. 1991. Native American medicine: Traditional healing. *Journal of the American Medical Association* 265: 2271–2273.

CAIRNS, J., and P. ARMSTRONG. 1994. Canadian Consensus Conference on Coronary Thrombolysis—1994 update. *Canadian Journal of Cardiology* 10: 517–521.

CANADIAN MEDICAL ASSOCIATION. 1986. Consensus Conference report: Indication for cesarean section: Final statement of the panel on the National Consensus Conference on Aspects of Cesarean Birth. *Canadian Medical Association Journal* 134.

CANADIAN MEDICAL ASSOCIATION. 1993. Medication use in the elderly. *Canadian Medical Association Journal* 149: 1152A–1152B.

CARR-HILL, R. A., P. DIXON, M. GRIFFITHS, M. HIGGINS, et al. 1995. The impact of nursing grade on the quality and outcome of nursing care. *Health Economics* 4: 57–72.

COAMBS, R. B., P. B. JENSEN, M. H. HER, and B. S. FERGUSON. 1996. Review of the scientific literature on the prevalence, consequences, and health costs of non-compliance and inappropriate use of prescription medication in Canada. A study prepared for the Pharmaceutical Manufacturers Association of Canada by the Centre for Health Promotion, University of Toronto.

DAVIDSON, W., and D. W. MOLLOY. 1994. Relation between physician characteristics and prescribing for the elderly in New Brunswick. *Canadian Medical Association Journal* 150: 917–921.

DREW, L. 1992. Health of Canada's Aboriginal People. *Canadian Journal of Public Health* 83: 163–164.

EISENBERG, D., R. KESSLER, C. FOSTER, F. NORLOCK, et al. 1993. Unconventional medicine in the United States. *The New England Journal of Medicine* 328: 246–252.

FRANZOSI, M., and A. P. MAGGIONI. 1994. GISSI update. Which patients with myocardial infarction should receive thrombolysis. *Chest* 101: 116S–123S.

GENTLEMAN, J., and G. F. PARSON. 1994. High and low surgical procedure rates in census divisions across Canada. *Health Reports* 6: 403–440.

HAN, J. 1982. Neurochemical basis of acupuncture analgesia. *Annual Review of Pharmacology and Toxicology* 22: 193–220.

HELEWA, M. 1995. Cesarean sections in Canada: What constitutes an appropriate rate? *J SOGC* 17: 237–246.

HINDLE, H., and J. K. NORHEIM. 1995. Rural Alberta thrombolysis study. Survey of practice patterns for managing acute myocardial infarction. *Canadian Family Physician* 41: 1180–1187.

HUTTEN-CZAPSKI, P. 1993. Thrombolytic therapy for myocardial infarction. Treatment introduced in Northern Ontario. *Canadian Family Physician* 39: 1071–1074.

INTERNATIONAL COUNCIL OF NURSES. 1993. *Nursing Support Workers: Position Statement and Guidelines.*

KASPAR, J., and A. G. MULLEY Jr. 1992. Developing shared decision-making programs to improve the quality of health care. *Quality Review Bulletin* 18: 183–190.

LECHKY, O. 1991. Transfer of health care to Natives holds much promise, lecturers say. *Canadian Medical Association Journal* 144: 195–197.

LEWITH, G., and J. KENYON. 1984. Physiological and psychological explanations for the mechanism of acupuncture as a treatment for chronic pain. *Social Science and Medicine* 9: 1367–1378.

LUCCHESI, G., and R. E. JACKSON. 1995. Sensitivity of the Ottawa Rules. *Annals of Emergency Medicine* 26: 1–5.

MATCHAR, D., and GOLDSTEIN. 1992. *Carotid Endarterectomy: A Literature Review and Ratings of Appropriateness and Necessity.* Santa Monica (CA): Rand.

MCCONNELL, J., and M. J. BARRY. 1994. Benign prostatatic hyperplasia: Diagnosis and treatment. *Clinical Practice Guidelines – Quick Reference Guide for Physicians* 8: 1–17.

MILLER, A., C. BAINES, and C. WALL. 1992. Canadian National Breast-Screening Study: 2. Breast cancer detection and death rates among women aged 50 to 59 years. *Canadian Medical Association Journal* 147: 1477–1488.

MILLMAN, B. 1977. Acupuncture: Context and critique. *Annual Review of Medicine* 28: 223–234.

MOORE, W., and H. J. BARNETT. 1995. Guidelines for carotid endarterectomy: A multidisciplinary consensus statement from the ad hoc committee, American Heart Association. *Stroke* 26: 188–201.

ONTARIO MINISTRY OF HEALTH. 1995. *Opportunities for Health: Immunization, The Next Steps.*

ORENSTEIN, W., and L. E. MARKOWITZ. 1994. Worldwide measles prevention. *Israel Journal of Medical Sciences* 30: 469–481.

PACHOS, C., and S. L. NORMAND. 1994. Trends in the use of drug therapies in patients with acute myocardial infarction: 1988 to 1992. *Journal of the American College of Cardiology* 23:1023–1030.

PHARMACEUTICAL INQUIRY OF ONTARIO. 1990. *Prescriptions for Health.*

PIGMAN, E., and R. K. KLUG. 1994. Evaluation of the Ottawa Clinical Decision Rules for the use of radiography in acute ankle and midfoot injuries in the emergency department: An independent site assessment. *Annals of Emergency Medicine* 24: 41–45.

RENFREW, M. M., and J. P. NEILSON. 1994. Overviews 03298, 03297, 032885, in pregnancy and childbirth module. In: *Cochrane Database of Systemic Reviews*, eds. M. ENKIN, and KEIRSE. Oxford, Cochrane Updates on Disk.

SHAPIRO, S. 1994. Screening: Assessment of current studies. *Cancer* 74: 231–238.

STIELL, I., and G. H. GREENBERG. 1992. A study to develop clinical decision rules for the use of radiography in acute ankle injuries. *Annals of Emergency Medicine* 21: 384–390.

STIELL, I., and R. D. MCKNIGHT. 1994. Implementation of the Ottawa Ankle Rules. *Journal of the American Medical Association* 271: 827–832.

TAMBLYN, R., and P. J. MCLEOD. 1994. Questionable prescribing for elderly patients in Quebec. *Canadian Medical Association Journal* 150: 1801–1809.

TULCHINSKY, T., and G. M. GINSBERG. 1993. Measles control in developing and developed countries: The case for a two-dose policy. *Bulletin of the World Health Organization* 71: 93–103.

VADEBONCŒUR, H. 1989. Une autre césarienne? Non merci. Montreal (QC): *Québec-Amérique.*

VAN DE WERF, F., and E. J. TOPOL. 1995. Variation in patient management and outcomes for acute myocardial infarction in the United States and other countries. Results from gusto trial. *Journal of the American Medical Association* 273: 1586–1591.

WAGNER, E., and P. BARRETT. 1995. The effect of a shared decision-making program on rates of surgery for benign prostatic hyperplasia: Pilot results. *Medical Care* 33: 765–770.

WESTON, C., and W. J. PENNY. 1994. Guidelines for the early management of patients with myocardial infarction. *British Medical Journal* 308: 767–771.

WOODARD, G., and L. EDOURD. 1992. Reaching out: A community initiative for disadvantaged pregnant women. *Canadian Journal of Public Health* 83: 188–190.

ZUBEK, E. 1994. Traditional Native healing: Alternative or adjunct to modern medicine? *Canadian Family Physician* 40: 1923–1931.

Decision Support Tools in Health Care

PAUL FISHER, PH.D.
University of Victoria and CPRN Health Network

MARCUS J. HOLLANDER, B.A. (HONS.), M.A., M.SC.
CPRN Health Network

THOMAS MACKENZIE, M.D., M.B.A.
Queens University

PETER KLEINSTIVER, PH.D.
Katalyst Professional Services Inc.

IRINA SLADECEK, B.A., B.SC.
PenDragon Consultants Ltd.

GAIL PETERSON, B.S.N., M.SC.
PenDragon Consultants Ltd.

SUMMARY

Introduction

This report provides a critical review and analysis of decision support tool (DST) use in health care. The findings of this study are based on a comprehensive international literature review, an international survey of DST developers and users, and the experience and expertise of the study team.

A wide range of instruments and/or tools can be referred to as aids to decision making. In order to clarify the boundaries of the aids included in this study, the following definition of DSTs was used:

> Decision support tools are intellectual instruments in which data, information, and knowledge related to a particular domain have been collected and structured in a way that directly supports the cognitive processes used in arriving at a particular domain-related decision.

The use of DSTs is believed to constitute a systematic and consistent way of improving the effectiveness of human decision making. The past 15 years have seen an explosive growth of DSTs that were expected to help solve perplexing real-world problems in a range of areas that included health care. Purported benefits of DST use were that it would reduce complexity; decrease response times for making decisions; improve problem solving; and provide greater consistency in the decisions that were made. It was also recognized that there were certain limiting factors associated with the use of DSTs, such as acceptability by users, and technical and cost limitations.

Given the amount of discussion regarding DSTs, initial impressions are that DSTs are in wide use, that they are effective, and that they have been extensively evaluated and proven to be effective. Based on the findings from this study, the above perceptions are only partially correct. There has been a significant effort to develop DSTs in the health sector. However, it does not appear that DSTs are in wide use or that their efficacy has been empirically demonstrated to any great extent. In addition, DST development appears to be proceeding on a limited scale in Canada compared with DST development in other countries.

Empirical Findings

An audit of the available literature shows that of the 86 DSTs analyzed, only 6 percent were from Canada, 50 percent were from the United States, and 44 percent were from jurisdictions outside North America. By far the majority of DSTs were developed for clinical applications (86 percent); however, only 24 percent of the clinical tools identified in the audit were actually being used.

Of the DSTs not in use, 90 percent were still under development. With regard to empirical evaluations, only a small proportion of DSTs have been subjected to independent external evaluations of effectiveness beyond validation against the experts on whose decision making the tools had been developed. Examples of DSTs that have been evaluated beyond validation and/or verification include a diagnostic support tool for clinical psychiatry (DSP) [5]* and a DST for pre-term birth risk assessment [55]. The use of these tools resulted in improved decision performance by nonexpert users as compared to their performance without the respective DST.

With regard to the survey of DST developers and users, clinical applications still predominated but a greater proportion of management- and policy-related tools were reported. This may reflect the fact that the articles in the audit represent DST developments two or more years in the past (i.e., the effect of the length of time it takes for articles to be published), while DSTs referred to in the survey may represent developments as recently as 1995.

In addition to the empirical assessment of DSTs by means of the audit and the survey, this report contains commentary and discussion of DSTs from three distinct perspectives: clinical practice and institutional management; the commercial marketplace; and policy and administration within different organizational contexts.

Commentary: The Clinical Practice and Institutional Management Perspective

An important conclusion reached in this project is that a more systematic approach is required for DST development. DST development should be driven by a systemic need and proceed in a more coordinated manner that sees development based on a wider vision of requirements than those which exist in any one given organization. A notable shortcoming of the current situation is that there is no systematic methodology for the development of DSTs.

An important contribution of this report is the formulation of 12 key steps for planning a successful DST development project.

1. Identify the purpose of the DST and determine if the problem it will address qualifies as a DST candidate.

---

* References that support statements made in the body of this document are found at the bottom of the page on which they are used and are indicated as footnote references (i.e., 26). References to DSTs included in the audit database and used as examples in this document are indicated by a number in square brackets (i.e., [26]). These references are found in the section "Articles Included in the DST Audit Database" of the document. Appendix 1 is a list of general references to DSTs and decision support that are not referred to specifically in the document or the DST Audit database.

2. *Scan the organizational environment to determine whether there is adequate support for the development of a DST.*
3. *Define the scope of decision making to be supported by the DST.*
4. *Identify the users of the DST.*
5. *Determine what data, information, and knowledge are required by the experts to make the best possible decision.*
6. *Define the output the DST will provide for all realistic combinations of inputs, including incomplete data.*
7. *Develop a data and information flow model for the decision-making processes to be addressed by the DST.*
8. *Build the DST.*
9. *Develop the interface to the DST.*
10. *Implement and refine the DST.*
11. *Conduct validation tests with experts and verification tests with users.*
12. *Conduct a systematic evaluation of the DST based on outcomes.*

Another major shortcoming identified in this report is the lack of specific guidelines or standards for the evaluation of DSTs. Such guidelines need to be developed and DSTs need to be subjected to properly conducted evaluations in order for their efficacy and efficiency to be demonstrated.

Commentary: The Perspective from the Marketplace

Several interrelated factors will influence the future commercial development of DSTs. Fiscal constraint in health care indicates that while budgets will continue to shrink, investment in information systems is anticipated to increase. This means that resources for in-house DST development may have to be reallocated from existing resources. The private sector may be a potential alternative source of funding. There are a number of reasons why commercial development may be a future trend.

The picture that emerges from the audit and the survey is one in which academics develop DSTs to test theoretical models while clinical researchers, technologists, and others develop DSTs to address particular practical problems within their own organizations. These DSTs may, at best, have limited success in any wider application. In addition, data on the costs of DST development may be hard to calculate in such settings because these costs are very seldom reported. If widespread acceptance of DSTs is to be achieved in today's economic climate, all development costs must be identified and published.

Another problem with current development practices is that DST developers typically focus on theoretical or institutionally limited applications for their DSTs. If DSTs are to be implemented on a wider basis, DSTs with wider applicability are required. Typical of any successfully marketed product or service is a clear business plan that identifies the potential market, core competencies, strengths and weaknesses, competitive positions, and development costs. Such plans are typically not made in the present DST development environment.

Another factor that will influence commercial development is the fact that decision makers currently find that existing information systems have little or no impact on the quality of care, the clinical and executive decision-making processes, cost containment, or operational productivity. Further investments in information technology must be cost effective and have demonstrable benefits and measurable results.

Commentary: The Organizational Behaviour Perspective

DSTs are developed and/or used in organizational settings. Currently, as with other decision rationales such as zero-based budgeting, DST developers, analysts, and others appear to assume an underlying model of organizational behaviour that is rational and scientific. In this model, data and information are key inputs into the decision-making process. Thus, DSTs are developed and/or purchased in order to provide better inputs into clinical practice, management and administration, and policy making.

The organizational theory literature, however, indicates that while this is one model, there are also other models that suggest that data and information have less importance in decision making or may be used as a tool for advocates advancing competing positions. Five models of organizational behaviour are presented in this report.

It must be realized that any one model of organizational behaviour does not represent every organization under all conditions. Therefore, one must recognize that different models or combinations of models may have primacy at different times in a given organization. A contingency model is presented that indicates which models of organizational behaviour are appropriate in which contexts. These contexts are framed within three dimensions: the extent of agreement about ideas/beliefs, the extent to which there are conflicts of interest, and the extent to which organizational reality is socially constructed.

The implication of this analysis, when applied to DST use, is that as decisions are made in different organizational contexts, the nature of the context might have a bearing on the extent to which DSTs can be successfully developed, implemented, and/or used. It concluded that DSTs can be developed and used more readily in contexts where there are relatively few conflicts of interest and where there is general agreement about the need, efficacy, and appropriateness of a rational and scientific approach that is embodied in the DSTs. It may be more difficult to introduce a DST into contexts where there are conflicts of interest and ideas (i.e., competing care models or value systems). For example, it is unlikely that a DST for policy formulation concerning abortion could be developed, because abortion is a highly charged issue with embedded value conflicts.

Recommendations

This report contains a number of recommendations, including:

- *DST development should be encouraged in environments where there is the opportunity and the willingness to integrate the DST with existing information systems.*
- *DST development should be encouraged in environments where there is systemic commitment to provide the intended users with access to the DST.*
- *The development of structured and systematic planning strategies and knowledge engineering methodologies should be actively supported.*
- *The development of methodologies for DST evaluation should be actively supported.*
- *Health care institutions and governance bodies should take the lead in guiding industry in DST development by clearly identifying and articulating the expectations of the users in terms of planning, development, and evaluation.*
- *DST development should be encouraged where that development focuses on systemic needs rather than the needs of an individual institution, organization, or program. This would allow for the DST to be more broadly marketed.*

TABLE OF CONTENTS

APPENDICES

LIST OF FIGURES

LIST OF TABLES

DECISION SUPPORT TOOLS IN HEALTH CARE

In 1994, the Canadian federal government created the National Forum on Health. The purpose of the Forum was to: find ways to improve the health of Canadians; improve the efficiency and effectiveness of health services; and provide the government with recommendations for action.

In order to offer practical advice based on research that is either completed or under way, the Forum has formed several working groups to identify and focus on issues or themes of national importance. The working group "Evidence-Based Decision Making" was created to find ways to ensure that decisions about health and health care are based on the best available evidence for all levels of providers, consumers, and policymakers.

One area of particular interest to this working group is that of decision support tools (DSTs) and how they can be applied to improve evidence-based health care decision making. This report deals with DSTs in four parts:

Part 1: A presentation of working definitions of evidence-based health care and DSTs, how DSTs are used in health care, and a framework for the categorization of DSTs within the health care domain.

Part 2: The results of an audit of articles from the academic and professional literature concerned with the design, development, implementation, and use of DSTs in health care.

Part 3: The results of a survey of DST developers and users concerning the current and future use of DSTs in health care settings.

Part 4: An analysis of the current state and future of DSTs for health care. The analysis is based on parts 1, 2 and 3 above as well as the accumulated experience of the authors in the area of decision support in health care. The analysis deals with health care provider[1] DSTs, management DSTs, policy-making DSTs, and integrated decision support systems that include DSTs. The discussion includes perspectives on the obstacles to DST development, dissemination, and use in health care and proposes measures that can be taken to overcome such barriers.

GUIDING STATEMENT

An emerging objective in the changing health care delivery environment is to make health care decision making more evidence-based. Achieving this objective will help address the provincial and nationally mandated goals of making health care delivery more efficient and more effective from the perspectives of the health care system, the care providers, and the consumers

---

1. The term health care provider includes clinical, management, and administrative/policy health care providers.

they serve. The widespread use of *appropriately* designed and implemented DSTs is one means of achieving this objective.

INTRODUCTION AND DEFINITION

The principal products of health care are decisions that have an impact on the wellness of patients or clients, the management of delivery institutions or organizations, and the administration of the system that supports health care at the provincial and national levels. The processes that produce these decisions require a high level of expertise and the consideration of a volume of data and/or information that is becoming beyond the capacity of individual providers to manage. Consequently, many decisions in health care run the risk of being made without supporting evidence. The body of data, information, and knowledge on which health care decisions are based is growing at an increasing rate and the decision-making environment can only deteriorate in the absence of a structured system of health care decision support.

Support for health care decision making has traditionally come from textbooks, learned papers, and consultations with experts. The decreasing amount of time available to health care providers to seek out and use this type of decision support, and the increasing volume and diversity of the support available in this format has fostered the development of DSTs. *DSTs are intellectual instruments in which data, information, and knowledge related to a particular domain have been collected and structured in a way that* directly *supports the cognitive* processes *used in arriving at a particular domain-related decision.* An evaluation of the availability, quality, and diversity of health care DSTs is the subject of this report.

EVIDENCE-BASED HEALTH CARE

A paradigm is a way of looking at the world that includes a definition of problems that can be addressed as well as a range of *admissible* evidence that may be used to arrive at solutions consistent with this world view. When defects or limitations in a paradigm accumulate to the extent that the world view is recognized as faulty or incomplete, a new paradigm is required. Decision making in health care delivery and management has reached such a level of incompleteness and now requires a new paradigm to guide it into the twenty-first century. While it is too early to suggest discarding the old paradigm completely, there is a new, evolving paradigm emerging referred to as evidence-based health care (EBHC).

Evidence-based medicine: What it is and what it isn't[2]

Evidence-based medicine is the conscientious, explicit, and judicious use of current best evidence in making decisions about the care of individual patients. The practice of evidence-based medicine means integrating individual clinical expertise with the best available external clinical evidence from systematic research. By individual clinical expertise we mean the proficiency and judgement that individual clinicians acquire through clinical experience and clinical practice. Increased expertise is reflected in many ways, but especially in more effective and efficient diagnosis and in the more thoughtful identification and compassionate use of individual patients' predicaments, rights, and preferences in making clinical decisions about their care. By best available external clinical evidence we mean clinically relevant research, often from the basic sciences of medicine, but especially from patient-centred clinical research into the accuracy and precision of diagnostic tests (including clinical examination), the power of prognostic markers, and the efficacy and safety of therapeutic, rehabilitative, and preventive regimens. External clinical evidence may invalidate previously accepted diagnostic tests and treatments and replace them with new ones that are more powerful, more accurate, more efficacious, and safer.

EBHC is health care delivery based on decisions made with correct, complete, appropriate, and current information and data. While modern health care providers strive to make evidence-based decisions, there appear to be many decisions made based on data and information that does not meet these conditions of data quality and quantity. This view may result from the belief that: the volume and complexity of data and information on which health care decisions are made is growing at a rate that challenges the ability of providers to keep abreast of developments; and the processes used in decision making are becoming too numerous and specialized for even dedicated providers to master completely.

These constraints augment the perception that some health care decisions are based on reasoning that may not be supported by the existing evidence. Complicating providers' efforts to make decisions more evidence-based is the suggestion[3] that many decisions may often be based more on values and beliefs and/or organizational and environmental constraints than on empirical evidence. This is not to suggest that health care decision making is deteriorating, rather it suggests that health care delivery may not be keeping

---

2. David L. Sackett et al., *Evidence-based medicine: What it is and what it isn't* (http://cebm.jr2.ox.ac.uk/ebmisisnt.html, 1996).
3. See the section "The Future of DSTs in Policy and Management: An Organizational Behaviour Perspective" of this document.

abreast of the decision-making potential provided by the expanding volume of available data, information, and knowledge.

Traditionally, the following assumptions were used to guide the type of data or knowledge collected when developing recommendations for clinical or policy decision making in health care:

- Unsystematic observations based on personal and/or professional experiences are a valid method for building and maintaining one's knowledge about health care.
- The study and understanding of basic mechanisms of health care principles are a sufficient guide for health care delivery and management.
- The combination of health care management training and common sense is sufficient to determine and/or evaluate the effects of health care delivery and/or management outcomes.
- Content expertise and experience are a sufficient basis for the generation of valid policies and guidelines for health care practices.[4]

The assumptions for a new EBHC paradigm include the following:

- Personal and professional experiences as well as intuitive knowledge are necessary for the development of personal expertise in a specific health care domain. However, systematic observation and reproducible and unbiased documentation are at least as important for ensuring that the information collected is valid and reliable.
- Studying and understanding basic principles of health care are prerequisites, but are insufficient by themselves for guiding health care decision making. These basic principles may be incorrect and, therefore, inadequate predictors of current and/or future performance.
- Understanding certain rules and/or types of evidence are necessary to correctly interpret health care literature.[5]

This new paradigm places a lower value on individual expertise or authority but recognizes that the individual responsible for health care delivery and/or management is able to make independent assessments of evidence and to evaluate the credibility of the evidence offered by experts. This paradigm is not a rejection of the knowledge that can be gained from colleagues or experts whose years of experience have provided them with valuable insights that could not be gained from formal scientific investigation, but it does assume that an individual who has developed an understanding of available evidence will provide superior care or decision making.[6]

4. Evidence-Based Medicine Working Group and the Health Information Research Unit, McMaster University (URL: http://hiru.mcmaster.ca/ebm/overview.htm, 1996).
5. Ibid.
6. Evidence-Based Medicine Working Group and the Health Information Research Unit, McMaster University (URL: http://hiru.mcmaster.ca/ebm/overview.htm, 1996).

EBHC is a concept that embraces the decision-making activities of all clinical, managerial, and administrative health care providers in institutional care, community care and health care governance settings. Accordingly, health care providers are actively promoting EBHC as a means of addressing the demands of health care clients for more effective care and the payers' demands for more efficient delivery.

The greatest challenge facing EBHC is the integration of the evidence base horizontally across the spectrum of health care delivery settings and vertically through the levels of health care activity. Given that the evidence for health care decisions is manifested in the form of data, information and knowledge, the means of achieving success in EBHC is in the development of appropriate, well-designed, and integrated information systems that include DSTs. DSTs differ from other information systems in that they are instruments designed to emulate the specific human cognitive and reasoning processes used in health care decision making.

DECISION SUPPORT TOOLS

Conceptual Model

DSTs are instruments[7] that support the decision-making process rather than tools that supply only the data and/or information required as inputs to a decision-making process. For example, a computerized patient record system that is simply an automated version of the hard copy is not a DST, while an instrument that uses patient signs and symptoms to provide a user with a set of diagnostic possibilities is a DST. The former system is used to record and communicate data and information to the user, while the latter supports human reasoning by aiding a user to determine the meaning of that data and information and, ultimately, arrive at a decision. Figure 1 provides a conceptual model of the decision-making environment.

The function of a DST is a reflection of what its name implies.

Decision[8] – the process of resolving a problem; the steps leading to an action;

Support – an aid; an enhancement;

Tool – an instrument to be used by a human and designed for a specific purpose or purposes.

---

7. The decision support instrument may be computer based or paper based and may take the form of tools such as guidelines or care maps.

8. In the context of a DST, *decision* is a verb since it is the process of deciding that is supported by using the tool. The *decision* product is supported by the design of the tool.

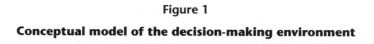

Figure 1

Conceptual model of the decision-making environment

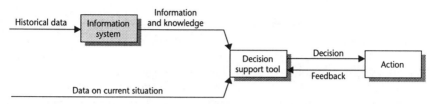

Note: Decisions are based on two inputs: historical data related to situations similar to the one currently being considered and data concerning the current situation in which a decision is required. The former provides the basis of a structured model of the process being applied to the current situation and the latter provides the data to be used in that process to arrive at a decision that is unique to the current situation. A critical aspect of these tools is the facility to accept feedback based on the action resulting from a decision. Without this, the decision and, consequently, the resulting action cannot be iteratively "tuned" to the current situation and the DST will not evolve to adapt to the changing reality of the health care environment.

The use of DSTs represents a systematic and consistent way of improving the effectiveness[9] of human decision making. A DST can be a descriptive tool that progressively guides the user in the decision-making process and/or a prescriptive tool that recommends an end solution to the user's problem. Users of a DST thus acquire information that assists them in the decision process and/or in making recommendations for final decisions from the system.

A DST is a means of accessing a decision model (defined as a logical abstraction of reality created to help someone make a decision). While there may be many inputs to a decision process, traditional decision making has usually relied on the use of a single measure to rank order preferences among alternative solutions. Through the use of a DST, a decision maker can improve the quality of decisions by being able to appropriately weight all *relevant*[10] variables or criteria that influence the decision.

A DST usually contains facts and rules but may also incorporate less tangible data items such as opinions, judgements, and/or educated guesses that may be explicit, logical, or heuristic in nature. A DST, therefore, may support decision makers faced with ill-structured problems by enhancing

---

9. This must be considered distinct from efficiency, which refers to decreasing the time and cost required to carry out a task. Management DSTs, however, can be designed and used for making more *effective* decisions regarding the *efficiency* of an activity.

10. *Relevant* is the operative word. *More* is not always *better* if the *more* is unrelated to the problem. In fact, it may degrade the quality of the decision if irrelevancies distract from the process required to achieve the objective—the best decision.

their understanding and judgement rather than by providing a unique *solution* to the problem.

DST design, development, and implementation requires people (knowledge engineers, analysts, designers, domain experts, and users); software (database management systems, simulation languages, application packages); hardware (computing platforms, graphics engines, transducers, and telecommunication systems); and a suitable problem.

The suitability of a problem for DST development depends on the structure of the decision process used to arrive at the solution. The *structure* of a decision is defined by intelligence (the definition of the problem), the problem statement, design (the enumeration of alternative solutions), and the choice (the identification of the best solution). If the problem can be definitely stated and all alternative solutions are known and the correct choice is clear, the decision is referred to as *structured*. If the problem is difficult to state and if the alternatives are unpredictable, the decision is referred to as *unstructured*.

All decisions occupy a position on a spectrum that includes these extremes. Problems for which the solution is arrived at through a structured or semistructured decision-making process are those that are considered *suitable* for the development and application of DSTs.

Problems for which the solution is highly unstructured are viewed as poor candidates for DST development, as the criteria used in the decision process are unclear or constantly changing and their relative weights are unpredictable. In these instances, it is therefore difficult to develop an analogue or model of the process of human reasoning used to arrive at a solution—a requirement for the development of a successful DST.

By way of illustration, reordering common supplies when the inventory falls below a certain threshold quantity is a simple and highly structured decision. Hiring a manager, however, depends on a combination of objective measures (experience, education, etc.) and subjective measures (personality, presence, etc.) and thus represents a semistructured decision. Formulating a policy governing access to abortion services depends almost entirely on subjective measures (popular opinion, political motivation, values, etc.) and is considered an unstructured problem and, therefore, unsuitable for DST development.

The output of a DST can vary from a single item of information to a complete decision analysis with recommendations. *Knowledge-based DSTs* (table 1, category 1) access and use databases addressing a specific problem area and provide factual information, while *situation-based DSTs* (table 1, categories 2–5) acquire data and information, generate inferences, and provide advice on the decision to be made. Situation-based DSTs can be further divided into tools that have to be *told* each step to carry out (table 1, categories 2–3) and definition systems, which read (and, in some sense, understand) the problem as a human would (table 1, categories 4–5). *Expert systems* fall into the last category and are the ultimate DSTs in that they mimic the behaviour of expert human decision makers. They usually accept and return natural language expressions, access external databases and use friendly graphical user interfaces to display results, computations, and recommendations. Examples of expert systems range from MIDAS [8], a very specific tool for the evaluation of pulmonary disease in HIV patients, to IMEX [18], a set of integrated DSTs for the diagnosis, treatment, and management of malaria.

Table 1

Taxonomic schema for DSTs according to logic of operation

DSTs category	Description
1. Specific retrieval	Returns knowledge item on file by specific request (e.g., care map or practice guideline system)
2. Selective retrieval	Manipulates, analyzes, and returns data according to case data input (e.g., case-mix costing system, clinical observational database)
3. Computational	Calculates and returns consequences of planned actions (e.g., institutional budgeting systems, radiotherapy dose calculation system)
4. Modelling	Predicts or extrapolates consequences on a *what-if* basis (e.g., risk analysis models, resource allocation models, accounting models, optimization models)
5. Inference	Proposes and/or makes decisions (e.g., diagnostic expert system)

Developmental History of Decision Support Tools

Growth of DSTs

When human expert knowledge can be packaged for a computer it becomes a resource that can be transported and then accessed by large numbers of nonexperts. It is this facility to extract and store knowledge that has inspired people to build DSTs. The success of such applications, however, is dependent on the selection of domains appropriate to the limitations of the technology. Examples of domains that fit current development criteria include
- deep space station design
- chemical synthesis planning
- rice disease diagnosis
- diagnosis of well-drilling problems
- weather forecasting

- cancer treatment management
- disease diagnosis[11]

In the past 15 years there has been an explosive growth of DSTs. DSTs were expected to help solve perplexing, real-world problems in specific engineering, scientific, and health care specialties.[12] The first DSTs were designed to manipulate and explore symbolically represented problems that human researchers found difficult to solve. What made these problems difficult was the increasing number of potential solutions that had to be examined as problem specifications increased in complexity. The larger the problem specifications, the greater the difficulty for humans to discover solutions or to be sure that the solutions they did determine represented all possible valid solutions. This *combinatorial explosion* far outstripped the abilities of human researchers and the result was the introduction of DST technologies that not only extended the types of problems that could now be solved, but solved these problems faster and cheaper than humans could.[13]

The Evolution of Information Technology and DSTs

The development and construction of a DST is similar to the development of other types of computer programs. As information systems (ISs) have evolved, however, important differences have arisen. This evolution of ISs can be viewed as existing on a continuum, as shown in figure 2.

On the left of the continuum are the IS development techniques that employed procedural languages[14] such as FORTRAN or COBOL as well as construction tools such as line editors and compilers. The data in these programs were explicitly specified and handled by resultant programs that had to specify precisely what was to be done to exactly what data and in what sequence. The important distinguishing feature of these programs was that the data and procedures were intertwined within the program.[15]

As one moved to the right of the continuum, the procedures and data began to be stored separately. Data could be stored in databases while the data management tasks were performed by database management systems

11. Partridge, D. 1986. *Artificial Intelligence: Applications in the Future of Software Engineering.* New York: Ellis Horwood Limited.

12. Barr, A., P. R. Cohen, and E. A. Feigenbaum. 1989. *The Handbook of Artificial Intelligence.* Vol. 4. California: Addison-Wesley Publishing Company, Inc.

13. Guidon, R. 1988. *Cognitive Science and Its Applications for Human-Computer Interaction.* New Jersey: Lawrence Erlbaum Associates, Publishers.

14. Procedural languages are languages where the user must define the procedures necessary to solve a problem.

15. Barr, A., and E. A. Feigenbaum. 1981. *The Handbook of Artificial Intelligence.* Vol. 1. California: Addison-Wesley Publishing Company, Inc.

Figure 2

The continuum of evolution of information systems development[16]

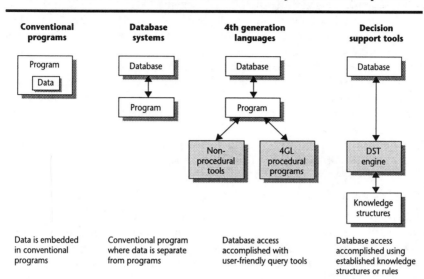

Conventional programs	Database systems	4th generation languages	Decision support tools
Data is embedded in conventional programs	Conventional program where data is separate from programs	Database access accomplished with user-friendly query tools	Database access accomplished using established knowledge structures or rules

(DBMS).[17] Progress in IS technology saw the development of fourth generation languages (4GLs)—high-level, nonprocedural languages[18] that could be used to access and manipulate data within a database. The main characteristic of 4GLs was that they made a database easier to use for both technical and non-technical users. Some 4GLs did not require the developer to specify the *sequence* in which data were to be manipulated and others did not require the developer to specify *how* the data were to be manipulated. This facility allowed programmers to specify the desired result and the software created the code required to achieve the result—a facility similar to the function of DSTs.

DSTs are found at the right end of the continuum. In most of these systems, the specification of *what* data were to be manipulated and the specification of *how* the manipulations were to be accomplished are stored separately. The data specified within the DST engine and the procedural manipulation of the data are handled by different system components.

---

16. Martin, J., and S. Oxman. 1988. *Building Expert Systems: A Tutorial.* New Jersey: Prentice Hall.

17. DBMS are software systems that provide all requisite data management services.

18. Nonprocedural languages are languages where the user states a problem to be solved, but not the procedures required to produce a solution.

Today, the information content of DSTs for health care have a wider context and more evolved nature than those used in other, related disciplines or systems. Management information systems (MISs), for example, deal with structured tasks with standard operating procedures, decision rules, and reliable information flows. Their goal is to increase efficiency. Operations Research (OR) and Management Science (MS) also deal with structured problems and aim to find better solutions through optimization techniques. DSTs, however, are thought to be distinguished by the fact that they address more judgmental decisions in an effort to increase effectiveness. The DST can be said to be a more evolved form of computer support, which goes beyond simple information retrieval and manipulation to not only provide broader support but also cover a range of decisions that are anticipated to provide more sophisticated output to the user.[19]

The Scope of Decision Support in Health Care

The users in health care settings today include individuals providing direct clinical care, individuals charged with managing the environments in which that care is provided, and individuals responsible for ensuring that a viable and efficient health care system exists to support organizational and operational health care activities. To this end, the following framework has been developed as the conceptual framework to define the content and scope of DSTs (figure 3).

The conceptual framework defines the categories of DSTs to be considered in this project according to three orthogonal aspects. The first criterion used in this categorization process was the *target application area* in which decisions are defined, as supported in clinical, management, and/ or policy domains.

The second criterion used was the *type of support* provided by the tool in the decision-making process. *Dynamic* or algorithmic tools interact with the decision maker, guiding the process progressively through each of the relevant criteria to a conclusion appropriate for the current decision-making event. Expert systems are examples of dynamic tools. *Static* tools are models developed from past, successful decision-making events that provide the user with a map of a decision path applicable to the particular decision-making event but not unique to that event. Clinical care maps, practice guidelines, and costing models are examples of static tools.

The third categorization criterion refers to the *type of implementation*. The DST may be implemented as a *manual system*, such as existing paper-based practice guidelines or policy and procedure manuals, or it may be implemented as part of a more comprehensive automated *computer-based system*.

---

19. Dalkir, K. 1990. *Intelligent Decision Support Systems: A Practical Approach.* Ontario: Government of Canada.

Figure 3

Conceptual framework for the audit and assessment of health care DSTs

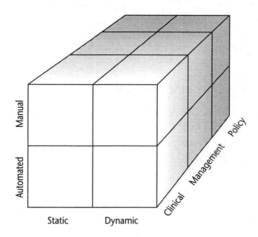

Purported Benefits to Be Derived from the Use of DSTs in Health Care

The complexity and frequency of today's health care decisions can overload even the most dedicated health care provider. The main challenge comes from the limited capacity humans have for considering and processing the increasing volume of data and information necessary for appropriate and effective decision making. It is unlikely that health care providers will continue to perform effectively in this environment without some form of decision support.

This challenge has led to the anticipation that DSTs could make more of the relevant information available to decision makers upon request. This would allow users to quickly consider and apply more *evidence-based* solutions to problems, thereby improving the quality of the decision. DSTs may, therefore, have a significant impact on decision making by providing a better problem solving environment—one that focuses on relevant items and separates facts from judgements.

The greatest anticipated benefit of a DST lies in the consistency and uniformity with which decision criteria are applied. Human decision makers have difficulty making decisions in today's environment because they cannot exhaustively consider *every* factor relevant to the decision. Decision makers also find it difficult to weigh each factor appropriately and to account for any synergy or interactions between criteria. Consequently, different decision makers frequently make different decisions under similar circumstances.

The potential contribution of DSTs is to shift the emphasis from the *nature* of the decision and/or the decision maker to the actual problem for which a solution is sought. By using DSTs, it becomes possible to tailor both data collection and data presentation to the needs of the decision maker and to process that data through more complex decision models. For example, heuristics—often used to evaluate consequences and to arrive at a set of possible strategies for solving a problem—can be included within the design of a DST.

Limitations of DSTs in Health Care

While different authors have suggested many unique and/or similar limitations associated with DST use, only the major issues are presented in this paper. These issues are discussed under the headings of theoretical, people-related, technical, evaluation, and cost limitations.

Theoretical Limitations

The delivery of health care typically requires that all types of health care providers be able to answer the following questions:
- What has happened in the past?
- What is happening right now?
- What will happen in the future?
- What do I need to create the future I want?

To effectively answer these questions, a user requires data that are:
- *factual;*
- *factual inferential*—data that requires interpretation;
- *causal inferential*—"why" questions; and/or
- *predictive*—"what if" questions.

While DSTs are expected to augment and/or compensate human decision making, there are limitations on how effectively they can meet this expectation. To date, the best assistance a well-designed DST can provide is data that answers factual and some forms of predictive questions.[20] DSTs cannot currently perform inferencing activities on information required to imitate human decision making. With no agreement or consensus on how humans *actually* reason and make decisions, it is unreasonable to expect a DST to effectively support or completely mimic human decision-making processes.[21]

---

20. Dalkir, K. 1990. *Intelligent Decision Support Systems: A Practical Approach.* Ontario: Government of Canada.

21. Glaser, R., and M. T. Chi. Eds. 1988. *The Nature of Expertise.* New Jersey: Lawrence Erlbaum Associated, Publishers.

People-Related Limitations

When compared to organizations in the private sector, health care organizations have been slow to accept the use of computers in their work environment. Computing in clinical health care continues to consist largely of auditing or monitoring systems rather than decision support.[22] The two basic constraints that continue to limit or delay the application of DSTs in clinical health care are that the use of computers constitutes a fundamental change in practice, and the fact that there is uncertainty associated with whether DSTs truly support the required human decision making.[23] To illustrate, a DST may be developed to solve predefined problems, but if it fails to help users solve the types of problems they encounter, the DST is of no use.

Health care providers involved in management and/or policy areas have no shortage of data available to them—in fact, it can be said that they are drowning in data. While the use of DSTs for domains such as general administration (i.e., financial general ledgers) and financial management and reporting (i.e., budgeting and forecasting) are widely used, there is a scarcity of DSTs that support the nonstandardized needs of managers. For example, combining utilization data with financial, clinical, and cost accounting data is not readily available, yet it is necessary for strategic planning. As a result, managers have not yet found currently available DSTs that are able to meet their more complex information needs.[24]

Technical Limitations

Technical problems are more likely to appear as DSTs become increasingly complex. While some are conventional hardware and software problems, such as exceeding memory capacity or program bugs, there may also be more basic, conceptual design problems that are not readily apparent. These can include problems such as inappropriate assumptions regarding the users or the development of a system that has addressed the wrong problem in the first place.

22. Miller, R. A. 1994. Medical diagnostic decision support systems—past, present and future: A threaded bibliography and brief commentary. *Journal of the American Medical Informatics Association* 1: 8–27.

23. Heathfield, H. A. 1993. Philosophies for the design and development of clinical decision support systems. *Methods of Information in Medicine* 32(1): 1–15.

24. Austin, C. J., J. M. Trimm, and P. M. Sobczak. 1995. Information systems and strategic management. *Health Care Management Review* 20(3): 26–33.

Evaluation Limitations

Two questions related to the effectiveness and efficiency of DST use are:
- Does the use of a DST improve the quality of decisions produced?
- Are there economic or other benefits attributable to the use of the DST?

The absence of a well-defined or universal evaluation methodology makes these questions difficult to answer, yet the need for answering these questions is unequivocal. The first question is important as it addresses the explicit goal of the DST—improving decision making. The second question is important because in many situations it is difficult to directly observe the benefits accrued from DST use. The present difficulties associated with clearly answering these questions points to the need for further research on the determinants of DST success.

Cost Limitations

The costs of technology can be divided into categories such as development, capital purchases, maintenance, and operation. The cost of DSTs under any of these categories varies and this information is rarely captured. These costs tend to be hidden and, therefore, it is difficult to assess the initial investment in a system. To date, an examination of available literature indicates that there is virtually no information available related to the costs or cost-effectiveness of DST use.

Scope of Present and Future Applications

Future trends in DSTs indicate an increase in expectations, increased technological awareness, and better quantitative skills on the part of decision makers, in addition to tremendous advances in the basic technology.[25] As familiarity with computers in general increases, the resistance to most computer systems will decrease. All this points to DST environments becoming more commonplace.

These changes may improve the effectiveness of DSTs and may perhaps radically transform the manner in which we make decisions. By expanding the variety and volume of information available to the decision maker, the quality of decisions made is expected to improve.[26] This, in turn, may accelerate the pace at which decisions are made and/or will be expected to be made.[27]

25. Dalkir, K. 1990. *Intelligent Decision Support Systems: A Practical Approach.* Ontario: Government of Canada.
26. Slatter, P. E. 1987. *Building Expert Systems: Cognitive Emulation.* England: Ellis Horwood Ltd.
27. Dalkir, K. 1990. *Intelligent Decision Support Systems: A Practical Approach.* Ontario: Government of Canada.

One possibility is that in the future, DST developers will be able to build their systems in a modular fashion by choosing required blocks of functions from a library. For example, standard packages would include report generators, statistical analysis kits, electronic mail, etc. These components could then be selected and routed through telephone networks to the particular application system being developed.[28]

Concurrent with decreases in hardware prices, costs are also decreasing for software. It is anticipated that this will result in a greater decentralization of decision making, improved quantitative analysis and, therefore, better decisions.[29] These technological advances, however, have not yet been matched by an increase in the human ability to monitor, filter, and selectively analyze large volumes of data.[30] Instead, an information overload has resulted—or has the potential to result—in the inefficient use of DSTs. What will be required from future DSTs are intelligent methods of processing information—knowledge management systems or intelligent DSTs (IDSTs).[31]

METHODOLOGY

Today, sample surveys have become the major method of conducting empirical research.[32] The use of sample surveys can provide data that range from the monitoring of trends to the testing of the current understanding of human processes. Using a well-designed sample survey is a relatively systematic, standardized approach to the collection of information.[33]

For the purposes of this project, the goal was to collect information related to the definition, application, and assessment of health care–related DSTs. To achieve this goal, the project was broken down into two phases designed to collect information related to an audit of DSTs based on the available literature, and a survey of the experiences of existing and/or potential health care DST developers and users.

28. Dalkir, K. 1990. *Intelligent Decision Support Systems: A Practical Approach.* Ontario: Government of Canada.

29. Glaser, R., and M. T. Chi. Eds. 1988. *The Nature of Expertise.* New Jersey: Lawrence Erlbaum Associated, Publishers.

30. Slatter, P. E. 1987. *Building Expert Systems: Cognitive Emulation.* England: Ellis Horwood Ltd.

31. Dalkir, K. 1990. *Intelligent Decision Support Systems: A Practical Approach.* Ontario: Government of Canada.

32. Rossi, P. H., J. D. Wright, and A. B. Anderson. Eds. 1986. *Handbook of Survey Research.* New York: Academic Press Inc.

33. Frankel, M. 1986. *Handbook of Survey Research,* eds. P. H. Rossi, J. D. Wright, and A. B. Anderson. New York: Academic Press Inc.

Audit of DSTs

Step 1

A descriptive database of health care–related DSTs—available or recommended—for clinical-, management-, or policy-related decision making was developed based on a survey of the existing academic and professional literature. The database field names created were as follows:

- DST name;
- precise target of tool (e.g., stroke prevention, surgical modelling, etc.);
- precise tool type (i.e., expert system, care map, observational database);
- mechanism of implementation (handbook, stand-alone PC, networked);
- clinical trial results;
- being used where;
- cost of development;
- estimated clinical benefits/costs;
- estimated organizational benefits/costs;
- tool class type (dynamic or static);
- decision target class of the tool (clinical, management, policy, client);
- implemented medium;
- evaluation results (for verifiability and validity);
- currently being used;
- why not being used;
- cost of implementation;
- cost of operation;
- barriers to dissemination.

Step 2

A survey of the MEDLARS, MEDLINE, HSSI, and HIRU databases was conducted using the following search parameters:

- decision support systems,
- decision support tools,
- management decision support systems, and
- management decision support tools.

The result was a list identifying 464 unique entries that required examination for determination of their suitability for inclusion in the DST Audit database. Based on a review of these 464 abstracts, 373 were selected for further examination as candidates for inclusion in the database.

The sole reason for rejection of an article was the absence of any reference to a DST. To illustrate, the following MEDLINE reference record was randomly chosen as an example of an article and its abstract:

TITLE: Nurse-midwives and the challenge of the information age.

SOURCE: J Nurse Midwifery 1995 May-June; 40(3): 313–4

NLM CIT. ID: 95318764

ABSTRACT: Rapid access to meaningful information is a corner stone to effective decision making in the Information Age. Computers are the tools for efficient and effective collection and analysis of data. As we enter an era of monumental change in the delivery of health care, our challenge as nurse-midwives is to use computer technology to support our goals and philosophy.

The theoretical nature of, and nonspecific reference to, computer technology in this abstract was the rationale used to exclude this reference from the DST Audit database.

Step 3

A new list identifying each of the 373 article names, authors, and journals was developed in order to determine which articles could be retrieved from the following libraries:
- The Royal Jubilee Hospital Medical Library;
- The University of Victoria;
- The University of British Columbia;
- The University of Waterloo;
- The University of Western Ontario; and
- Queen's University.

Of the 373 articles selected (based on information contained within the article abstracts), only 193 were able to be retrieved and are listed in the list of general references to DSTs and decision support (appendix 1).

Step 4

Following their retrieval, each of the 193 articles were reviewed in detail. It was found that only a subset of these articles met the criteria for inclusion in the database (i.e., the article addressed a specific DST). This subset contained 87 articles about 86 different DSTs.[34] Details about each DST were then entered into the DST Audit database. This database was used as the basis for the analysis of the literature.

Survey of Health Care DST Use

Step 1

A survey tool was designed to elicit data from individuals identified as key players in the design, development, implementation, and/or use of health

---

34. Some articles were about more than one DST and there was more than one article for some single DSTs.

care–related DSTs (see appendix 1 for a copy of the covering letter and complete survey tool). The types of data required were organized under the following categories:
- respondent information;
- DST information;
- DST effects;
- DST evaluation;
- obstacles to implementation of the DST; and
- future of the DST.

Step 2

The names of potential survey respondents were obtained from the following sources:
- authors whose articles were included in the DST Audit database;
- DST vendors (selection based on investigators' personal knowledge);
- researchers (selection based on investigators' personal knowledge);
- health care administrators listed in the manual, Canadian Hospital Executive 1995–1996; and
- individuals included in COACH's Scientific and Research Special Interest Group (SARSIG) mailing list.

It is important to note that time constraints prevented a more systematic selection of potential respondents, yet the authors of this report believe this list is an adequate representation of clinicians, researchers, and administrators involved in health care delivery and/or DST use.

Step 3

Once an address list was compiled, the survey tool was e-mailed or faxed[35] to North American vendors, North American health care administrators, and international academics/researchers.

The individuals contacted as potential survey respondents are listed in appendix 3. Responses of this survey are not published because they must be considered confidential in accordance with the respondents' explicit requests.

Each respondent was encouraged to send a copy of the survey tool to any persons they viewed as potential respondents. While each respondent was asked to keep a log of who they passed the survey to, no data are available on who or how many additional persons have been sent a survey.

---

35. Due to the length of the survey tool, respondents preferred not to complete it by phone. The preference was to read and answer as *their* time permitted.

Step 4

As each survey response was received, the results were entered into the survey database. The contents of the database were used as the basis for the survey results analysis.

RESULTS

DST Audit Results

The DST Audit database contains a record for each of the 86 unique DSTs described in the 87 articles identified from the original list of 193 articles. They range in publication date from 1991 to 1996 and are drawn from 47 different journals. These papers describe 86 different DSTs, classified according to the *working definitions* listed in table 2, and form the foundation for the interpretation of the results in this section.

Table 2
Working definitions used for the DST audit

Clinical decision support tools	– tools intended to support a health care provider[1] in decisions related to diagnosis, therapy, and care planning of individual patients.
Management decision support tools	– tools intended to support a health care provider in decisions related to the operation of a health care facility or program, or a part thereof.
Policy decision support tools	– tools intended to support a health care provider in decisions related to the planning, development, implementation, and/or modification of the operations of a health care facility or program, or a part thereof.
Teaching decision support tools	– tools designed to instruct health care providers in the process of decision making regarding the health care of individual patients or the operation of health care facilities or programs. (All DSTs will, in fact, instruct users in the process of decision making. This tool class is limited to those tools whose primary intent is instruction in decision making.)
Manual decision support tools	– tools that are implemented on paper or other hard-copy media.
Electronic decision support tools	– tools that are implemented on computer systems.

Table 2 (cont.)

Dynamic decision support tools	– tools in which the decision support output results from progressive interaction between the user and the tool. The result is focused on the particular case or situation for which the user is seeking support. Diagnostic expert systems usually fall into this category since the consultation is comprised of a series of questions issued by the system that the user answers. Each of the user's answers determines the nature of the subsequent question.
Static decision support tools	– tools in which the decision support output results from a *best fit* pattern of responses. The result is focused on the particular type of class, case, or situation for which the user is seeking decision support. Care map systems usually fall into this category since the decision support is a fixed guideline for the response to a case or situation that best fits the criteria entered by the user. The existence of one criterion does not dynamically affect the consideration or weighting of other criteria.

1. A health care provider is any individual responsible for making decisions that impact the health care of individuals or the operation of facilities and programs through which health care is provided.

The content of this audit database was then analyzed for particular trends and the results are described below.

The distribution of audited DSTs, by country of origin (based on the paper in which each DST is described), is shown in table 3.[36]

The distribution of DSTs by *target class* (as shown in figure 4) is consistent with the ease with which DSTs can be developed for each class. As described in the section "Conceptual Model," clinical decisions are highly structured and the variables used in clinical decision making are more predictable and less subject to dispute. In management and policy areas of decision making, this process becomes progressively less structured and the variables less predictable and more subject to dispute among decision makers. Input variables to policy decisions are also more likely to be influenced by unpredictable political factors or popular opinion than are clinical and management decisions. The regulation of pharmaceuticals is currently a controversial area in which this problem can be seen. While DSTs such as

---

36. All percentage figures in the tables and figures in this section of the report are based on N = 86 DSTs unless otherwise stated.

Table 3

Distribution of audited decision support tools by country of origin and DST percentage distribution by 4 categories: Canada, United States, Other, and Unknown

United States	43	China	2	Croatia	1
United Kingdom	7	Denmark	2	Greece	1
Canada	5	Germany	2	Malaysia	1
Finland	4	Japan	2	Poland	1
France	3	Sweden	2	Spain	1
Italy	3	Australia	1	Unknown	1
Netherlands	3	Belgium	1	N =	86

Percentage distribution of audited decision support tools	
Canada	6
United States	50
Other	44
Unknown	1

"RXPERT" [68] can be used for making objective indexing decisions based on empirical evidence, there is a strong tendency among physicians and the public to resist such regulation.

While not arbitrary, the boundaries between the target classes are ill defined. The only tool that could be classified as a policy DST was "Design-a-Trial" [27]. This is a tool intended to assist decision makers in designing clinical trials and, consequently, has clinical and management implications as well as policy implications. The management DSTs vary widely in scope, from "Transition I" [24], a comprehensive tool that applies traditional business principles to hospital planning and management, to a Lotus 1-2-3–based tool [61] designed to support nurse managers when they are making staffing decisions based on changing patient loads in a ward.

These results lead to the conclusion that at this early stage in the evolution of DSTs, developers tend to work in areas of less environmental uncertainty in order to focus on the challenges of design and development. This may change with time as analytic methods and development protocols stabilize and become more uniformly accepted among DST designers and developers respectively.

Automated DSTs (those designed to be used on a computer system) accounted for 97 percent of the audited DSTs (figure 5). Given the complexity of the health care decisions being supported by DSTs and, in particular, dynamic DSTs, manual implementation of a tool would likely have made the time required by a user to obtain complex decision support

Figure 4

Distribution of audited DSTs according to decision target class

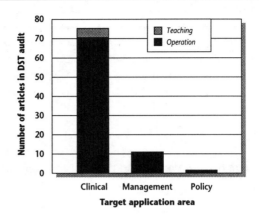

	Operation (%)	Teaching (%)
Clinical	80	6
Management	13	
Policy	1	

Note: Tools intended solely for *teaching* purposes have been isolated. Tools specifically intended for both teaching and operation have been included under *operation* as all tools have instructional value whether it is a design intent or not.

unworkable in most health care operations. Health care providers report that the printed policy and procedure manuals found in every hospital ward and department are rarely consulted because the sheer volume of these manuals prevents timely access to the required information.[37] Consequently, computer-based implementation remains the only practical way of providing these tools to their intended users.

In relative terms, there are more dynamic implementations of clinical DSTs than there are management and policy DSTs (figure 6). This may be due in part to the more predictable structure of decision processes and the more stable nature of the variables used in making clinical decisions, as clinical decision making tends to be a more iterative or step-by-step process than management- or policy-related decision making. For example, "ASURE" [21] is considered a static tool through which parts of a patient record are

---

37. Peterson, G. M. 1995. Knowledge engineering in nursing: Knowledge engineering methods for a pressure ulcer expert system. M.Sc. thesis, University of Victoria.

Figure 5

Distribution of audited DSTs according to decision target class and tool class type

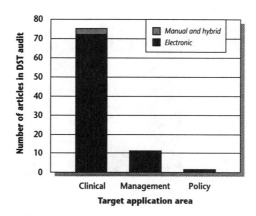

	Electronic (%)	Hybrid (%)	Manual (%)
Clinical	83	1	2
Management	13		
Policy	1		

identified that *may* indicate inappropriate utilization. However, the ASURE user is left to process the decision, one in which variables not considered in the structure of the DST may be more important than those that are considered. Contrast the latter with "MEDUSA"[56], a dynamic DST that provides diagnostic proposals on acute abdominal pain. While MEDUSA is still being evaluated, validation results indicate 80 percent accuracy in decision output compared to human experts in the field.

In management and policy areas, simple pattern recognition tends to be a more effective means of decision support. For example, in clinical areas, the value of one or more variables may affect how additional variables are considered in the decision-making process. In management and/or policy areas, the weight of individual variables tends to be more independent. To illustrate, in the assessment of patient risk for pressure ulcer development, the variables *patient has no sensory impairment* and *patient is able to move independently* makes the presence of other important variables such as *low body weight* and *dehydration* virtually irrelevant, thereby eliminating the

Figure 6

Distribution of audited DSTs according to decision target class and the mode of interaction between the user and the DST

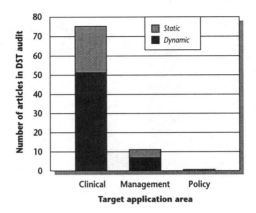

	Dynamic (%)	Static (%)
Clinical	60	28
Management	6	5
Policy		1

need to consider these or any other variables.[38] Alternatively, a management decision for a capital purchase must include consideration of variables such as *available budget* and *expressed need.* Changes in *expressed need* may impact or drive the budgeting process, but at some point the available budget remains unaffected by *expressed need* and vice versa.

Most audited tools have not been developed past the prototype stage and thus are not in use. Of the DSTs covered in the audit, only 25 percent were reported to be in current use, over 50 percent were not in use, and the status of the remaining DSTs was unknown (figure 7).

If an assumption is made that the distribution of the variable *unknown* is similar to the distribution of the variables *being used* and *not being used,* and that data contained in figure 7 is a representative sample of all DSTs, then over 70 percent of DSTs in existence are not in current use.

38. Peterson, G. M. 1995. Knowledge engineering in nursing: Knowledge engineering methods for a pressure ulcer expert system. M.Sc. thesis, University of Victoria.

Figure 7

Distribution of audited DSTs according to their operational status

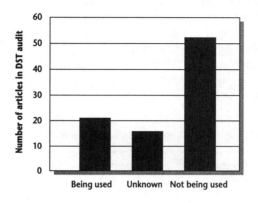

Being used **(%)**	24
Unknown **(%)**	17
Not being used **(%)**	59

The two main reported reasons for DSTs *not being used* was that the tool was either still under initial development or that it required further development after its initial evaluation (table 4). Only a small percentage of DSTs had either been abandoned or had no reported plans for continued development.

Table 4

Reason DST not being used

	Proportion of audited DSTs (%)
Under initial development	90
Need further development after initial trials	4
Unknown status	4
Developed but not implemented	2

There is a significant difference between the number of DSTs in current use and the number of DSTs that have been evaluated (table 5). Over 60 percent of all papers reviewed gave no indication of whether the DST had been subjected to any formal DST evaluation process. Less than 25 percent of all DSTs identified as *being in use* have been subjected to any evaluation indicating positive results; 40 percent of the tools reported as *not being used* indicate positive evaluation results.

Most of the evaluations that were performed were simply validation and verification tests against the experts on whose decision making the systems had been modelled. Only a few DSTs were subjected to the systematic evaluation required for clinical trials. Among these are "HEPAR" [87], a diagnostic DST for liver disorders, and "DAFODILL" [2], also a liver disorder diagnostic tool that uses MRI images. The figures shown in table 5 lead one to question what criteria are being used to determine whether a DST is put into use or not.

Table 5

DSTs status vs. validation/verification results

	Positive (%)	Equivocal (%)	Unknown (%)	In progress (%)
Not being used	18	2	32	6
Being used	5		17	2
Unknown	5		13	
Total	**28**	**2**	**62**	**8**

The methodologies used for evaluating DSTs are inconsistent and the objectives of the evaluations are unclear. The most common tests reported were validation and/or verification against the experts on whose decision making the DST was modelled. While verification and validation processes are aspects of a complete evaluation methodology, they do not *and should not* constitute the single rationale to be used for determining whether a DST should be implemented for routine use in the health care environment.

It is not surprising that the performance of most DSTs evaluated was reported to be unequal to that of the experts on whom they were modelled. Most DSTs operated at about 70 to 80 percent of the level of the human experts and were deemed clinically unusable on that basis. Korpinen et al. reported that even though their Epilepsy Expert [34] performed "... very close to the level of experts," the system was "... not suitable for clinical use."

Few of the papers acknowledged that the DST in question was intended to support nonexpert users in decision-making activities normally performed by human experts. Berner et al. reviewed the performance of four DSTs intended for decision support in internal medicine [65]. While DST performance was assessed against 10 expert physicians and found to be inferior, they emphasized that there was a clear difference between the *accuracy*, which they claim to have measured, and the clinical *usefulness* of the DSTs. They acknowledged that "the most common seekers of such consultations were considered to be primary care physicians or subspecialists needing assistance outside their area of expertise."

Clearly, validation and verification of DSTs against the experts whose consultation they are intended to replace must be followed by an evaluation of the decision performance of the intended user group with and without the aid of the DST in question. It may be unreasonable to expect a *robot* like a DST to perform at the level of an expert, but if it enhances the decision-making performance of nonexperts it may be unreasonable to reject that DST as unsuitable.

Given the scarcity of formal evaluation results for the DSTs examined in the audit, it is difficult to assign much quantitative credibility to the reported benefits attributed to the use of DSTs (table 6). However, even if one dismisses the quantitative credibility of their claims on the grounds that a proper evaluation of the tool was not conducted, the range of *anticipated* benefits still warrants comment.

While the bulk of the DSTs were targeted at clinical decision making, many authors reported or inferred anticipated benefits in the area of management as well as in the targeted clinical area of decision support. This is reflected in table 7. While the majority of the DSTs audited were targeted at clinical decision making, most of the articles reported benefits that clearly lie in the area of management. For example, OCIS [62] is a cancer patient information system that provides both clinical and management decision support based on a single but comprehensive data set and knowledge base. This finding is consistent with the emerging acknowledgement that the *evidence* for management decisions must include clinical data such as the *consequences* of health care decisions.

Table 6

Reported benefits of audited DSTs

Reported benefits of audited DSTs	Proportion of audited DSTs (%)	Example tool [ref.]
Management benefits		
Resource analysis/management	34	Lotus 1-2-3 [61]
Cost control/efficiency	32	Automated Antibiotic Consultant [84]
Clinical instruction	28	Breast Cancer DST [49]
Other	4	Apache [72]
Clinical care benefits		
Patient care quality/specificity	26	Hepar [86] [87]
Patient care management	18	Pediatric Asthma Guideline [79]
Patient care uniformity/specificity	16	Assure [21]
Patient satisfaction	4	Computerlink [81] [82]
Clinical diagnosis benefits		
Diagnostic uniformity/specificity	30	Sleep Expert [35] [36]
Diagnostic quality/availability	30	AIDA [7]

The barriers to dissemination and use of the DSTs reported in the audited publications (table 7) are consistent with identified reasons for DSTs not being in current use (table 4). That is, the DSTs require further development and, more specifically, the content of the database, knowledge base, or rule base with which the DST operates is as yet incomplete. As a consequence, the DST was found to be "not yet suitable for routine use." As in the previous example, one must question the process and interpretation of the evaluations that lead the authors to these conclusions.

Table 7

Reported barriers to dissemination and use of audited DSTs

Reported barriers to dissemination and use of audited DSTs	Proportion of audited DSTs (%)	Example tool [ref.]
Needs further development	44	Sleep Expert [35] [36]
DB/KB/RB[1] content	30	HFP [33]
Decision support output quality	28	Apache [72]
Evaluation pending	20	Pediatric Asthma Guideline [79]
User interface	16	Cartes [32]
User resistance	8	Transition I [24]
User's computer literacy	8	Computerlink [81] [82]
Time dependency	6	Medusa [56]
Cost	6	Titrator [19]
Other	4	LIED [29]

1. Database/knowledge base/rulebase—these are the different structures within which models of human expertise are stored and made available to the user through the DST interface.

It can be assumed that reports of user resistance and computer unfamiliarity largely overlap as the later tends to be a major cause of user resistance. It is worth noting, however, that this was not reported as a leading factor preventing the dissemination and use of the DSTs audited; it appears to be second to the quality of the user interface through which the tool is accessed. While ergonomics has figured prominently as an influential factor in interface design, developers are only beginning to acknowledge the importance of psychophysics and psychometrics in the construction of the human-machine interface. A user interface must be considered the "language" that a program uses to communicate with the user and, as such, the interface must conform as closely as possible to the human language and the communication logic of the professional user. Systematic approaches to the development of user interfaces that take these factors into account are only now beginning to emerge.

A few authors reported that the lack of consideration of the time dependency of some input criteria compromised the output validity of the DSTs they examined and was, therefore, a barrier to use and dissemination [56]. This may become an important factor in future DST development since it may account for a large part of the difference between the performance of a DST and that of the human expert. Most DSTs are designed to consider criteria present at a fixed point in time while human experts tend to include time-based changes in those criteria when arriving at a decision.

Survey Results

To date, only 31 of 106 known[39] possible respondents have returned the survey (29 percent return rate). The known possible respondents were individuals identified specifically through the DST audit or known to the investigators to be active in DST development, use, or evaluation. Some potential respondents declined to participate due to either the length of the survey or because the systems they were working on did not fit the operational definition of DSTs being used for the survey.[40] As a result, the number of responses is low, thereby limiting the significance of any statistical analysis. However, the figures in tables 8 and 9 indicate that the sample is comprised of respondent types and DST target classes in representative proportions. The trends indicated are, therefore, worthy of comment and are consistent with the results of the DST audit. All percentages shown in the results tables in this section are based on N = 31.

Table 8 presents the proportion of respondents according to their role in the design, development, and implementation of the DST with which they were involved. Most of the respondents were the project directors and/ or developers/analysts of the DST in question and were, therefore, able to speak broadly about that DST. A minority of respondents were users and evaluators. This finding is consistent with the fact that very few of these DSTs are in use or have been evaluated. It should be noted that in table 8, as in subsequent tables, the percentages do not total 100 percent. In many cases the respondents had multiple roles in the DST project and/or the DST was designed for multiple targets. The numbers as presented reflect this fact.

---

39. The survey was distributed via a number of mail list servers. The numbers of subscribers to these lists is not included in the *known* contacts, but is estimated at 1,000.

40. Correspondence with the HIRU group at McMaster University revealed that while the systems they were working on or had developed could be considered as information systems useful in decision making, none of them qualified as a DST according to the definition used for this project.

Table 8

Respondent involvement with DST

	Proportion of respondents (%)
Project director	63
Developer/analyst	41
User	19
Evaluator	4

Table 9 describes the distribution of the surveyed DSTs according to their intended user target. Of the DSTs surveyed only five targeted physicians exclusively by offering, for example, a DST for diagnosis and treatment of epilepsy and a DST for diagnosis of liver lesions based on MRI images. Two of the DSTs surveyed targeted nurses exclusively by offering a nursing research utilization framework and a DST for pressure ulcer risk assessment, diagnosis, and treatment.

Even fewer DSTs were targeted exclusively at managers and/or policy-makers. One described a population-based service utilization DST intended for resource management and policy development. In addition, only one DST, a clinical care planning tool, was targeted directly at patients.

Most of the DSTs surveyed were targeted at more than one type of clinical provider by offering, for example, a nutrition expert system intended for use by physicians and nutritionists in patient care planning, a psychiatric DST intended for use by physicians and therapists, and a neonatal ventilation DST intended for use by physicians and nurses. Others were targeted at clinical providers and their managers/administrators by offering, for example:
- a stroke patient management DST intended for use by care providers, managers, and researchers;
- a managed care appropriateness DST intended for use by physicians and managers; and
- a collaborative acute care planning DST for use by care providers, managers, and administrators.

Many of the DSTs surveyed included an educational/training component for instructors and/or students. Examples include a DST for the assessment of general diagnostic competence, and a community health program planning tool.

As anticipated, the distribution of areas for which the surveyed DSTs were targeted (table 10) is consistent with the distribution of the intended users. Only a few of the DSTs surveyed were intended for use in a single location. These include:
- a ventilation management DST intended for use in neonatal ICUs;
- a hip replacement patient care map intended for use on surgical wards; and

Table 9

Intended user targets of the surveyed DSTs

	Proportion of respondents (%)
Clinician	81
Technologist/therapist	48
Manager	44
Planner (policy)	37
Clinical instructor	30
Student	11
Other	11

- a liver lesion DST for MRI images intended for use in diagnostic imaging departments.

Some of the DSTs surveyed were intended for use in multiple clinical venues (e.g., an acute care planning DST intended for use on wards, and in diagnostic and therapy departments) or, more often, for use in both clinical and in management/administration venues. These include:

- a stroke patient management DST intended for clinical patient care, clinical service management, and clinical research; and
- a managed care appropriateness DST intended for clinical patient care, utilization management, and quality assurance.

Again, only a few of the DSTs were intended for use only in management and administration areas (e.g., a population-based, service utilization DST intended for resource management and policy development.

Table10

Intended target area of the DST

	Proportion of respondents (%)
Ward	59
Management	41
Therapeutic service	37
Administration	30
Support service	30
Diagnostic service	26
Rehabilitation service	7
Education	7
Other	11

The distribution of targeted users and areas reported in the survey (tables 9 and 10) does not agree with the distribution of DSTs according to the target class observed in the audit (figure 4). Table 11 shows that the DSTs included in the survey are targeted more at managers and policymakers than are the DSTs included in the audit. This discrepancy in findings may reflect an emerging trend in the purpose of DSTs. Given delays in publication, it is possible to conclude that the results of the audit represents thinking about DSTs from two or three years ago, while the survey responses represent current thinking. This change is consistent with the increasing focus on responsible fiscal management in health care and the recognition of the emerging need to integrate clinical systems with management systems in the support of decision making. It is worth noting that only two tools, DAFODILL [2] and Computerlink [81] [82], are included in both the audit and the survey.

Table 11

Comparison of relative distribution of DST target areas between the audit and the survey

	Audit (%)	Survey (%)
Clinical	86	72
Management and administration	14	28

Nearly one-half (48 percent) of the survey respondents indicated that the time users required to arrive at a decision was reduced through the use of the DSTs surveyed. This benefit, combined with the information from the survey respondents who answered the question regarding the effect of their DST on decision quality, indicated that decisions made with the support of the DST were more appropriate, accurate, consistent, and/or effective compared to decisions made without the DST (table 12).

Table 12

Effect of DST decision quality

	Proportion of respondents (%)
Appropriate	37
Accurate	11
Consistent	11
Effective	7
Other	19
None	7

The users of one of the surveyed DSTs, a care planning advisor linked to a clinical database, reported that decisions were clinically more accurate and effective using the DST and that this resulted in a marked decrease in patient length of stay as well as improved resource utilization.

Another DST, one targeted at infection control in hospitals, is reported to have improved the response time to infection incidents and the efficiency with which the infections are subsequently managed. This, in turn, is reported to have decreased the continuing cost of providing infection control services in the respondent's hospital. Variability in clinical decisions is also reported to have decreased as a consequence of DST use; the use of a care map tool for patients that have had a total hip replacement apparently increased the consistency and improved the "continuity of data" for patients in this condition.

It cannot be concluded, based on the survey results, that the use of DSTs leads statistically to more effective and/or efficient decision making. As with the audited DSTs, most of the surveyed DSTs have either not been subjected to formal outcomes-based evaluations or such evaluations have not yet been completed (table 13). The figures in tables 13 and 14 add up to less than 100 percent because many of the articles did not refer to any evaluation for the DST(s) they described.

Table 13

Results of formal DST evaluation

	Proportion of respondents (%)
Positive	19
Pending	11
Equivocal	7
Positive but needs work	7
No formal evaluation reported	56

Of those evaluated, most were not evaluated beyond the validation/verification phase, and only 37 percent had been subjected to quantitative or baseline evaluations (table 14). One exception to this is the total hip replacement care map for which quantitative data were formally collected for a three-month trial. The results of this study include significant reductions in patient length of stay and practice variation.

Given the limits of the tests to which most of the other DSTs surveyed were subjected, it is safer to conclude that the respondents *anticipate* the effects of DST use on health care decision making. Having said this, the expectation that DSTs may have a positive effect on the targeted decision-making processes is probably not unreasonable. For example, the use of a "research utilization framework" for nursing practices is reported to have reduced decision-making time, increased the evidence-based component of nursing decisions, and improved patient care based on anecdotal feedback from the users as well as individual patient outcomes (the outcome criteria were not specified). This particular respondent, however, acknowledged the need for more formal evaluation of this DST.

Table 14

DST evaluation method

	Proportion of respondents (%)
Quantitative	22
User survey	15
Baseline comparison	15
Qualitative	11

Unlike the results of the audit in which user resistance ranked sixth in the barriers to the dissemination and use of the DST (table 7), the survey respondents reported that user resistance was the major factor limiting the implementation of DSTs (table 15). It is conceivable, however, that user resistance is manifested as the "need for further development" or "limitations to the knowledge base content" concerns shown in the audit results. While these are legitimate and important reasons for users to resist the use of the DSTs, the survey respondents listed "loss of control" and "fear of comparison" as reasons why users resist using DSTs, in 19 percent and 11 percent of the surveys respectively (table 16).

This indicates that some of the user resistance reported in table 15 may result from users' legitimate concerns regarding the quality of decision support output from the tools and/or the scope of the tools. Some user resistance may also be attributable to human factors, such as fear of technology, resistance to change, and professional independence.

Table 15

Factors limiting the implementation of DSTs

	Proportion of respondents (%)
User resistance	37
Access to tool	29
Scope of tool	26
Cost	22
Output reliability	7
Other	22

It is worth noting that while the respondents listed *access* to the DST as a major limiting factor, this variable was not identified as a barrier to the dissemination and use of DSTs during the audit. This may be because the publications reviewed for the audit focused more on the development and performance of the DSTs in question rather than on implementation issues.

Our survey provided the opportunity to make inquiries related to more practical issues. The lack of access to a DST indicates that the availability of hardware and software to support the use of these tools continues to be a limiting factor in the dissemination and use of DSTs regardless of how well they perform compared against human experts or how useful nonexperts find them.

Table 16 lists who supported and who resisted the use of the surveyed DSTs before and after implementation. These results may be misleading, as it appears that DST use received less support after implementation than before. These results are displayed in this format in order to remain true to the respondents' answers to the survey questions. It may be of more value to compare the ratio of support and resistance in each user category. These results show that clinical personnel were the principal source of user resistance both before and after implementation, but that there was a notable reduction in resistance, compared to support, after implementation. This may be due to a marked reduction in apprehension about output quality, a fear of loss of control of clinical decision making, and a fear of having their decisions compared to the recommendations of the DST in question.

The figures reported in table 16 concerning why users supported the DSTs are consistent with previously noted observations that the focus on management and administration appears to have increased. The main sources of support driving implementation of the DSTs include cost and quality controls, which are also drivers for evidence-based health care. This is in agreement with the anticipated departmental (efficiency, cost control, resource management) and institutional (resource utilization, cost control) benefits reported by survey respondents (tables 17 and 18).

While clinical providers are the principal source of resistance to the development and use of DSTs, for the reasons cited above, they are also the foremost champions of DSTs even before implementation (table 16). This indicates that among the identified users/stakeholders, the development and use of DSTs is most contentious among clinical providers. This is typified by the responses noted in one survey describing an interdisciplinary care map tool for clinical care planning. The respondent reported that clinicians were the principal source of both support and resistance both before and after implementation, but that the ratio of support over resistance had definitely increased after implementation. Before implementation "anticipated reduced LOS (length of stay) and improved care" and "fear of losing control of practice, fear of cookbook medicine" were cited as the reasons for support and resistance respectively. After implementation "improved

Table 16

Support for and resistance to DSTs before and after implementation

	Before implementation		After implementation	
	Who supported (%)	Who resisted (%)	Who supported (%)	Who resisted (%)
Clinicians	41	33	37	26
Management	37	7	22	4
Administration	19	4	11	7
Researchers	11		4	
Other	11	4	4	

	Before implementation		After implementation	
	Why supported (%)	Why resisted (%)	Why supported (%)	Why resisted (%)
Output quality	23	19	26	7
User control	4	19		7
Computer literacy		7		4
System cost	4	4		7
Cost control	23		7	
Quality control	26		22	
Knowledge transfer	10			
Reliability	10			
Fear of comparison		11		
Other		11	11	4

patient care," "improved communication with nurses and support services" and production of "reliable clinical reporting data" were cited as the reasons for support, and "fear of losing control" and "discomfort of having practice under scrutiny by peers" were offered as the reasons for continued user resistance. While resistance remains significant, there appears to be growing clinical support for DSTs driven by a desire to provide as high a quality of care for patients as possible. While the rate at which DSTs are subjected to formal evaluations remains low, providers must be realizing some benefits or must be anticipating that a benefit is forthcoming from the use of DSTs if one is to justify their expressed levels of confidence.

One of the emerging challenges faced by health care providers as DSTs and other information systems are adopted, is working through the apparent conflicts associated with the users' fear of loss of decision control to automated systems (table 16), the professional understanding among health care providers of the need to control the costs and quality of care, and the need to manage resources of all types (tables 17 and 18). These conflicts may be resolved by educating clinical providers on the intended and appropriate role of DSTs in decision making and by bringing clinical providers more into the planning and design phases of DST development. The latter will inevitably give clinical providers a greater sense of *ownership* of the tools, thereby reducing the perceived threat of having to relinquish clinical decision-making control to a machine.

Table 17

Departmental benefits of DSTs

	Proportion of respondents (%)
Efficiency	19
Cost control	19
Communication	19
Resource management	7
Other	15

Table 18

Institutional benefits of DSTs

	Proportion of respondents (%)
Resource utilization	15
Cost control/reduction	15
Reporting	15
Evidence-based decision making	11
Efficiency	7

Table 19

Clinical benefits of DSTs

	Proportion of respondents (%)
Clinical standards	26
Practice patterns	19
Diagnosis and treatment	7
Other	26

The need for fiscally responsible standardization and improvement of health care is becoming more and more apparent to all stakeholders in the health care community. It is also becoming more widely recognized that these goals may be accomplished using appropriately designed and implemented DSTs. Furthermore, there is a trend to bridge the gap between clinical, management, and policy decision making in health care.

Health management consists mainly of making decisions that result in present or future actions. The effectiveness of these decisions, in terms of extent and timing, depend on two types of information: the correct appraisal of quantitative elements of a situation and an accurate assessment of the consequences of the action decided upon. While the first type of information is reasonably well accepted, the second is only just beginning to be appreciated. In industry, the feedback of outcome information through the initial stages of action in order to control systems is advanced. In this manner, discrepancies and variation can be noted immediately, allowing *smarter* decisions to be made.

DISCUSSION

The Future of DSTs: The Clinical Practice and Institutional Management Perspective

Today, researchers represent the majority of those building DSTs.[41] The purpose of developing these systems is usually to explore theoretical issues and, consequently, the intent is to evaluate the performance of a theoretical model (such as how closely the DST mimics human decision making). This type of DST development often neglects issues such as user acceptability, system performance, cost, and maintenance.[42] It is not surprising, therefore, that the majority of DSTs have not progressed beyond the prototype phase.[43]

DSTs do, however, have a future in clinical practice and institutional management due to the:
- increasing volume and complexity of the data, information, and knowl-edge that health care providers are expected to consider in decision making;
- trend toward integration of health care across health care environments (the continuity of care or managed care concept);

---

41. Lilford, R. J. 1990. Limitations of expert systems: Intuition versus analysis. *Bailliere's Clinical Obstetrics and Gynaecology* 4(4): 851–856.
42. Marcot, B. Testing your knowledge base. *Validating and Verifying Knowledge-Based Systems*, ed. Uma Gupta. pp. 214–218.
43. Heathfield, H. A. 1993. Philosophies for the design and development of clinical decision support systems. *Methods of Information in Medicine* 32(1): 1–15.

- increasing demand by public and private payers for fiscal and clinical accountability; and
- increasing support for the concept of evidence-based health care.

Despite decades of research and millions of dollars in expenditures on DSTs, few are in widespread use within health care environments.[44] While this statement remains true in the sense that few single DSTs are in use, it is misleading with regard to the state of development of these systems. DSTs are ubiquitous and research on DST use in health care is growing.[45] The current results indicate that providers operating at all levels of health care are recognizing the *potential* of DSTs to enhance decision-making processes. The anticipated result of DST use is that health care providers will be able to devote more time to the more complex, unstructured problems that can only be addressed and/or resolved by a human decision maker.

As discussed in the section "Purported Benefits to Be Derived from the Use of DSTs in Health Care," the current health care environment has generated large volumes of data and information structured in ways that would be useful for decision making were it not for the time required to identify and access the relevant data and information. Since the data and information required for operational, management, and policy-making decision support overlap, an appropriately structured DST should have the facility to provide clinical, management, and administrative decision support within that DST's functional domain.

Human knowledge required to identify, access, and process the data and information required for a particular decision is the essential component of any DST. In future, DST developers must first define and then make the DST decision-processing model conform to the decision-making processes exhibited by domain experts rather than vice versa. Ideally, therefore, the process should reflect the best decision-making practices possible that encompass the best evidence possible. As a result, future DSTs may be seen as mechanisms that support the practice of evidence-based health care. Their development as potential adjuncts to health care decision making should be encouraged. Realizing the benefits of DSTs in terms of evidence-based health care will require a concerted effort on the part of institutions and organizations to develop a comprehensive, *integrated* information infrastructure devoted to health care communication.

To date, however, most health care organizations continue to epitomize the term "islands of information," with departments operating with differing information systems or with no automation at all. Yet, when measured as a percentage of operational costs, the information needs of health care are

---

44. Ibid.

45. Gottinger, H. W., and H. P. Weiman. 1990. *Artificial Intelligence: A Tool for Industry and Management.* London: Ellis Horwood.

among the most intense and complex of all service industries. Examples abound in industries such as air travel and banking of successfully achieved integration. To illustrate, the introduction and increasingly widespread use of ATM interfaces has resulted in banks being able to not only link their own multiple branch transactions, but has also facilitated the timely and accurate communication between different banking establishments. Most industries have developed an infrastructure that enables the feedback of end-result information to the initial stages or actions of a DST or other information technologies. Discrepancies and variations can, therefore, be detected and acted on immediately, allowing for better decision making. [46]

Despite a growing awareness of the importance of information as a management resource, "there is little empirical evidence that hospital executives have used information systems effectively."[47] Canadian hospitals continue to lag behind industries of similar financial scale in comprehensively applying information management techniques to their data resources. While other information-intense industries such as banking, retailing, and insurance allocate as much as 10 percent of their annual budgets to information systems, health care organizations such as hospitals devote only 2 to 4 percent.[48] Although some hospitals now operate with updated technology that has grown around the facility's information needs, many commercial products remain limited, restricting rather than enhancing information access by hospital managerial, clinical and operational staff. While the DST survey indicates that this may be changing, the bulk of DSTs developed to date target single user groups of health care professionals, such as clinicians only. What continues to be missing are the "electronic linkages of clinical and financial data... that tie patients and providers together across the continuum of care from the patient's home to the work setting, to the many possible sites of contact within the delivery system."[49]

While this type of information linkage has not yet occurred within the Canadian health care environment, the Chedoke-McMaster Hospitals and the Peel Memorial Hospital are "currently reviewing their information systems for evolution within their respective established... organizational structures" in order to bridge the *islands of information* through enhanced information

46. Harber, B. W., and S. A. Miller. 1994. Program management and health care informatics: Defining relationships. *Healthcare Management FORUM* 7(4): 28–35.

47. Austin, C. J., J. M. Trimm, and P. M. Sobzak. 1995. Information systems and strategic management. *HealthCare Management Review* 20(3): 26–33.

48. Harber, B. W., and S. A. Miller. Program management and health care informatics: Defining relationships. *Healthcare Management FORUM* 7(4): 28–35.

49. Austin, C. J., J. M. Trimm, and P. M. Sobzak. 1995. Information systems and strategic management. *HealthCare Management Review* 20(3): 26–33.

access by all key health care stakeholders.[50] It remains to be seen how successful their approach will be in integrating users and information.

The Ideal DST Project

While no perfect DST exists, it is possible to define the ideal DST project based on the results of the current project, the methodological literature on information systems development, and the collective experience of the authors. The following describes the 12 steps that should be part of an "ideal" DST project. This may be a bold statement but, in the absence of any accepted standards for DST project planning, it is appropriate.

1. *Identify the purpose of the DST and determine if the problem it will address qualifies as a DST candidate.*
   Any DST must have the objective of supporting decision making and, therefore, the development project must satisfy that objective. The problem for which the decision is required should meet the following criteria if the project is to proceed:
   - it must be a problem for which the absence of support affects the decision quality of those individuals most often called upon to deal with the problem;
   - human decision support in the problem area must be rare, difficult to access, and/or expensive. There must be an anticipated benefit to using the DST that cannot be easily realized any other way;
   - the decision-making process must be structured or semistructured (given the current DST technology). There should be no unpredictable variables (political or popular opinion) that affect the course of the decision process. Developers must be able to model the decision process as precisely as possible;
   - there must be expert decision makers in the area in which the DST is to be used. They must be available for the knowledge engineering, validation, and verification phases of the project; and
   - there must be general agreement among the experts about what variables constitute legitimate input to the decision, what weight is assigned to each of those variables, and in what order those variables are considered in the process. The DST must represent the best available decision-making standard.

2. *Scan the organizational environment to determine whether there is adequate support for the development of a DST.*
   It is likely that DST development will be difficult if there is strong resistance to its development and/or use. This may be the case in

---

50. Harber, B. W., and S. A. Miller. Program management and health care informatics: Defining relationships. *Healthcare Management FORUM* 7(4): 28–35.

situations in which objective data and information do not serve as the primary inputs to the decision-making process.

3. *Define the scope of the decision making to be supported by the DST.*
Decisions are interdependent due to input requirements and knowledge bases that overlap. The range of decisions to be addressed by the DST must be precisely defined so that the development process has focus. For example, developers have to ask if a clinical DST will be a diagnostic tool only, or if it will include care planning and management support for decisions that stem from the diagnosis. Based on the DST survey, clinical, management, and policy decisions in a given problem area can be addressed by a single tool.

4. *Identify the users of the DST.*
Anticipated users must be defined as precisely as possible (e.g., pediatric ward nurse, manager of nutritional services, vice-president of finance etc., rather than as a nurse, manager, or executive). The defined users are those responsible for the decision making defined within the decision scope of the DST.

5. *Determine what data, information, and knowledge are required by the experts to make the best possible decision.*
This includes the weight experts assign to each criterion as well as the order in which they consider them. This is referred to as knowledge engineering and requires a systematic methodology that has been the subject of much debate among developers. This should also be the longest and most exhaustive phase of the project.

6. *Define the output the DST will provide for all realistic combinations of inputs, including incomplete data.*
The output will form the basis of the verification tests. The decisions based on that output will be the basis of the validation tests.

7. *Develop a data and information flow model for the decision-making processes to be addressed by the DST.*
In this area, at least, there are a variety of valid, systematic methodologies that can be used.

8. *Build the DST.*
This phase is the simplest and will generally be the shortest phase of the project.

9. *Develop the interface to the DST.*
The interface design must be consistent with both the decision process model and with the manner in which the users are accustomed to handling the data.

10. *Implement and refine the DST.*

11. *Do validation tests with the experts and verification tests with the users.*
The decision support product of the DST must be evaluated against that of the experts. The quality/utility of the interaction between the

DST and the users must be evaluated against what the users would expect from human decision support.

12. *Do a systematic evaluation of the DST based on outcomes.*

This may be a clinical trial or some other form of baseline study and the outcome variables should include all that are impacted by decisions supported by the DST (e.g., clinical results, costs, patient satisfaction, LOS, professional confidence, etc.).

The Future of DST Development: The Market Perspective

In Canada, health care spending represents a business in excess of $72.5 billion per year. In 1994, this represented 9.7 percent of Canada's annual gross domestic product, or $2,478 per person. Nationally, the annual rate of increase of total health care expenditures slowed to 1.0 percent in 1994—down from 2.5 percent in 1993 and 5.6 percent in 1992.[51] These fiscal constraints are responsible for momentous transformations in the current and future delivery of health care. Reduction and/or elimination of certain services, the privatization of others (e.g., laser surgery clinics), multitiered access ("Fears for Tiers"), disease management (managed care) and video/telemedicine are but a few of the innovative methods currently under discussion and/or implementation. What is a key component of any change, however, is the need for quality information delivered efficiently and effectively.

As shown in table 20, the percentage distribution of national health care expenditures from 1975 to 1994 reveals several important trends. The cost of physician services, as a percentage of total health care spending, has remained constant over this time period. Secondly, spending on drugs has steadily increased since 1975. Capital spending peaked around 1987 and has declined steadily since. Finally, relative spending on hospital services has constantly declined throughout the entire period in question.[52] These last two trends are particularly significant from the perspective of DST development. The major barrier for any meaningful development and implementation of DSTs is to determine who is going to pay.

Investment in a cohesive health information infrastructure that includes DSTs, will play a major role in the process of health care reform. In their report *Advice to Government: Focusing on the Levers for Change in Health Care*, the Ontario Joint Policy and Planning Committee identified the need for sophisticated management information systems as the number one issue for the role of the physician.[53]

---

51. National Health Expenditures in Canada, 1975–1994.

52. National Health Expenditures in Canada, 1975–1994.

53. Advice to government: Focusing on the levers for change in health care. Sponsored by the restructuring subcommittee of the Joint Policy and Planning Committee. April 1995.

Table 20

**Percentage distribution of national health care
expenditures 1975–1994**

Year	1975	1980	1985	1990	1994
Hospitals	45.0	41.9	40.9	39.1	37.3
Other institutions	9.2	11.3	10.2	9.4	9.8
Physicians services	15.0	14.7	15.1	15.2	14.2
Other health services	7.4	8.5	8.2	8.5	8.5
Drugs	8.8	8.4	9.5	11.3	12.7
Capital	4.4	4.7	4.6	3.7	2.9
Other	10.3	10.5	11.5	12.9	14.6

Source: National Health Expenditures in Canada, 1975–1994.

Population health, outcomes measurement, and the efficiency of interventions will depend upon fast, accurate, and reliable integrated information. As electronic networking and the accessibility of distributed databases grow, DSTs will be essential to research, analyze, synthesize, and translate primary data into meaningful information and knowledge for effective and efficient patient care. However, despite the proliferation of technological developments in medical computing, health care providers have been slow to incorporate computers for patient data management and clinical decision making. In part, this may be due to the awkwardness of initial programs, poor integration with the work habits of providers, nonexistent graphical user interfaces, lack of integration among applications, and a general mistrust of computers.

Skepticism regarding the utility of medical informatics also plays a role. In an editorial, Dr. Stewart Cameron stated: "We cannot assume that every novel computer application will be an improvement over existing practice … we may discover that the considerable trouble of computerizing did not provide any benefits."[54] Indeed, Cameron cites two studies that demonstrated little or no benefit from computer-aided diagnosis.

This skepticism is further supported by findings in a report commissioned by the Canadian Organization for the Advancement of Computers in Health for the Eighth World Congress on Medical Informatics, conducted by Deloitte & Touche.[55] Although the respondent profile was

54. Cameron, S. 1995. Evidence-based informatics. *Canadian Medical Informatics* (May–June).

55. Deloitte & Touche. Emerging trends in information technology. *International Health Industry Results* (Med-Info '95).

international, 60 percent of the 125 respondents were Canadian. As illustrated in figure 8, the most remarkable finding of the survey was that the responding organizations felt that their respective investments in information technology had little or no impact on improving the quality of care, the timeliness of clinical and executive decision making, cost containment, decrease in length of stay, or operational productivity. Clearly, further investment in information technology must be cost effective, with demonstrable benefits and measurable results.

Figure 8

Improvement via IT investment

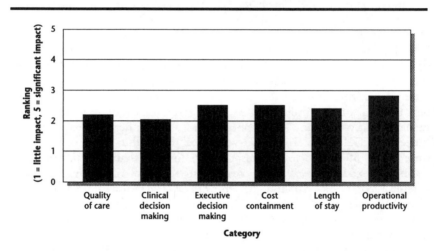

The results of our DST audit also support these findings. Although the use of DSTs is anticipated to improve the quality of decision making, the available literature is unclear on the impact of DSTs from a clinical, organizational, or systemic (entire health care system) perspective. In fact, of the DSTs examined, the anticipated benefits from clinical, organizational, or systemic perspectives were unknown in 66 percent, 70 percent, and 88 percent of the cases respectively.

As shown earlier in this report, the primary developers of DSTs are individuals who develop DSTs for academic reasons or for specific applications in their host organizations. However, of the DSTs identified in the decision support tools audit, most have not progressed beyond the prototype phase and, thus, are not in widespread use. Only 24 percent were reported to be in use in at least one location. There are several reasons for this apparent lack of success. Typical of any successfully marketed product or service, a comprehensive business plan that identifies potential markets, core competencies, strengths and weaknesses, competitive positions, development costs, etc., is mandatory. Business planning and marketing, however, is not a strength of academia—their focus is on theoretical issues. The DST audit revealed that development and implementation costs were only occasionally identified. In addition, in none of the DSTs examined were operating costs mentioned. These costs must be identified and published in order to obtain widespread acceptance of DSTs in today's economic climate. In contrast, commercially developed software necessarily identifies and projects these costs prior to initiating development. Further, many of the DSTs identified in the audit have been developed with a specific target user in mind. For example, in many cases DSTs have been developed for a specific institution and, therefore, lack broader applicability.

In comparison, and for obvious competitive reasons, few data exist on industrial development of DSTs. However, in the Sixth Annual HIMSS/ Hewlett-Packard Leadership Survey, 92 percent of U.S.-based respondents believed that information management technology would play either a significant or somewhat significant role in health care delivery.[56] Although the information is U.S. based, it also indicated that 29 percent of the respondents would invest 50 percent more in information systems over the next two years. In our opinion, there is no reason to believe that information management will be any less important to Canadian health care providers. Indeed, the Deloitte & Touche survey found that within the same two-year time frame, 58 percent of the respondents forecast that their information technology expenditures would increase by an average of 47 percent. As shown in table 20, of the $72.5 billion spent in 1994 on total health care expenditures, Canadians spent 37.3 percent, or $27 billion, on hospitals. Current estimates indicate that 1.5 percent to 2.0 percent of total hospital spending is directed to information systems. This means that in 1994, approximately $410 to $540 million was spent on information systems. Assuming no increase in total expenditures, but extrapolating based on the above forecast data, information system expenditures in each of the next two years could exceed $1.0 billion. Since no increases from either the federal (transfer payments) or the provincial (ministry budgets) levels are expected, these expenditures will necessarily have to be reallocated from other sources.

We believe these findings are of paramount importance. The results of this report appear to indicate a strong trend toward requiring commercial development of DSTs, and also indicate that significant growth in information technology expenditures is expected in this sector. In addition, health care providers need to be targeted as one of the primary users of DSTs and, therefore, excellent graphical user interfaces are required.

---

56. Hewlett-Packard. 1995. Trends in health care computing. Sixth annual HIMSS, Hewlett-Packard Leadership Survey.

The Future of DSTs in Policy and Management: An Organizational Behaviour Perspective

Introduction

With regard to the area of DSTs application, this section focuses on management- and policy-related tools. The primary purpose of this section is to provide what is essentially informed speculation about the future of DSTs from an analysis of theories of organizational behaviour and examples of what happened to other rational initiatives in the past. This section will introduce the reader to a number of basic concepts and theoretical models from the administrative and policy sciences that have considerable application to the health sector but that appear to be used relatively infrequently by health researchers and analysts.

Administration and policy are combined in this section as policy formulation takes place in an organizational context and, as such, is influenced by organizational constraints and behaviours. In addition, models of organizational behaviour are discussed as relevant conceptual models for understanding the policy-making process in texts on policy.[57, 58]

Relevant Concepts from the Administrative and Policy Literature

Current theories of organizational behaviour have evolved through a number of phases and have been informed by actual practice and by writers from other disciplines. The following presents a brief and, therefore, somewhat incomplete, overview of these issues. Interested readers are referred to current texts on organizational theory and policy for more in-depth discussion.[59, 60, 61, 62, 63] Five models of organizational behaviour are presented. These models

57. Crichton, A. 1981. *Health Policy Making*. Ann Arbor (MI): Health Administration.
58. Doern, G. B., and R. W. Phidd. 1988. *Canadian Public Policy*. Scarborough (ON): Nelson Canada.
59. Bolman, L. G., and T. E. Deal. 1987. *Modern Approaches to Understanding and Managing Organizations*. San Francisco: Jossey Bass Publishers.
60. Hoy, W. K., and C. G. Miskel. 1987. *Educational Administration: Theory Research and Practice*. New York: Random House.
61. Shafritz, J. M., and J. S. Ott. 1987. *Classics of Organization Theory*. Chicago: The Dorsey Press.
62. Doern, G. B., and R. W. Phidd. 1988. *Canadian Public Policy*. Scarborough (ON): Nelson Canada.
63. Kernaghan, K., and D. Siegel. 1987. *Public Administration in Canada*. Toronto: Methuen.

will serve as the basis for the development of hypotheses about the possible future evolution of DSTs.

1. The Rational/Scientific Model

In organizational theory, the rational model posits a unitary organizational actor. This means that goals are clearly stated and understood by individuals in the organization and that all actors within the organization share the same goals and work toward the same ends. There is a clear division of labour and a hierarchical chain of command. A rational scientific problem-solving approach is used to meet the challenges of the organization. Goals are established, alternate means are identified to achieve set goals and objectives, each of these means is subjected to dispassionate empirical scrutiny, and the most effective of these means is adopted and implemented. The outcome of this process is evaluated to ensure that the original goals and objectives have been achieved. The rational model is often referred to as the classical model of organizational theory and is based on the work of Max Weber, Frederick Taylor,[64] and other writers. This model has also been referred to by Allison[65] in public administration literature as the rational policy model.

2. The Pluralistic/Increment Model

The rational model was criticized as not accurately representing organiza-tional behaviour. The model was challenged by the human relations model that derived from studies of the motivation and behaviour of workers. This model is essentially a pluralistic model that says that organizations are composed of numerous subunits, each with their own roles and respon-sibilities.[66] These subunits have intragroup loyalties, are in competition with each other for resources and responsibilities, and develop their own nego-tiated order. Decisions are essentially incremental as managers satisfice (adopt the first satisfactory answer to a problem) rather than maximize (adopt the ideal solution) due to constraints on time and resources.[67] Also, maintaining

64. Stoner, J. A. F. 1978. *Management.* Englewood Cliffs (NJ): Prentice Hall, Inc.
65. Allison, G. T. 1969. Conceptual models and the Cuban missile crisis. *Political Science Review* 63(3): 689–718.
66. Ibid.
67. Simon, H. A. 1976. *Administrative Behaviour.* New York: The Free Press.

the negotiated balance of power between subunits means that only modest adjustments to the existing order will be accepted by the organization.[68, 69]

3. The Power/Conflict Model

The power model is sometimes also referred to as the bureaucratic politics model.[70] In this model, organizations are seen as being composed of a set of powerful players, each occupying a critical position within the organization. These players have different degrees of power and may have competing interests. A player's position within the system defines a player's advantages and handicaps as well as what that player may do, and must do, to be successful within the organization. The way a player defines issues and takes action is coloured by his position in the organization. This view of organizations posits an environment of competing actors who selectively choose the issues in which they will become involved. Organizational decisions and actions are outcomes of struggles among powerful actors.

4. The Public Choice Model

Another analytical approach to receive active attention in Canada in the 1980s has been the public choice model. Public choice consists essentially of the application of economic principles of analysis to political behaviour. It posits a self-interested utility-maximizing *economic man*. Rather than an economic market for goods and services, there is a political market for votes and a bureaucratic market for the expansion of staff and budgets. The public choice literature began to emerge in the 1970s as part of the neoconservative critique of liberal pluralism and is based on the economic man of the rational model but incorporates some of the dimensions of the power approach.

Public choice is generally acknowledged to stem from the work of James Buchanan, Anthony Down, William Niskanen, and others. Canadian writers[71] have developed a Canadian brand of public choice theory. They posit four key groups that interact to maximize their own advantage: politicians, bureaucrats, special interest groups, and the media. Politicians

---

68. Lindblom, C. E. 1959. The science of muddling through. *Public Administration Review* 19(2): 79–88.

69. Lindblom, C. E. 1973. Rational policy through mutual adjustment. In *Social Change: Sources, Patterns and Consequences*, eds. A. Etzioni, and E. Etzioni-Halevy. New York: Basic Books.

70. Allison,G. T. 1969. Conceptual models and the Cuban missile crisis. *Political Science Review* 63(3): 689–718.

71. Hartle, D. G. 1988. *The Expenditure Budget Process of the Government of Canada: A Public Choice–Rent-Seeking Perspective.* Toronto: The Canadian Tax Foundation.

are seen as being primarily interested in obtaining enough votes to win the next election while bureaucrats are interested in expanding their staff and budgets. Interest groups seek to receive funding for projects from government, and the media is interested in the increased advertising and circulation revenues that arise as a result of interesting news.

5. The Organizational Culture/Symbolic Model

In recent years, a new model of organizational behaviour has emerged that will be referred to as the organizational culture/symbolic model. Bolman and Deal[72] note that symbols are important to bring to life an overall corporate culture. This culture is based on matters such as shared values and beliefs, heroes and heroines, rituals and ceremonies, and a cultural network of priests and priestesses, storytellers, gossips, and spies.[73]

If organizational life is subjective, then the role of impression management becomes much more important to administrators in public organizations. Gardner and Martinko[74] note that organizational success is related to the degree to which an actor's performance is perceived as being congruent with the audience's definition of the situation and beliefs about what constitutes appropriate behaviour. When the congruence is high, the actor elicits a favourable response. Culbert and McDonough[75] also make the point that in a contest between two actors in an organization, one triumphs by winning over the audience of the other organizational actors who witness the contest.

Discussion

How can the above models help us to hypothesize about the future use of DSTs in management and policy formulation in the health sector? Figure 9 provides a typology of different contexts in organizational life. These contexts, in turn, determine the norms, values, and strategies of organizational behaviour and policy making. An understanding of these models and their contexts will, in turn, allow us to hypothesize about the future development of DSTs.

---

72. Bolman, L. G., and T. E. Deal. 1987. *Modern Approaches to Understanding and Managing Organizations.* San Francisco: Jossey Bass Publishers.
73. Ibid.
74. Gardner, W. L., and M. J. Martinko. 1988. Impression management in organizations. *Journal of Management* 14(2): 321–338.
75. Culbert, S. A., and J. J. McDonough. 1980. *The Invisible War: Pursuing Self-Interests at Work.* New York: John Wiley & Sons.

Figure 9

A contextual model of organizational relations

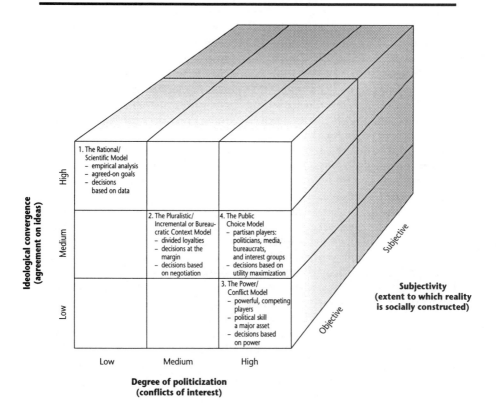

In figure 9, organizational realities and relations are framed according to three dimensions: the degree of congruence in ideology (agreement on ideas); the degree of politicization (conflicts of interest); and the degree of subjectivity (the extent to which reality is socially constructed). Most organizational theory assumes an objective reality; four of the five models of organizational theory shown in figure 9 assume that reality is objective.

Subjective theories are not yet well enough developed to enable them to be clearly placed in figure 9. In addition, the processes of constructing new symbols, beliefs, or realities are often used as strategies in the other four models. It is most likely that DSTs can be developed in an environment that allows for a scientific and rational approach and in which there is a belief that reality is objective. In this situation there are no fundamental conflicts over values (i.e., high ideological congruence) and no political/ bureaucratic conflicts about the issue for which DSTs are being developed.

Thus, key actors will agree to abide by the results derived using a scientific/ technological methodology. This situation pertains, at least to some degree, to clinical practice, in which the models of care, and the scientific bases on which they have been developed, are not problematic. In clinical situations one can resist by questioning the validity of the tool—but not the clinical practice that it is designed to aid—and the use of technology (the familiarity with computers and the relevance of computers in clinical judgement). Resistance by clinicians would be based on the technical issue of whether computers can actually complement clinical decision making and make it more effective. This resistance may come from clinicians who are less familiar with the use of computers as a tool in clinical practice. If the tool is in fact not a good one, resistance may come from a larger group of clinicians because the tool is not effective. In cases where there are competing notions of what is correct clinical practice, it may be more difficult to implement DSTs and they may become tools in a fight for dominance between proponents of different models of care.

It is most likely that, in regard to management and policy, DSTs will be developed, and find acceptance in the context of the rational/scientific model. DSTs could be developed in areas such as finance (e.g., projections of anticipated expenditures) where there is general agreement on the acceptability and rationality of accounting practices. In addition, DSTs may be developed in clearly operational areas such as staff scheduling, projections of the usage of supplies (e.g., number of sterile bandages), or operational processes (e.g., projections of laundry volumes). This is indeed what appears to be happening. The above hypotheses about DSTs are, in fact, fairly congruent with the empirical findings from this study. Over time, it is hoped that clinical and operational DSTs will be subjected to cost-effectiveness evaluations and will have to survive on their ability to produce objectively valuable results.

It is clear from the foregoing analysis of DSTs that the vast majority of DSTs developed to date have been developed for clinical applications. The DSTs on management focus primarily on basic operational, workload, or financial issues. Management DSTs included applications for predicting the optimal allocation for helicopter pads [63], staffing patterns and costs related to managing nursing services [61], cost control [84], auditing clinical practice and costs [20], monitoring and evaluation of clinical engineering departments [26], and formulary decision making [68]. Thus, management DSTs focused on basic operational issues that could benefit from an empirical analysis.

With regard to the survey of DST developers and users, there are a number of relevant findings. A number of developers noted in the section on implementation that there was some user resistance, but these same responders typically chose not to expand on this point in the sections that dealt with who resisted the adoption of DSTs and why. The DSTs noted in the survey, for both clinical and management applications, also focused on fairly operational issues. Some respondents did discuss whether or not there were persons who were resistant to, or did not support, the introduction and use of DSTs. These resistors were typically clinicians on the front lines who were older, who were not yet comfortable with computers, and who questioned the validity of the outputs produced. For some applications, the supporters were the clinicians themselves and for others the supporters were senior managers and information system personnel.

There were a few fairly significant findings that were consistent across both the audit and the survey:

- many DSTs are fairly expensive to develop and it typically takes two to three years, if not longer, to develop a DST;
- at present, most DSTs are still in the prototype stage and have not yet passed the major hurdle of actual implementation;
- at present, there has been little formal evaluation, let alone cost-benefit analysis, of DSTs.

The Projected Future of DSTs

There are several possible scenarios of the future of DSTs. One is that not enough DSTs deliver the goods and they come to fall out of favour over time. It is hypothesized that it would take at least three to five years before this would happen, even if most DSTs are not effective aids to decision making. This is because DSTs will, in all likelihood, go through a honeymoon phase in which they will be highly advertised by vendors and supported by managers who will want to adopt them for their symbolic value. They will fall out of favour for purposes other than straight operational issues because they are based on a rational conceptual model and do not incorporate the other factors that come into play in decision making in a more conflict-prone environment. The three- to five-year time frame is based on the rise and fall of other rational approaches such as zero-based budgeting.

If DSTs prove to be effective tools for clinicians and for operational matters, managers, systems experts, and others may try to apply this technology to a broader range of issues. It is hypothesized that there will be a heyday of "DST mania" as managers and systems experts climb on board the DST train. Using or developing a DST will become a new status symbol in health organizations and will be deemed to be evidence of good managerial practice. Similar patterns of symbolic status evolved when cellular phones and laptop computers were introduced into organizations. There will probably be a high premium on the symbolic value of DSTs. This will result in a lag in actual empirical evaluations of efficacy because DSTs will be deemed to be a good thing—and good things are typically not evaluated because: "Why would something that is deemed to be good need to be evaluated?" In addition, the failures of DSTs, such as current and past failed attempts at developing executive information systems (EISs), may be papered over for some period of time because of the cognitive dissonance between the reality of a marginally useful tool and the positive belief in the utility of such tools as well as in their symbolic value. Over time, DSTs may be overtaken by new emerging approaches and their use will retrench to the more traditional areas of clinical practice and operational activities. Readers who are skeptical about this scenario are referred to the rise and fall of other objective methods such as zero-based budgeting, value-for-money auditing, and other rational approaches to planning and decision making.

A variation on the above scenario could be that DSTs will have a resurgence, perhaps under another name, when developments in artificial intelligence are such that they can capture and model the true complexity of organizational life. However, that time is still yet to come. If it comes sooner rather than later, the rise in more sophisticated DSTs may occur before the completion of the anticipated demise in their popularity, resulting in a resurgence of interest in DSTs.

The conceptual model presented in figure 9 shows that decisions are made on the basis of values, relative power, competing interests and other such factors, as well as on the basis of data and information. An attempt to begin to discuss the range of data that go into the decision-making process has been made by Hollander and Prince,[76] who present an extended table of information requirements for decision making.

Formulations that prove to be effective but that are based on empiricism and assume a rational model of organizational behaviour, can find a home in organizational activities that take place in a context consistent with the rational/scientific model of organizational behaviour. However, such formulations will fall short in other contexts because they typically do not account for satisficing, mutual adjustment, and other forms of bureaucratic behaviour that shape the decision-making process. Such formulations will clearly fail where there are fundamental conflicts over ideas and conflicts of interests. It is unlikely that a DST will be developed that will aid decision making in areas of fundamental value conflicts such as abortion. It should, however, be remembered that policy making can be based on values as well as on facts.

Conclusion

It should be noted that the above scenarios are simply projections based on theoretical foundations and, as such, are at best informed speculation. Some

76. Hollander, M. J., and M. J. Prince. 1993. Analytical units in federal and provincial governments: Origins, functions and suggestions for effectiveness. *Canadian Public Administration* 36(2): 190–224.

precedents for this speculation have been noted, but there is currently no empirically based methodology to accurately project the future use of DSTs. However, it is hoped that decision makers will consider properly evaluating any DSTs that are slated for wider usage.

In addition, it is hoped that this paper will give some pause to those who may wish to develop or adopt DSTs, making them think about the organizational context into which they plan to introduce their tool. Effective DSTs can indeed be helpful in the right organizational contexts. It is the matter of context that will be critical for the effective proliferation of DSTs.

RECOMMENDATIONS

System-Level Support for DST Development

The analyses of the audit and survey indicate that DSTs are being developed in relative isolation from developers/departments and those people and/or departments who may be affected if the DST is implemented. This isolation can occur within the same institutions or organizations in which the DST is intended for use. This means that they are being developed apart from the resident body of data and information. Less than 5 percent of the audited and surveyed tools have any integration with an institution's information system and for those that are integrated, the integration is only partial. However, many of the survey respondents indicated that integration with existing information systems is an important feature for the continued development and use of their DSTs.

The performance of a DST relies on access to current and relevant bodies of knowledge yet, in health care, that body of knowledge changes continuously. If DSTs are developed in isolation from this body of knowledge, they will either be unsuccessful or quickly become obsolete. *It is recommended that DST development be encouraged in environments where there is the opportunity and the willingness to integrate the DST with the institution's or organization's existing information systems.* This will encourage use and dissemination of DSTs and provide a better foundation for the systematic evaluation of DSTs based on outcomes.

DSTs are intended to provide decision support to nonexpert users working throughout the health care system. The anticipated systemic benefits of DST use cannot be assessed unless these users can access the DST. *It is recommended that DST development be encouraged in environments where there is an institutional or systemic commitment to provide access to the DST for the intended users.* This is the only way that the DSTs can be evaluated beyond the validation and verification stage. The lack of systemic commitment is most likely the reason that many of the tools that have been developed are not being used.

Methodological Issues in DST Development

There is no comprehensive, systematic methodology for the knowledge engineering phase of DST development. In fact, planning and knowledge engineering are only briefly mentioned in DST publications, despite the fact that they are the most important phases of DST development. *It is recommended that the development of structured and systematic planning strategies and knowledge engineering methodologies be actively supported.* These methodologies should be rigorously tested as they emerge so that developers have access to established techniques to successfully fulfil the planning and knowledge engineering requirements of any DST project.

As mentioned throughout this report, most DSTs are subjected to some form of validation/verification testing, but almost none are subjected to an objective and systematic outcomes-based evaluation such as a clinical trial. Part of the reason for this is that the lack of systemic commitment precludes opportunities to do such trials. Even if the systemic commitment is present, however, there are no established methodologies available to DST developers to perform systematic evaluations. *It is recommended that the development of methodologies for DST evaluation be actively supported.* The use of standardized methodologies would allow health care providers to objectively assess and compare DST technologies.

Industrial/Commercial Partnerships

The most likely industrial developers of DSTs are the same ones currently producing information systems for health care. Changing trends in health care will force these companies to move from institutional to regional systems that must include an integrated set of policy, management, and clinical data for management effectiveness. This provides an opportunity to integrate DSTs into strategic and changing trends. *It is recommended that health care institutions and governance bodies take the lead in guiding industry in DST development by clearly identifying and articulating the expectations of the users in terms of planning, development, and evaluation of DSTs.* In this way, industry will be fulfilling a *real* rather than *perceived* need, which in turn should stimulate the growth of an information-based health industry in Canada.

Furthermore, with the progressive integration of health care institutions, organizations, and programs into regional jurisdictions, it is likely that the information system and decision support needs will become more focused on health care function rather than on a given service venue. *It is recommended that DST development be encouraged where that development focuses on systemic needs rather than the needs of an individual institution, organization, or program in order for that DST to be more broadly marketed.* DSTs developed with a focus on function will be more easily disseminated to locations beyond that in which the development occurred (i.e., the product will be more marketable).

ARTICLES INCLUDED IN THE DST AUDIT DATABASE

[1]   McREA, J. D., et al. 1989. A controlled evaluation of diagnostic criteria in the development of a rheumatology expert system. *British Journal of Rheumatology* 28(1): 13–17.

[2]   TOMBROPOULOS, R., S. SHIFFMAN, and C. DAVIDSON. 1993. A decision aid for diagnosis of liver lesions on MRI. *Proceedings of the Annual Symposium on Computer Applications in Medical Care.* pp. 439–443.

[3]   XU, L. D. 1994. A decision support system for AIDS intervention and prevention. *International Journal of Biomedical Computing* 36(4): 281–291.

[4]   DAVIS, G. E., W. E. LOWELL, and G. L. DAVIS. 1993. A neural network that predicts psychiatric length of stay. *Clinical Computing* 10(2): 87–92.

[5]   AMARAL, M. B., et al. 1995. A psychiatric diagnostic system integrating probabilistic and categorical reasoning. *Methods of Information in Medicine* 34(3): 232–243.

[6]   KRUSINSKA, E., et al. 1993. Statistically rule-based decision support system for the management of patients with suspected liver disease. *Medical Informatics* 18(2): 113–130.

[7]   LEHMANN, E. D., et al. 1994. AIDA: An interactive diabetes advisor. *Computer Methods and Programs in Biomedicine* 41(3–4): 183–203.

[8]   SONNENBERG, F. A., C. G. HAGERTY, and C. A. KULIKOWSKI. 1994. An architecture for knowledge-based construction of decision models. *Medical Decision Making* 14(1): 27–39.

[9]   SUERMONDT, H. J., and G. F. COOPER. 1993. An evaluation of explanations of probabilistic inference. *Computers and Biomedical Research* 26(3): 242–254.

[10] BRAI, A., J. F. VIBERT, and R. KOUTLIDIS. 1994. An expert system for the analysis and interpretation of evoked potentials based on fuzzy classification: Application to brainstem auditory evoked potentials. *Computers and Biomedical Research* 27(5): 351–366.

[11] FRASE, R. B., and S. Z. TURNEY. 1990. An expert system for the nutritional management of the critically ill. *Computer Methods and Programs in Biomedicine* 33(3): 175–180.

[12] BARRIERE, S. L., and S. F. LOWRY. 1995. An overview of mortality risk prediction in sepsis. *Critical Care Medicine* 23(2): 376–393.

[13] BERMAN, L., M. CULLEN, and P. L. MILLER. 1993. Automated integration of external databases: A knowledge-based approach to enhancing rule-based expert systems. *Computers and Biomedical Research* 26(3): 230–241.

[14] CHANG, P. L., et al. 1994. Clinical evaluation of a renal mass diagnostic expert system. *Computers in Biology and Medicine* 24(4): 315–322.

[15] WEBER, J. E., and P. H. BARTELS. 1989. Colonic lesion expert system: Evaluation of sensitivity. *Analytical and Quantitative Cytology and Histology* 11(4): 249–254.

[16] ASTRUC, J., et al. 1993. Comparative study of human expertise and an expert system: Application to the diagnosis of child's meningitis. *Computers and Biomedical Research* 26: 383–392.

[17] FUGLEBERG, S., A. GREULICH, and D. I. STENVER. 1991. Computer-assisted diagnosis of acute azotaemia: Diagnostic strategy and diagnostic criteria. *Computers in Biology and Medicine* 21(6): 399–406.

[18] SUAN, O. L. 1990. Computer-aided diagnosis and the treatment of malaria: The IMEX system. *Computers in Biology and Medicine* 20(5): 361–372.

[19] EAST, T. D., et al. 1955. Computers in critical care. *Critical Care Nursing Clinics of North America* 7(2): 203–217.

[20] TAYLOR, J. C., W. T. MCGIVNEY, and A. J. STEINBERG. 1994. ComuniCare: Case management and clinical decision support systems. *Proceedings of the Annual Symposium on Computer Applications in Medical Care.* p. 1063.

[21] NELSON, B. D., and R. M. GARDNER. 1993. Decision support for concurrent utilization review using a HELP-embedded expert system. *Proceedings of the Annual Symposium on Computer Applications in Medical Care.* p. 176–182.

[22] LINNARSSON, R. 1993. Decision support for drug prescription integrated with computer-based patient records in primary care. *Medical Informatics (London)* 18(2): 131–142.

[23] KOKOL, P., et al. 1994. Decision trees based on automatic learning and their use in cardiology. *Journal of Medical Systems* 18(4): 201–206.

[24] VIAN, T., S. VERJEE, and R. B. SIEGRIST Jr. 1993. Decision support systems in health care: Factors influencing the development and transfer of technology. *International Journal of Technology Assessment in Health Care* 9(3): 369–379.

[25] HANSON, A. C., et al. 1994. Design and development of an expert system for student use in a school of nursing. *Computers in Nursing* 12(1): 29–34.

[26] MARSHALL, J. C., and J. D. BRONZINO. 1994. Development of a clinical engineering knowledge-based system to facilitate departmental decision making. *Biomedical Instrumentation and Technology* 28(6): 448–454.

[27] WYATT, J. C., et al. 1994.Development of design-a-trial, a knowledge-based critiquing system for authors of clinical trial protocols. *Computer Methods and Programs in Biomedicine* 43(3–4): 283–291.

[28] JOHNSON, B., et al. 1994. Discern—an integrated prospective decision support system. *Proceedings of the Annual Symposium on Computer Applications in Medical Care.* p. 969.

[29] MOLINO, G., et al. 1990. Educational applications of a knowledge-based expert system for medical decision making in hepatology. *Italian Journal of Gastroenterology* 22: 97–104.

[30] HATANO, T., et al. 1991. Entering data into expert system for lower urinary tract pressure – flow studies. *Urologia Internationalis* 47, suppl.(1): 48–51.

[31] HOOPER, J. A., et al. 1993. EquipTeach: A computer-aided instruction to teach users how to operate specific medical equipment. *Biomedical Instrumentation and Technology* (Sept.–Oct.): 394–399.

[32] WIGREN, T., and P. KOLARI. 1994. Evaluation of a decision support system for inoperable non-small cell lung cancer. *Methods of Information in Medicine* 33(4): 397–401.

[33] LONG, W. J., S. NAIMIL, and M. G. CRISCITIELLO. 1994. Evaluation of a new method for cardiovascular reasoning. *Journal of the American Medical Informatics Association* 1(2): 127–141.

[34] KORPINEN, L., et al. 1994. Evaluation of Epilepsy Expert—a decision support system. *Computer Methods and Programs in Biomedicine* 45(3): 223–231.

[35] KORPINEN, L., et al. 1994. Evaluation of Sleep Expert —a computer-aided decision support system for sleep disorders. *Medical Informatics (London)* 19(3) (July–Sept.): 247–252.

[36] KORPINEN, L., and H. FREY. 1993. Sleep Expert—an intelligent medical decision support system for sleep disorders. *Medical Informatics (London)* 18(2): 163–170.

[37] GARDNER, R. M., and H. P. LUNDSGAARDE. 1994. Evaluation of user acceptance of a clinical expert system. *Journal of the American Medical Informatics Association* 1(6) (Nov.–Dec.): 428–438.

[38] HUFF, S. M., et al. 1994. HELP the next generation: A new client-server architecture. *Proceedings of the Annual Symposium on Computer Applications in Medical Care.* pp. 271–275.

[39] MACERATI, R., et al. 1989. Expert systems and the pancreatic cancer problem: Decision support in the pre-operative diagnosis. *Journal of Biomedical Engineering* 11: 489–510.

[40] SCHREINER, A., and T. CHARD. 1990. Expert systems for the prediction of ovulation: Comparison of an expert system shell (Expertech Xi Plus) with a program written in a traditional language (BASIC). *Methods of Information in Medicine* 29(2): 140–145.

[41] KOCH, B., and J. MCGOVERN. 1993. EXTEND: A prototype expert system for teaching nursing diagnosis. *Computers in Nursing* 11(1): 35–41.

[42] BOHREN, B. F., M. HADZIKADIC, and E. N. HANLEY Jr. 1995. Extracting knowledge from large medical databases: An automated approach. *Computers and Biomedical Research* 28(3): 191–210.

[43] LAU, F., and D. D. VINCENT. 1993. Formalized decision support for cardiovascular intensive care. *Computers and Biomedical Research* 26(3): 294–309.

[44] KAHN, C. E. Jr. 1993. Graphical knowledge presentation in a MUMPS-based decision support system. *Computer Methods and Programs in Biomedicine* 40(3): 159–166.

[45] VAN DEN HEUVEL, J., et al. 1990. GUUS an expert system in intensive care unit. *International Journal of Clinical Monitoring and Computing* 7(3): 171–175.

[46] BONADONA, F. 1990. Hypershell: An expert system shell in hyper-media environment: Application in medical audiology. *Medical Informatics (London)* 15(2): 105–114.

[47] ORPHANOUDAKIS, S. C., C. CHRONAKI, and S. KOSTOMANOLAKIS. 1994. I2C: A system for the indexing, storage, and retrieval of medical images by content. *Medical Informatics (London)* 19(2): 109–122.

[48] HUDSON, D. L., M. E. COHEN, and P. C. DEEDWANIA. 1994. Information integration in a decision support system. *Proceedings of the Annual Symposium on Computer Applications in Medical Care.* p. 1051.

[49] VAN DIEST, P. J., et al. 1994. Integrated decision support system/image archive for histological typing of breast cancer using a relation-oriented inference system. *Histopathology* 25(3): 253–259.

[50] JOHANSSON, B., and Y. BERGQVIS. 1993. Integrating decision support, based on the Arden Syntax, in a clinical laboratory environment. *Proceedings of the Annual Symposium on Computer Applications in Medical Care.* pp. 394–398.

[51] RUTSCHER, A., E. SALZSIEDER, and U. FISCHER. 1994. KADIS: Model-aided education in type I diabetes; Karlsburg Diabetes Management System. *Computer Methods and Programs in Biomedicine* 41(3–4): 205–215.

[52] VINGTOFT, S., et al. 1993. KANDID: An EMG decision support system—evaluated in a European multicenter trial. *Muscle Nerve* 16(5): 520–529.

[53] SANDS, W. 1994. Kinesiological motion expert system. *Computer methods and programs in Biomedicine* 45: 261–263.

[54] HAMILTON, J. 1994. Labour management software provides decision support system for obstetric units. *Canadian Medical Association Journal* 150(6): 967–968.

[55] WOOLERY, L. K., and J. GRZYMALA-BUSSE. 1994. Machine learning for an expert system to predict preterm birth risk. *Journal of the American Medical Informatics Association* 1(6): 439–446.

[56] FATHI-TORBAGHAN, M., and D. MEYER,1994. MEDUSA: A fuzzy expert system for medical diagnosis of acute abdominal pain. *Methods of Information in Medicine* 33(5): 522–529.

[57] KERAVNOU, E. T., et al. 1994. Modeling diagnostic skills in the domain of skeletal dysplasias. *Computer Methods and Programs in Biomedicine* 45(4): 239–260.

[58] FACKLER, J., and I. KOHANE. 1994. Monitor-driven data visualization: SmartDisplay. *Proceedings of the Annual Symposium on Computer Applications in Medical Care.* pp. 939–943.

[59] FRANCO, A., et al. 1990. Neonate – An expert application for the HELP system: Comparison of the computer's and the physician's problem list. *Journal of Medical Systems* 14(5): 297–306.

[60] CHOW, J. L., K. N. LEVITT, and G. J. KOST. 1993. NMRES: An artificial intelligence expert system for quantification of cardiac metabolites from phosphorus nuclear magnetic resonance spectroscopy. *Annals of Biomedical Engineering* 21(3): 247–258.

[61] MARTORELLI, R. D. 1994. Nurse manager's use of Lotus 1-2-3 template as support for decision making for nursing hours, staffing and direct nursing costs per day. *Proceedings of the Annual Symposium on Computer Applications in Medical Care.* p. 963.

[62] ENTERLINE, J. P., et al. 1994. OCIS: 15 years' experience with patient-centered computing. *MD Computing* 11(2): 83–91.

[63] CLARK, D. E., et al. 1994. Optimal location for a helicopter in a rural trauma system: Prediction using discrete-event computer simulation. *Proceedings of the Annual Symposium on Computer Applications in Medical Care.* pp. 888–892.

[64] JOUSIMAA, J., and I. KUNNAMO. 1993. PDRD: A computer-based primary care decision support system. *Medical Informatics (London)* 18(2): 103–112.

[65] BERNER, E. S., et al. 1994. Performance of four computer-based diagnostic systems. *The New England Journal of Medicine* 330(25): 1792–1796.

[66] MATABAN, B. A. M. 1994. Prototype expert system for infusion pump maintenance. *Biomedical Instrumentation and Technology* (Jan.): 19–29.

[67] ZIELSTORFF, R. D., et al. 1993. Providing clinicians with problem-based access to knowledge: Troubleshooting pulmonary artery catheter waveforms. *Proceedings of the Annual Symposium on Computer Applications in Medical Care.* pp. 351–355.

[68] GREER, L. 1992. RXPERT: A prototype of expert system for formulary decision making. *Annals of Pharmacotherapy* 26(2): 244–250.

[69] DARMONI, S. J., et al. 1994. SETH: An expert system for the management of acute drug poisoning in adults. *Computer Methods and Programs in Biomedicine* 43: 171–176.

[70] LAU, F., H. KWOK, and K. S. BAY. 1993. Some computer-based decision support tools for the rehabilitation manager. *Physiotherapy Canada* 45(1): 29–38.

[71] PROBST, C. L., and J. RUSH. 1990. The careplan knowledge base: A prototype expert system for postpartum nursing care. *Computers in Nursing* 8(5): 206–213.

[72] VASSAR, M. J., and J. W. HOLCROFT. 1994. The case against using the APACHE system to predict intensive care unit outcome in trauma patients. *Critical Care Clinics* 10(1): 117–134.

[73] SIEBEN, G., et al. 1994. The development of a decision support system for the pathological diagnosis of human cerebral tumors based on a neural network classifier. *Acta Neurochirurgica* 129(3–4): 193–197.

[74] STITT, F. W. 1994. The problem-oriented medical synopsis: Coding, indexing, and classification sub-model. *Proceedings of the Annual Symposium on Computer Applications in Medical Care.* p. 964.

[75] WONG, W. S. F., K. S. LEUNG, and Y. T. SO. 1990. The recent development and evaluation of a medical expert system (ABVAB). *International Journal of Biomedical Computing* 25(2–3): 223–229.

[76] HOUSTON, A. S., R. J. IORNS, and M. A. MACLEOD. 1991. The use of induction in the design of an expert system for thyroid function studies. *Nuclear Medicine Communications* 12(6): 497–506.

[77] DEUTSCH, T., et al. 1994. Time series analysis and control of blood glucose levels in diabetic patients. *Computer Methods and Programs in Biomedicine* 41(3–4): 167–182.

[78] HECKERMAN, D., E. J. HORVITZ, and B. N. NATHWANI. 1992. Toward normative expert systems: Part I: The Pathfinder Project. *Methods of Information in Medicine* 31(2): 90–105.

[79] SHIFFMAN, R. N. 1994. Towards effective implementation of a pediatric asthma guideline: Integration of decision support and clinical workflow support. *Proceedings of the Annual Symposium on Computer Applications in Medical Care.* pp. 797–801.

[80] GILLIS, P. A., et al. 1994. Translating traditional principles of system development into a process for designing clinical information systems. *International Journal of Technology Assessment in Health Care* 10(2): 235–248.

[81] BRENNAN, P. F., S. M. MOORE, and K. A. SMYTH. 1995. The effects of a special computer network on caregivers of persons with Alzheimer's disease. *Nursing Research* 44(3): 166–172.

[82] BRENNAN, P. F., and S. RIPICH. 1994. Use of a home care computer network by persons with AIDS. *International Journal of Technology Assessment in Health Care* 10(2): 258–272.

[83] VERDAGUER, A., et al. 1992. Validation of the medical expert system PNEUMON-IA. *Computers and Biomedical Research.* pp. 511–526.

[84] EVANS, R. S., et al. 1994. Improving empiric antibiotic selection using computer decision support. *Archives of Internal Medicine* 154(8): 878–884.

[85] EVANS, R. S., et al. 1993. Development of an automated antibiotic consultant. *Clinical Computing* 10(1): 17–22.

[86] KORVER, M., and P. J. LUCAS. 1993. Converting a rule-based expert system into a belief network. *Medical Informatics (London)* 18(3): 219–241.

[87] LUCAS, P. J. F., and A. R. JANSSENS. 1991. Second evaluation of HEPAR, an expert system for the diagnosis of disorders of the liver and biliary tract. *Liver* 11: 340–346.

Paul Fisher *joined the School of Health Information Science in 1990 after five years as a consultant to the Great Vancouver Health Service and the British Columbia Ministry of Health in the implementation and evaluation of digital radiography and picture archiving and communications systems (PACS). He teaches courses in database, network and information system design. Dr. Fisher's current interests include integrated community health information systems, clinical decision support systems, and telemedicine. He lectures frequently on the use of database and telecommunications technologies, especially the Internet, for health care delivery and management in Canadian and international settings.*

APPENDICES

APPENDIX 1

List of General References to DSTs and Decision Support

ADLER, D., A. ISRAELI, and Y. MAHLER. 1995. Clinical information systems: Considerations in selecting the hospital department with primary responsibility. *Biomedical Instrumentation and Technology.* pp. 97–105.

AHLFELDT, H., et al. 1994. Data-driven medical decision support based on Arden Syntax within the HELIOS environment. *Computer Methods and Programs in Biomedicine* 45 suppl.: S97–S106.

AINSWORTH, J., and P. WILSON. 199?? Would your judgement stand up to scrutiny? *British Journal of Nursing* 3(19): 1023–1025.

AUDET, A. A., S. GREENFIELD, and M. FIELD. 1990. Medical practice guidelines: Current activities and future directions. *Annals of Internal Medicine* 113: 709–714.

AXT-ADAM, P., J. C. VAN DER WOUDEN, and E. VAN DER DOES. 1993. Influencing behaviour of physicians ordering laboratory tests: A literature study. *Medical Care* 31(9): 784–794.

BAETE, G. 1994. Development of a computerized equipment management system using an IBAX health care system platform. *Biomedical Instrumentation and Technology* (July–Aug.): 282–300.

BARAHONA, P. 1994. EPISTOL: The future of knowledge-based systems and techniques for the health sector. *Computer Methods and Programs in Biomedicine* 45(1–2): 51–54.

BARTON, A. J. 1994. Data needs for decision support of chief nurse executives. *Journal of Nursing Administration* 24(4 suppl.): 19–25.

BERRIOS, G. E., and E. Y. CHEN. 1993. Recognising psychiatric symptoms. Relevance to the diagnostic process. *British Journal of Psychiatry* 163: 308–314.

BIGOS, M., et al. 1994. Pattern sorting: A computer-controlled multidimensional sorting method using k-d trees. *Cytometry* 16(4): 357–363.

BOES, R. 1989. Choosing computer-based tools for facilities management. *Health Facilities Management* (Feb.): 23–24.

BONFILS, P., et al. 1994. Auditory threshold evaluation by distortion-product oto-acoustic emissions using decision support system. *Acta Otolaryngol (Stockh)* 114(4): 360–365.

BUTLER, T. W. 1995. Management science/operations research projects in health care: The administrator's perspective. *Health Care Management Review* 20(1): 19–25.

CANFIELD, K. 1994. Clinical resource auditing and decision support for computerized patient record systems: A mediated architecture approach. *Journal of Medical Systems* 18(3): 139–150.

CANNATACI, J. A. 1989. Liability for medical expert systems: An introduction to the legal implications. *Medical Informatics* 14(3): 229–241.

CASPER, G. R., and P. F. BRENNAN. 1993. Improving the quality of patient care: The role of patient preferences in the clinical record. *Proceedings of the Annual Symposium on Computer Applications in Medical Care.* pp. 8–11.

CERNE, F. 1988. Information management: Executive systems give CEOs management tools. *Hospitals* (Nov. 20): 80–81.

CHUDLEIGH, M. F. 1994. Hazard analysis of a computer-based medical diagnostic system. *Computer Methods and Programs in Biomedicine* 44: 45–57.

DAS, A. K. 1994. A temporal-abstraction mediator for protocol-based decision support systems. *Proceedings of the Annual Symposium on Computer Applications in Medical Care.* pp. 320–324.

DAS, A. K., and M. A. Musen. 1994. A temporal query system for protocol-directed decision support. *Methods of Information in Medicine* 33(4): 358–370.

DEGOULET, P., et al. 1994. The component-based architecture of the HELIOS medical software engineering environment. *Computer Methods and Programs in Biomedicine* 45 (suppl.): S1–S11.

DICKERSIN, K., Y. MIN, and C. L. MEINERT. 1992. Factors influencing publication of research results. *Journal of the Americal Medical Association* 267(3): 374–378.

EDDY. 1990. Guidelines for policy statements: The explicit approach. *Journal of the American Medical Association* 263(16): 2239–2243.

EDITORIAL. 1995. Evidence-based medicine, in its place. *The Lancet* 346(8978): 785.

ELLIS, J., et al. 1995. Inpatient general medicine is evidence based. *The Lancet* 346: 407–410.

EVIDENCE-BASED MEDICINE WORKING GROUP (CANADA). 1992. Evidence-based medicine. *Journal of the American Medical Association* 268(17): 2420–2425.

FELDMAN, P., M. GOLD, and K. CHU. 1994. Enhancing information for state health policy. *Health Affairs* 13(3): 236–250.

FILE, P. E., P. I. DUGARD, and A. S. HOUSTON. 1994. Evaluation of the use of induction in the development of a medical expert system. *Computers in Biomedical Research* 27(5): 383–395.

FINK, R. 1994. Safety assessment of data management in clinical lab. *Computer Methods and Programs in Biomedicine* 44: 37–43.

FORSSTROM, J. J., et al. 1995. Using data preprocessing and single layer perceptron to analyze laboratory data. *Scandanavian Journal of Clinical Laboratory Investigation: Supplement* 222: 75–81.

FROST, R. D., and M. L. GILLENSON. 1993. Integrated clinical decision support using an object-oriented database management system. *Methods of Information in Medicine* 32(2): 154–160.

GAO, X., et al. 1993. Pre-compiling medical logic modules into C++ in building medical decision support systems. *Computer Methods and Programs in Biomedicine* 41(2): 107–119.

GIUSE, N. B., et al. 1994. Information needs of health care professionals in an AIDS outpatient clinic as determined by Cart Review. *Journal of the American Medical Informatics Association* 1: 395–403.

GORDON, C., Q. JACKSON-SMALE, and R. THOMSON. 1994. DILEMMA: Logic engineering in primary care, shared care and oncology (AIM Project A2005). *Computer Methods and Programs in Biomedicine* 45(1–2): 37–39.

GRAHAME-SMITH, D. 1995. Evidence-based medicine: Socratic dissent. *British Medical Journal* 310(6987) (April 29): 1126–1127.

GREEN, C. G., M. A. KHAN, and R. BADINELLI. 1993. Use of the Delphi research technique to test a decision model in food service systems: A case study in food production. *Journal of the American Dietary Association* 93(11): 1307–1309.

GRONROOS, P., et al. 1995. Using computerized individual medication data to detect drug effects on clinical laboratory tests. *Scandanavian Journal of Clinical Laboratory Investigation: Supplement* 222: 31–36.

GUYATT, G. H., D. L. SACKETT, and D. J. COOK. 1994. User's guides to the medical literature. *Journal of the American Medical Association* 271(1): 59–63.

HAMMOND, P., et al. 1994. Safety and decision support in oncology. *Methods of Information in Medicine* 33(4): 371–381.

HARD, R. 1991. Information overlaod: CEOs seek new tools for effective decision making. *Hospitals* (Oct. 20): 24–32.

HATCHER, M. 1994. Voting and priorities in health care decision making ; portrayed through a group decision support system ; using analytic hierarchy process. *Journal of Medical Systems* 18(5): 267–288.

HAUG, P. J., et al. 1994. Decision support in medicine: Examples from the HELP system. *Computers in Biomedical Research* 27(5): 396–418.

JACOBS, S. M., and S. PELFREY. 1995. Decision support systems. Using computers to help manage. *Journal of Nursing Administration* 25(2): 46–51.

JAESCHKE, R., G. GUYATT, and D. L. SCKETT. 1994. User's guides to the medical literature. *Journal of the American Medical Association* 272(5): 389–391.

JOHNSTON, M.E., et al. 1994. Effects of computer-based clinical decision support systems on clinician performance and patient outcome. A critical appraisal of research. *Annals of Internal Medicine* 120(2): 135–142.

KAY, S., et al. 1994. SAPPHIRE: Scenarios, architecture, and process. *Computer Methods and Programs in Biomedicine* 43(3–4): 217–225.

KORPINEN, L. 1993. Computer-aided decision making for epilepsy and sleep diagnostics. *Acta Neurol. Scand. Suppl.* 144: 1–101.

KOURI, T., et al. 1995. Reliability and adequacy of discharge diagnosis databases in the production of reference values. *Scandanavian Journal of Clinical Laboratory Investigation: Supplement* 222: 69–73.

KUILBOER, M. M., et al. 1993. Knowledge reuse: Temporal-abstraction mechanisms for the assessment of children's growth. *Proceedings of the Annual Symposium on Computer Applications in Medical Care.* pp. 449–453.

KUNCHEVA, L. 1993. An aggregation of pro and con evidence for medical decision support systems. *Computers in Biology and Medicine* 23(6): 417–424.

KURZWEIL, R. 1989. Beyond pattern recognition. *BYTE* (Dec.): 277–288.

LAVELLE, S. M. 1994. The intelligent decision-mapping patient record (IDMR). *Computer Methods and Programs in Biomedicine* 45(1–2): 97–99.

LILFORD, R. J. 1990. Limitations of expert systems: Intuition versus analysis. *Bailliere's Clinical Obstetrics and Gynaecology* 4(4): 851–856.

LUMSDON, K. 1993. Pioneering protocols. Hospitals test the computer's use in patient care decisions. *Hospitals* 67(9): 18–21.

MACDOUGALL, E. B. 1993. Decision support systems for diabetes management [letter ; comment]. *Diabetes Care* 16(4): 663–664.

MAJIDI, F., et al. 1993. Chemotherapy and treatment scheduling: The Johns Hopkins Oncology Center outpatient department. *Proceedings of the Annual Symposium on Computer Applications in Medical Care.* pp. 154–158.

MARCHESE, A. L. 1993. A flexible information system. *Biomedical Instrumentation and Technology* (May–June): 210–215.

MATTHEUS, R. 1994. European integrated picture archiving and communication systems ; CEC/AIM. *Computer Methods and Programs in Biomedicine* 45(1–2): 65–69.

MAYNARD, C., et al. 1995. The exclusion of women from clinical trials. *Medical Decision Making* 15(1): 38–43.

MCDONALD, C. J., S. L. HUI, and X. H. ZHOU. 1994. Analyzing computer-based decision support systems [letter ; comment]. *Annals of Internal Medicine* 121(6): 469.

MCFADDEN, E. T., et al. 1995. Approaches to data management. *Controlled Clinical Trials* 16(2 suppl.): 30S–65S.

MCNANUS, S. M., and J. V. PEARSON. 1993. Nursing at a crossroads: Managing without facts. *Health Care Management Review* 18(1): 79–90.

MILLER, R. A. 1993. Taking inventory of medical decision support software development. *Methods in Medical Informatics* 32: 9–11.

_____. 1994. Medical diagnostic decision support systems—past, present, and future: A threaded bibliography and brief commentary [published erratum appears in the *Journal of the American Medical Informatics Association* 1(March–Apr.): 160]. *Journal of the American Medical Informatics Association* 1(1): 8–27.

MOCK. N., et al. 1993. Development of information-based planning in Niger. *International Journal of Technology Assessment in Health Care* 9(3): 360–368.

MONTBRIAND, M. J. 1995. Decision tree model describing alternate health care choices made by oncology patients. *Cancer Nursing* 18(2): 104–117.

MORRISSEY, J. 1994. Spending more on computers to help keep costs in line. *Modern Health Care* (Feb. 14): 63–70.

_____. 1995. Information systems refocus priorities. *Modern Health Care* (Feb. 13): 5–72.

MUN, S. K., et al. 1995. Teleradiology/telepathology requirements and implementation. *Journal of Medical Systems* 19(2): 153–164.

MYKYTYN, K., P. P. MYKYTYN Jr., and C. W. SLINKMAN. 1990. Expert systems: A question of liability? *MIS Quarterly* (March): 27–42.

NAJI, S. A., et al. 1993. Improving the selection of patients for upper gastrointestinal endoscopy. *Gut* 34(2): 187–191.

NELSON, B. D., et al. 1994. Computerized decision support for concurrent utilization review using the HELP system. *Journal of the American Medical Informatics Association* 1(4): 339–352.

ORNSTEIN, S. M., R. B. OATES, and G. N. FOX. 1992. The computer-based medical record: Current status [see comments]. *Journal of Family Practice* 35(5): 556–565.

OXMAN, A. D., D. L. SACKETT, and G. H. GUYATT. 1993. User's guides to the medical literature. *Journal of the American Medical Association* 270(17): 2093–2097.

OZKARAHAN, I. 1994. A scheduling model for hospital residents. *Journal of Medical Systems* 18(5): 251–265.

PLASSCHAERT, A. J., et al. 1995. Decision making in restorative dentistry: Intuition or knowledge based? [editorial]. *British Journal of Dentistry* 178(9): 320–321.

ROCHA, R. A., et al. 1994. Designing a controlled medical vocabulary server: The VOSER project. *Computers in Biomedical Research* 27(6): 472–507.

ROOS, N. P., and M. BROWNELL. 1994. Introducing data into the health policy process developing a report on the efficiency of bed use in Manitoba. *Health Care Management Forum* 7 (summer): 46–50.

SAILORS, R. M., and T. D. EAST. 1994. A model-based simulator for testing rule-based decision support systems for mechanical ventilation of ARDS patients. *Proceedings of the Annual Symposium on Computer Applications in Medical Care*. p. 1007.

SALAMON, R. 1989. Expert systems in medicine. *World Health* (Aug.–Sept.): 2–3.

SHAHAR, Y., and M. A. MUSEN. 1993. RESUME: A temporal-abstraction system for patient monitoring. *Computers in Biomedical Research* 26: 255–273.

SHARPE, P. K., and P. CALEB. 1994. Artificial neural networks within medical decision support systems. *Scandanavian Journal of Clinical Laboratory Investigation: Supplement* 219: 3–11.

SUJANSKY, W., and R. ALTMAN. 1994. Towards a standard query model for sharing decision support applications. *Proceedings of the Annual Symposium on Computer Applications in Medical Care*. pp. 325–331.

TIERNEY, W. M., et al. 1995. Computerizing guidelines to improve care and patient outcomes: The example of heart failure. *Journal of the American Medical Informatics Association* 2(5): 316–322.

TIMPKA, T., and M. JOHANSSON. 1994. The need for requirements engineering in the development of clinical decision support systems: A qualitative study. *Methods of Information in Medicine* 33(2): 227–233.

VAN DER LEI, J. 1993. Experience from computer-based patient records for computer-assisted decision making. *Methods of Information in Medicine* 32: 14–15.

VAN GENNIP, E. M., J. L. TALMON, and A. R. BAKKER. 1994. ATIM: Accompanying measure on the assessment of information technology in medicine. *Computer Methods and Programs in Biomedicine* 45(1–2): 5–8.

VON HANWEHR, R., et al. 1995. Interventional telemedicine for noninvasive neuroradiosurgery: Remote-site high-performance computing, mathematical optimization, and virtual scenario simulation. *Journal of Medical Systems* 19(3): 219–262.

WEIR, C. J., et al. 1994. Poor accuracy of stroke scoring systems for differential clinical diagnosis of intracranial haemorrhage and infarction [see comments]. *The Lancet* 344(8928): 999–1002.

WHITMORE, K., and S. MOUSSARI. 1993. A clinical engineering information system incorporating Ecri-Hecs ; Hecslink ; and DBase. *Biomedical Instrumentation and Technology* (Jan.–Feb.): 33–41.

WILLARD, K. E., B. H. SIELAFF, and D. P. CONNELLY. 1995. Integrating legacy laboratory information systems into a client-server world: The University of Minnesota Clinical Workstation (CWS) project. *Methods of Information in Medicine* 34(3): 289–296.

WILSON, R., M. S. ROWAN, and J. HENDERSON. 1995. Core and comprehensive health care services. 1. Introduction to the Canadian Medical Association's Decision-Making Framework. *Canadian Medical Association Journal* 152(7): 1063–1066.

WONG, E. T., et al. 1994. Interfacing a stand-alone diagnostic expert system with a hospital information system. *Computers in Biomedical Research* 27(2): 116–129.

WULFMAN, C. E., et al. 1993. Graphical access to medical expert systems. V. Integration with continuous-speech recognition. *Methods of Information in Medicine* 32(1): 33–46.

ZEIDE, J. S., and J. LIEBOWITZ. 1987. Using expert systems: The legal perspective. *IEEE Expert* 2(1): 19–21.

ZIELSTORFF, R. D. 1995. Capturing and using clinical outcome data: Implications for information systems design. *Journal of the American Medical Informatics Association* 2(3): 191–196.

APPENDIX 2

Cover Letter and Survey Tool

Decision Support Tools in Health Care Survey
being conducted for
the National Health Forum
Working Group on Evidence-Based Decision Making
being conducted by
Canadian Policy Research Networks: Health Network and
PenDragon Consultants Limited

In 1994, the Canadian federal government created the National Forum on Health. The purpose was to find ways to improve: (1) the health of Canadians, (2) the efficiency and effectiveness of health services, and (3) to provide the government with recommendations for action.

In order to offer practical advice based on research that is either completed or under way, the Forum has formed several working groups to identify and focus on issues or themes of national importance. The working group "Evidence-Based Decision Making" was created to find ways to ensure that decisions about health and health care are based on the best available evidence at all levels of decision-making providers, consumers, and policymakers.

One area of particular interest to this working group is that of decision support tools (DSTs) and how they can be applied to improve health care decision making.

As a researcher involved in the design, development, and/or implementation of DSTs, we are asking for your support by participating in the following survey. The purpose of this survey is to elicit information based on your experiences in the field of DSTs. As we are under a tight deadline, please fax the completed survey to (604) 592-6439.

Thank you for your time.

Decision Support Tools in Health Care Survey
being conducted for
the National Health Forum
Working Group on Evidence-Based Decision Making
being conducted by
Canadian Policy Research Networks: Health Network and
PenDragon Consultants Limited

1. Respondent information

1.1 Name of respondent: ————————————————

1.2 Mailing address: ——————————————————

1.3 Phone: —————————————————————————

1.4 Fax: ——————————————————————————

1.5 E-mail address: ——————————————————

1.6 Respondent's area of specialty: ——————————

1.7 Respondent's academic and professional qualifications (please include year in which achieved):

degree	year	degree	year	degree	year

1.8 Respondent's current position

    1.8.1 Title: ————————————————————————

    1.8.2 Number of years in current position: ——————

    1.8.3 Location (if different from above):

    1.8.4 Type of facility (hospital, clinic, health unit, etc.):

    1.8.5 Facility specialty (acute care, long-term care, psychiatric, etc.):

2. Decision support tool information

2.1 Decision support tool name: ————————————

2.2 Respondent's involvement in development (project director, analyst, user, etc.): _____

_____

_____

2.3 Does the respondent use this decision support tool directly? Y/N
     If no, who does?   _____

_____

2.4 Intended user group:

Physician   ☐
Nurse   ☐
Therapist   ☐
Technologist   ☐
Manager   ☐
Administrator   ☐
Instructor   ☐

Other (please specify) _____

2.5 Intended functional area of decision support tool:

Ward (surgical, paediatric, general, obstetric, etc.)   ☐

Diagnostic service (laboratory, imaging, EDS, etc.)   ☐

Administrative (officers, section chiefs, chief of departments, etc.)   ☐

Management (unit managers, personnel officers, etc.)   ☐

Therapeutic service (surgical, chemotherapy, respiratory, etc.)   ☐

Support service (nutrition, pharmacy, security, etc.)   ☐

Other (please specify)   ☐

2.6 Platform of decision support tool (choose all that apply):

PC/DOS   ☐
PC/WIN   ☐
UNIX workstation   ☐
Mainframe   ☐

Other (please specify) _____

2.7 Method of access to decision support tool (choose all that apply):

Stand alone [PC, workstation]

Mainframe

Networked—Client server

Networked—File server

Other (paper, video, etc.) (please specify)_____

2.8 If said decision support tool is networked, does it share data and information with other resident information systems?   Y/N

3. Decision support tool effects

3.1 Has use of this tool affected the time required for the user to reach an decision? (More or less? By how much?)

_____

_____

3.2 Has use of this tool affected the quality of the decision reached by the user? (Are the decisions more or less appropriate and effective?)

_____

_____

3.3 How did you/do you measure this change/improvement?

_____

_____

3.4 Benefits of decision support tool with use

3.4.1 Clinical: _____

_____

_____

3.4.2 Departmental: _____

_____

_____

3.4.3 Institutional: _____

_____

_____

3.4.4 Health care system:_____

_____

_____

3.4.5 Other (specify): _____

_____

_____

3.5 Costs of decision support tool

   3.5.1 How was this tool acquired (developed in-house, purchased, acquired for free)?_____

_____

   3.5.2 Can you identify the cost of this tool? Y/N

   3.5.3 If purchased

      3.5.3.1 What was the total price of the tool? $ _____

      3.5.3.2 If new hardware and/or software had to be purchased what did it cost? $ _____

_____

      3.5.3.3 When was it purchased? _____

   3.5.4 If developed in-house

      3.5.4.1 When did the project start?_____

      3.5.4.2 What did development cost? $ _____

      3.5.4.3 How long did development take?

_____

      3.5.4.4 What did implementation cost?

$ _____

      3.5.4.5 How long did implementation take?

_____

      3.5.4.6 What did evaluation cost? $ _____

      3.5.4.7 How long did evaluation take?

_____

      3.5.4.8 When was the project completed?

_____

3.5.5 What are the operating costs of this tool?

    3.5.5.1 User training (include user time): $ _____

    3.5.5.2 Licensing fees (include system software if only application): $ _____

    3.5.5.3 Maintenance (equipment, analyst, operator, etc.): $ _____

    3.5.5.4 Other (specify: e.g., space): $ _____

4.   Decision support tool evaluation

4.1 Has this tool been subjected to formal evaluation or clinical trials? Y/N

4.2 What was the setting of the trials conducted (hospital, clinic, university, other [specify])? _____

_____

4.3 In evaluating the decision support tool what was the methodology used?

_____

_____

_____

4.4 Results obtained from evaluation(s) conducted:_____

_____

_____

_____

4.5 Have the results of the evaluation(s) been published? If so, please specify the reference(s): _____

_____

    4.5.1 If yes, would you provide a copy of the article(s)? Y/N

5.   Obstacles to implementation and use of this tool

5.1 Factors limiting implementation and use of this tool

    Limited in scope

    Limited access

    Unreliable access

    Unreliable output

    Operating and capital costs

Difficult to use

User resistance

Other (please specify) _____

5.2 Before implementation

5.2.1 Who supported the implementation and use of this tool (MDs, nurses, managers, administrators, etc.)? _____

_____

_____

5.2.2 Why did they support its implementation and use (cost, reliability, quality control, etc.)? _____

_____

_____

5.2.3 Who resisted the implementation and use of this tool (MDs, nurses, managers, administrators, etc.)? _____

_____

_____

5.2.4 Why did they resist its implementation and use (cost, reliability, quality control, etc.) _____

_____

_____

5.3 After implementation

5.3.1 Who supported the implementation and use of this tool (MDs, nurses, managers, administrators, etc.)? _____

_____

_____

5.3.2 Why did they support its implementation and use (cost, reliability, quality control, fear, etc.)? _____

_____

_____

5.3.3 Who resisted the implementation and use of this tool (MDs, nurses, managers, administrators, etc.)? _____

_____

_____

5.3.4 Why did they resist its implementation and use (cost, reliability, quality control, fear, etc.)?

_____

_____

6. Dissemination of this decision support tool

6.1 Has this tool been distributed to other sites?   Y/N

6.2 Where has this tool been disseminated to? (space for multiple entries)

    6.2.1 Site name: _____

    6.2.2 Has it been used at this site?   Y/N

    6.2.3 Has it been tested at this site?   Y/N

    6.2.1 Site name: _____

    6.2.2 Has it been used at this site?   Y/N

    6.2.3 Has it been tested at this site?   Y/N

    6.2.1 Site name: _____

    6.2.2 Has it been used at this site?   Y/N

    6.2.3 Has it been tested at this site?   Y/N

    6.2.1 Site name: _____

    6.2.2 Has it been used at this site?   Y/N

    6.2.3 Has it been tested at this site?   Y/N

7. Future of decision support tool

7.1 What is the future of this tool (further development, discontinued use, integration with information system, etc.) and why?

_____

_____

_____

_____

7.2. What is the future of decision support tools in health care? Independent of considerations of any current tools, what functions or domains of health care do you think decision support tools would be most useful for, and why?

_____

_____

_____

_____

8.   Who else should we survey?

_____

_____

_____

_____

APPENDIX 3

Contact List for Survey Distribution

Those labeled in bold are respondents.

Aldrich, John
Department of Radiology
Faculty of Medicine
University of British Columbia
Vancouver Hospital and Health
Sciences Centre, Heather Pavilion
(604) 875-4158
aldrich@unixg.uB.C..ca

Babcock, Gary
President/CEO
HTN Inc.
146 Lakeshore Road East
Oakville, Ontario
L6J 1H4
(905) 845-3005
(905) 842-9206

Berube, Jacques
President
Med 2020
2025 Lanthier Drive
Orleans, Ontario
K4B 1M2
(800) 461-2020
(613) 830-5992

Bichindaritz, Isabelle
LIAP 5, UFR de Math Info
Université René-Descartes, Paris 5
45, rue des Saints-Pères
75006 Paris, France
33-1-44-55 35 63
33-1-44-55 35 36
bici@mathinfo.univparis5.fr

Billard, Patrick
Industry Manager Health
IBM Canada Ltd.
3600 Steeles Avenue East
Markham, Ontario
L3R 9Z7
(905) 316-6185
(905) 316-4660

Birnbaum, David
Applied Epidemiology
609 Cromar Road
Sidney, B.C.
V8L 5M5
(604) 656-5881
(604) 656-5881
david.birnbaum@uB.C..ca

Brennan, Patti
Case Western Reserve University
Cleveland, Ohio
44106 4904, U.S.A.
(216) 368-5130
(216) 368-3542
pfb@po.cwru.edu

brent.nelson@m.cc.utah.edu

Brien, Carol
CBRIEN@HealthVISION.ca

Brogan, Tom
Brogan Consulting Inc.
2301 Carling Avenue, Suite 202
Ottawa, Ontario
K2B 7G3
(613) 596-5042
(613) 596-5040

Broudo, Marc
#401-2194 Health Sciences Mall
Vancouver, B.C.
V6T 1Z3
(604) 822-5921
(604) 822-2495
mbroudo@unixg.uB.C..ca

Carruthers, Robert J.
Wellington Medical Systems
1651 Broadway Avenue
Nanaimo, B.C.
(604) 753-9111
(604) 753-4911
robertc@island.net OR
compro@island.net

Carter, Anne
Canadian Medical Association
1867 Alta Vista Drive
Ottawa, Ontario
K1G 3Y6
(613) 731-9331
(613) 731-1779
nstn1629@fox.nstn.ca

Chang, Betty
School of Nursing
University of California at Los Angeles
ilz1blc@mvs.oac.ucla.edu

Chesnick, Kathy
Kingston General Hospital
76 Stuart St.
Kingston, Ontario
K7L 2V7
(613) 548-3232 ext. 4232
(613) 548-6077
chesnick@post.queensu.ca

Clark, Justin S.
Department of Medical Informatics
University of Utah
7NE LDS Hospital
325 8th Avenue
Salt Lake City, Utah
84112 U.S.A.
(1-801) 585-6781
Justin.Clark@m.cc.utah.edu

Clarke, Heather F.
2855 Arbutus Street
Vancouver, B.C.
V6J 3Y8
(604) 736-7331 ext. 318
(604) 738-2272
clarke@rnabc.bc.ca

clarsen@unixg.ubc..ca

Copping, Anthony R.
Quilchena Consulting Ltd.
205 3347 Oak Street
Victoria, B.C.
V8X 1R2
(604) 475-4996
(604) 475-3278
Quilchena@pinc.com

Coward, Patricia
Greater Victoria Hospital Society
Victoria, B.C.
pcoward@gvhs.gov.B.C..ca

david.bandon@crpht.lu

denier@sunaimed.univ rennes1.fr

DeSanctis, Geraldine
Fuqua School of Business
Box 90120
(919) 660-7700
gd@mail.duke.edu

Doige, Doris
Toronto General Hospital
(416) 340-3111
(416) 340-3641

Dojat, Michel
INSERM Unité 296
Faculté de Médecine
8, rue Général-Sarrail
94010 Creteil Cedex
France
33-1-48-98 46 03
33-1-48-98 17 77
dojat@laforia.ibp.fr
http://www.laforia.ibp.fr/~dojat/

Ducharme, Francine M.
Departments of Pediatrics and of
Epidemiology and Biostatistics
McGill University and
Montreal Children's Hospital
2300 Tupper Street
Montreal, Quebec
H3H 1P3
(514) 934-4400 ext. 2649
(514) 934-4351
Francind@Epid.lan.McGill.ca

Erica_Harris@ccmail.gov.B.C..ca

Evans, G. Dewey
B.C. Children's Hospital
Room 403B, Oak Street
Vancouver, B.C.
V6H 3V4
(604) 875-2243
(604) 875-3186
devans@wpog.childhosp.B.C..ca

Fay, Donald
Queen Elizabeth II Health Sciences
Centre
Halifax, Nova Scotia
B3H 2Y9
(902) 453-5585
(902) 492-3770

Fox, John
Imperial Cancer Research Fund
jf@acl.lif.icnet.uk

Frankish, James
Institute of Health Promotion
Research
University of British Columbia
2206 East Mall, LPC building
Room 308
Vancouver, B.C.
V6T1Z3
(604) 822-9205
(604) 822-9201
frankish@unixg.uB.C..ca

Gardner, Reed
Department of Medical Informatics
University of Utah
7NE LDS Hospital
325 8th Avenue
Salt Lake City, Utah
84112 U.S.A.
reed.gardner@m.cc.utah.edu

Garlatti, Serge
ecom Bretagne
LIASC
ZI de Kernevent
BP 832
29285 BREST Cedex
France
33-98-00 14 53
33-98-00 10 30
Serge.Garlatti@enst.bretagne.fr OR
serge@liasc.enst.bretagne.fr

Georges.weil@imag.fr

Gibaud, Bernard
Laboratoire SIM
Gibaud@sim3.univ rennes1.fr

Girard, Roger
#600 - 6600 Chemin Côte des Neiges
Montreal, Quebec
H3S 2A9
(514) 737-3201
(514) 737-1918
rgirard@iscdn.mcgill.ca

gkassel@hds.univ compiegne.fr

Gordon, Dan
Information Services
Sunnybrook Health Science Centre
Toronto, Ontario
(416) 480-6100 ext. 3301
(416) 480-4080.
danielg@ibme.utoronto.ca

Green, Lawrence W.
Institute of Health Promotion
Research
University of British Columbia
2205 East Mall (LPC building 324)
Vancouver, B.C.
V6T 1Z3
(604) 822-5776
(604) 822-9210
lgreen@unixg.uB.C..ca

Guerriere, Michael
Toronto Hospital
Toronto, Ontario
MGUERRIERE@torhosp.toronto.on.ca

Hanson, Anne
School of Nursing
Ball State University
Muncie, Indiana
U.S.A.
(317) 285-5763
ahanson@bsu.edu

Harasym, Peter H.
University of Calgary
Health Sciences Centre
Office of Medical Education
3330 Hospital Drive NW
Calgary, Alberta
T2N 4N1
(403) 220-4256
(403) 270-2681
harasyn@acs.ucalgary.ca

Hatfield-Jones, Richard
College of Family Physicians

Haynes, R. Brian
Health Information Research Unit
Clinical Epidemiology and
Biostatistics
Faculty of Health Sciences
Health Sciences Centre, room 3h7
McMaster University
(605) 525-9140 ext. 22311
(905) 546-0401
bhaynes@fhs.csu.McMaster.CA

Hayward, Robert
Health Information Research Unit
Clinical Epidemiology and
Biostatistics
Faculty of Health Sciences
Health Sciences Centre, room 3h7c
McMaster University
(605) 525-9140 ext. 22311
(905) 546-0401
haywardr@fhs.csu.McMaster.CA
Health Information Systems
Salt Lake City, Utah
(1-801) 265-4400

healthnet listserv
814 recipients

Holbrook, Anne
Centre for Evaluation of Medicines,
St. Joseph's Hospital, and
Department of Medicine, McMaster
University, Room 4X1
(905) 522-1155 ext. 5269 (SJH) or
(905) 521-2100 ext. 3371 (MUMC)
(905) 521-6136 (SJH) or
(905) 521-4971 (MUMC)
holbrook@fhs.csu.mcmaster.ca

Hucko, Paula
Senior Vice-President
IST Group Inc.
100 York Blvd., Suite 300
Richmond Hill, Ontario
L4B 1J8
(905) 886-8521
(905) 886-8411

Inkster, Mark
Marketing Director
Stentor Resource Centre Inc.
1535 Lakeshore Rd. East
Suite 510
Mississauga, Ontario
L5E 3E2
(416) 353-1873
(905) 591-3875

Jadad, A. R.
Health Information Research Unit
Clinical Epidemiology and
Biostatistics
Faculty of Health Sciences
Health Sciences Centre, room 3h8a
McMaster University
(605) 525-9140 ext. 22166
(905) 546-0401
jadada@fhs.csu.McMaster.CA

jaulent@hbroussais.fr

Jennett, Penny
Office of Medical Education
Faculty of Medicine
Health Sciences Centre
University of Calgary
3330 Hospital Dr. NW
Calgary, Alberta
T2N 4N1
jennett@med.ucalgary.ca

Jeselon, Pat
Greater Victoria Hospital Society
Victoria, B.C.
pjeselon@LOKI.GVHS.GOV.B.C..CA

Kaczorowski, Ron
General Manager Medical Products
Group
Hewlett Packard (Canada) Ltd.
5150 Spectrum Way
Mississauga, Ontario
L4W 5G1
(905) 206-3249
(905) 206-4121

Kapur, Rajiv
SoftMed
(301) 897-3400

Kerr, Sandra
GVHS
2101 Richmond Ave.
Victoria, B.C.
V8R 4R7
(604) 370-8000 ext. 2450
(604) 370-8556

Koch, Bill
Department of Nursing Practice and
Management
Faculty of Nursing
Royal Melbourne Institute of
Technology
Bundoora Campus
Bundoora, Australia
9468-2445
9467-5286
BILL@rmit.edu.au

Konig, Sergio Alberto
postmaster@nimcba.sld.ar

Lane, Christi
Strategic Information Services
IMS Canada
5770 Hurontario Street, 10th Floor
Mississauga, Ontario
L5R 3G5
(905) 712-5059 OR (905) 712-5000
(905) 712-5125
LaneC@imsint.com

Lau, Francis
3030D Business Building
Faculty of Business
University of Alberta
Edmonton Alberta
T6G 2R6
(403) 492-5828
(403) 492-3325
flau@gpu.srv.ualberta.ca

Leonard, Pierre
#1600 - 2 Place Alexis Nihon
3500 Boul. de Maisonneuve Ouest
Westmount, Quebec
H3Z 3C1
(514) 934-6703
(514) 934-6751

Lobato, Amado Espinoza
Autonomous University of
Guadalajara
aelr@uagunix.gdl.uag.mx

MacNaught, Donald
SHL
Ottawa, Ontario

MacPherson, D. W.
Regional Parasitology Laboratory
St. Joseph's Hospital
50 Charlton Ave. E.
Hamilton, Ontario
L8N 4A6
(905) 522-1155 ext. 4011
(905) 521-6090
dmacpher@fhs.csu.mcmaster.ca

Mailloux, Terry
Theratechnologies
Montreal, Quebec

Mailloux, Terry
Chairman and CEO
Theratechnologies
7701 17th Avenue
Montreal, Quebec
H2A 2S5
(514) 729-7904
(514) 593-8142

Mann, Kelly
National Sales Manager
3M Health Information Systems

Marcus, Robert
Picis
401 2nd Avenue South, Suite 630
Seattle, WA
98104-2837 U.S.A.
(206) 368-4093
(206) 682-8467

Maria.Malek@imag.fr

McCloy, Lynda
Director of Therapy Services
The Arthritis Society
895 W. 10th Ave.
Vancouver, B.C.
V6K 1L7
(604) 879-7511
(604) 871-4500
Lynda_McCloy@tasvan.arth.gov.B.C..ca

McCombs, Barrie
Director, Medical Information Service
University of Calgary
(403) 220-8551
(403) 270-2330
bmccombs@acs.ucalgary.ca

McDonnell, Elaine
Ottawa Grace Hospital
Ottawa, Ontario

mehddeb@hbroussais.fr

Metcalf, Joy
St. Mary's General Hospital
911 Queens Boulevard
Kitchener, Ontario
N2M 1B2
(519) 744-3311 ext. 22514
(519) 749-6426

Michael Pluscauskas
XMAN@MGCHEO.MED.UOTTAWA.CA

Miller, Perry
Department of Anesthesiology
Faculty of Medicine
Yale University
(203) 785-6753
perry.miller@yale.edu

Nathwani, Bharat N.
Department of Pathology
Faculty of Medicine
University of Southern California
Los Angeles, CA
(213) 226-7064
(213) 226-7119

Oppenheimer, Becky
HBO & Company
301 Perimeter Center North
Atlanta, Georgia
30346 U.S.A.
(404) 393-6532

Otto Rienhoff
haegar@mdv.gwdg.de

Patel, Vimla
Department of Psychology
McGill University
pa@hebb.psych.mcgill.ca

Pedraza, Luis M
pedraza@sida.fmedic.unam.mx

Pepe, Matthew
Manager, Health Information Systems
3M Canada Inc.
P.O. Box 5757
London, Ontario
N6A 4T1
(519) 452-6057

Pharmacare
CLVERMAN@B.C.SC02.GOV.B.C..CA

Ramos, Igor
Autonomous University of
Guadalajara
IRAMOS@UDGSERV.CENCAR.UDG.MX

Reese, Bernie
Vice-President Sales & Marketing
Canada
HBO & Company
301 Perimeter Center North
Atlanta, Georgia
30346 U.S.A.
(1-800) 662-9030

Rosenal, Tom
Division of Health Informatics
Office of Medical Education
Faculty of Medicine
Room 1651, Health Sciences Centre
University of Calgary
3330 Hospital Dr. NW
Calgary, Alberta
T2N 4N1
rosenal@acs.ucalgary.ca

Ruland, Cornelia
Case Western Reserve University
cmr8@po.cwru.edu

Ryan, Shelia
School of Nursing
University of Rochester
Rochester, New York
U.S.A.
shry@davinci.nursing.rochester.edu

Sawsan.Elkassar@laforia.ibp.fr
Scientific and Research Special Interest
Group of COACH
sarsig@critcare.vichosp.london.on.ca

Seroussi, Brigitte
Service d'Informatique Médicale
91, Boulevard de l'Hôpital
75634 Paris, Cedex 13
France
33-1-45-86 56 84
33-1-45-86 56 85
bs@biomath.jussieu.fr

Shams, Kamrudin
President/CEO
The Shams Group
1430 Valwood Pkwy
Suite 120
Carrollton, TX
75006, U.S.A.
(214) 484-9393
(214) 484-6840
tsg@shams_group.com

Sharples, Mike
School of Cognitive and Computing
Sciences
University of Sussex
Brighton, U.K.
BN1 9QH
44-273-678393
44-273-671320
mike@cogs.sussex.ac.uk
http://www.cogs.susx.ac.uk/users/
mike/index.html

Shiffman, Smadar
Stanford University School of
Medicine
Stanford, CA
94305 U.S.A.
(415) 725-6699
shiffman@camis.stanford.edu

Smith, Bev
Acquired Intelligence
205 1075 McKenzie Avenue
Victoria, B.C.
V8P 2L5
(604) 479-8646
(604) 479-0764

Tam, Julie
Professional and Scientific Affairs
Canadian Drug Manufacturers
Association
4120 Yonge Street
North York, Ontario
M2P 2B8
(416) 223-2333
(416) 223-2425

Tan, Joseph
Department of Health Care and
Epidemiology
Faculty of Medicine
University of British Columbia
James Mather Building
5804 Fairview Avenue
Vancouver, B.C.
V6T 1Z3
(604) 822-2737
(604) 822-4994
josepht@unixg.ubc.ca OR
joseph.tan@mtsg.ubc.ca

Thomson, Alan D.
Medical Consultant
Regional Services Division
B.C. Ministry of Health
62, 1515 Blanshard Street
Victoria, B.C.
V8W 3C8
(604) 952-1862
adthomso@BCsc02.gov.BC.ca

Tranner, Joan
Oshawa General Hospital
24 Alma St.
Oshawa, Ontario
L1G 2B9

Uyeno, Dean
Department of Health Care and
Epidemiology
Faculty of Medicine
University of British Columbia
James Mather Building,
5804 Fairview Avenue
Vancouver, B.C.
V6T 1Z3
(604) 822-2366
(604) 822-4994

Wall, Joe
Regional Manager
Meditech Inc.
Meditech Circle
Westwood, Mass.
02090 U.S.A.
(617) 329-5300
(617) 329-9977

Weber, Jean
Department of Statistics
University of Arizona
weber1@CCIT.Arizona.edu

Weinstein, Judith
Coordinator, Case management
Oshawa General Hospital
24 Alma St.
Oshawa, Ontario
L1G 2B9
(905) 576-8711 ext. 3981
(905) 433-4363
caseman@hospital.oshawa.on.ca

Won, Raymond
Senior Sales Executive
HBO & Company
1195 Glenora Drive
London, Ontario
N5X 2P6
(519) 432-4764
(519) 432-2808

Yamada, Ronald H.
Information Strategies and Corporate
Affairs
MDS Health Group Limited
100 International Blvd.
Etobicoke, Ontario
M9W 6J6
(416) 675-7661 OR (416) 213-4224
(416) 213-4222

Zitner, David
Medical Quality Consultant
Queen Elizabeth II Health Sciences
Centre
Halifax, Nova Scotia
B3H 2Y9
(902) 428-2853
(902) 428-2850
dzitner@ac.dal.ca
zweig@biomath.jussieu.fr

Building a National Health Information Network

CHARLYN BLACK, M.D., SC.D.

Department of Community Health Sciences
Faculty of Medicine
University of Manitoba

SUMMARY

This project was conducted to identify an approach or combination of approaches that can optimally be used to transform population-based data into information useful for managing the health care system.

Out of 52 current initiatives identified for consideration, 18 were classified as population-based health information systems and reviewed in detail. This involved assessment of general orientation, content areas covered, comparative focus, reporting mechanisms, data sources, and relative strengths and weaknesses. In addition, information was obtained about the extent to which each system has been used in policy and planning processes.

An important finding was the discovery of a great deal of activity in the development and implementation of information systems across the country. All the initiatives reviewed have important strengths, many of which deserve consideration for implementation at a national level. Detailed analysis of the 18 health information systems revealed that they have very different "personalities." While all have adopted a population health framework for presentation of indicators, they use this framework and choose indicators within it in a somewhat different manner. The emerging patchwork of information does not support an understanding of population health across Canadian settings.

An additional observation from the review is that in adopting a population health framework, most of the information systems focused more directly on measuring health status and the determinants of health that fall outside the medical care system than has previously been possible. As a result, aspects of usage of medical care and elaboration of the contribution of medical care to population health remain underdeveloped in all but a few of the initiatives.

During the review, it became apparent that most of the 18 initiatives were at a very early stage in the process of developing links to support decision making. It is clear that much remains to be learned about how to make health information systems relevant to the policy process. Several characteristics were identified as central to a system's ability to support the decision-making process in the current environment. These include a focus on comparative analysis across planning areas, with analyses to highlight an understanding of the relative contributions of nonmedical and medical care inputs to health, and linkage of information to current funding and delivery perspectives. Finally, flexibility to provide focused responses to well-articulated policy questions enhances a system's capability to contribute meaningful information from the perspective of policymakers. Over time, different types of evidence will likely be required from health information systems to support policy decision making.

This review provides strong support for a national initiative to permit assessment of population health and to provide information to support important policy decisions that face Canada in trying to maximize the health of its population. Such an initiative should clearly draw on the strengths of various systems that have been reviewed for this report and, to some extent, build on work already done. The initiative should be national in scope, with a major focus on providing information to support decision making at national, provincial, and regional jurisdictional levels. It should provide population-based information within a comprehensive population health framework, incorporating information about determinants of health that fall both within and outside the health care system. Initially, comparative analyses of indicators should be conducted to highlight differences and similarities across populations, using relevant policy and program (i.e., geographic) jurisdictions. Because provinces have different capabilities in terms of available data, the initiative should be flexible to accommodate different strengths and weaknesses. Finally, it should link information to funding and service delivery perspectives to provide information about policy directions that arise from a population health perspective.

In structuring a national information system, emphasis should be placed on analytic comparisons and interpretation of comparative data. It is clear that much work has gone into developing individual health information systems. On the other hand, the systems that appear to be having an influence are those that present comparative data in an integrated format that raises issues from the perspective of population health. Integrated and comparative analysis across the nation would likely be beneficial to advancing concepts of using evidence to support decision making in a manner that is congruent with a population health framework.

Over the longer term, other approaches deserve emphasis. These include measuring trends over time, measuring progress toward goals, and including international comparative data. In addition, comprehensive comparative national information systems should be developed with a focus on vulnerable populations such as children, Aboriginal people, and persons living in poverty. Other analyses could include pre- and postevaluations of major reforms and comparisons of effects across jurisdictions that have chosen different policy options to address population health. Finally, there should be an assessment of which approaches provide the most useful information for decision making to improve population health at various levels of jurisdiction (i.e., federal, provincial, and regional authority).

The differing personalities of the 18 health information systems reviewed for this report reflect different data capabilities, conceptual models, and perceived requirements for information. While it is possible to identify general approaches that might be incorporated into implementation of a national initiative, co-operation and partnerships will be required to move such an agenda forward.

Based on these findings, the following recommendations are made.

Recommendation 1

It is recommended that the National Forum on Health champion investment in information systems that go beyond data warehousing and are designed to provide evidence to support policy and health services decision making within the context of a population health perspective.

Recommendation 2

It is recommended that the National Forum on Health encourage and support the development of a national population-based health policy information network.

Such an initiative should draw on the best aspects of systems that have been developed and have proven useful in the policy process, but should be flexible enough to incorporate strengths from emerging initiatives. A modular approach would permit development of a core set of analyses for all jurisdictions but would also support development of more in-depth comparative analyses, depending on data availability and interests. After production of an initial report, information should be updated and a new report produced on a regular basis, possibly every two or three years, to monitor change.

Ideally, a national initiative should recognize the priorities and specificities of different jurisdictions but also be structured to allow comparisons and minimize unnecessary duplication. The creation of a national population-based health policy information network will require cooperation and partnerships, but a single entity should take responsibility to direct its development. Agencies that could potentially move such an initiative forward include Statistics Canada, the Canadian Institute for Health Information (CIHI), a cooperative venture involving the applied health services research units (Centre for Health Services and Policy Research at the University of British Columbia, the Manitoba Centre for Health Policy and Evaluation at the University of Manitoba, the Institute for Clinical and Evaluative Sciences and the Health Intelligence Units in Ontario, the Interdisciplinary Research Group on Health and researchers from the Laval University, Quebec City, and the Population Health Research Unit at Dalhousie University) and ministries of health in remaining provinces; or the Federal/Provincial/Territorial Conference of Deputy Ministers.

TABLE OF CONTENTS

APPENDICES

LIST OF TABLES

INTRODUCTION

This project was conducted to identify an approach or combination of approaches that can optimally be used to transform population-based data into information useful for managing the health care system. The intent is to shift the focus of health policy perspectives from one that emphasizes health care to one that incorporates the concepts of population health. This information can then be used as a basis for planning and decision making about policies and programs related to health and health care.

Many different population-based health information initiatives have developed useful and valid indicators of socioeconomic determinants of health, personal behaviours that influence health, use of health care resources, supply and capacity of the health care system, or expenditures on health care. Most initiatives also combine information from several of these perspectives. However, to manage the health care system effectively, it is essential to understand the linkages of each of these components to the other and, ultimately, to producing population health. A population-based health information infrastructure that will link these factors together to facilitate understanding of the determinants of health has potential for improving population health and achieving greater efficiency in the expenditure of health care dollars.

Numerous initiatives are under way in the area of health information in Canada, primarily at the provincial level. Some initiatives in the United States also address the use of population-based data to support decision making in public policy and health. These can play an instrumental role in restructuring the health system in Canada to improve its quality, effectiveness, and efficiency. A national strategy which uses a population-based health information infrastructure, with standards and information relevant to planning and policy making at the levels of national, provincial and regional health authorities, has the potential to prevent duplication of effort and provide a systematic method for evidence-based decisions.

This document summarizes analyses of current information systems and their ability to support evidence-based decision making in the Canadian context. On the basis of this information, recommendations are made about approaches that can be used to enhance evidence-based policy making using population-based data.

Objectives

Objective 1

To provide an overview of major initiatives relevant to developing a population-based health information infrastructure (to include information about the host organization, its mandate, and sources of funding).

Objective 2

To identify specific characteristics and linkages of a population-based health information infrastructure necessary to support evidence-based decision making in five areas: population health, health services use, health outcomes, resource allocation, and policy development.

Objective 3

To recommend a population-based health information infrastructure model that will support decision making in public policy and health care at the level of national, provincial, and regional health authorities.

Objective 4

To identify strategies and partnerships required for implementation of this population-based health information infrastructure at the various levels.

METHODS

Identification of Initiatives

An inclusive approach was taken to identify health information initiatives for consideration and analysis in this report. A number of initiatives known to the principal investigator served as a starting point. Contacts were made with key sources in each province to assist with further identification of initiatives and to seek clarification on the development and orientation of the various information systems.

Screening of Initiatives for In-Depth Review

Two criteria were used to screen the health information initiatives to identify a subset that represented population-based health information systems (table 1). First, a given initiative had to function as a health information system, and second, it had to be population based. Only those initiatives that represented population-based health information systems were considered for in-depth review and detailed presentation in the final report. Other initiatives were reviewed informally to gain a general understanding of the area.

A health information system, the first criterion, was defined as one in which the primary goal is to transform data into information useful for planning, and decision making about, policies and programs related to health and health care. To perform this function, an information system must provide a broad picture rather than respond only to specific questions. The system must also have access to data about the region in question and, possibly, other regions.

Table 1

Criteria used to identify population-based health information systems

---

CRITERION 1:

Is the initiative a health information system?

A health information system has as a primary goal the transformation of data into information useful for planning, and decision making about, programs and policies related to health and health care.

CRITERION 2:

Is the initiative population based?

A population-based perspective provides an understanding relevant to all members of a population or defined group of persons.

Initiatives at the proposal stage (e.g., Manitoba's Population Health Assessment Template and Newfoundland's Improved Health for Newfoundland and Labrador through Improved Health Information) were excluded, as were surveys of undetermined periodicity (e.g., Quebec, Ontario, and Alberta health surveys). It was noted, however, that such surveys, while not considered as health information systems for this report, may provide useful input to such systems. The provincial "smart health" initiatives were also excluded because, while they use data, they are oriented to providing on-line information useful for managing direct service provision (e.g., Prince Edward Island's "Island Health Information System"). As with health surveys, they may provide important input for health information systems but, by themselves, do not represent an information system.

The second criterion, a population-based orientation, was defined as one that provides an understanding relevant to all members of a population or defined group of persons. Specifically, its perspective must go beyond that of service users. Initiatives that focused on services provided, or that focused only on users of services, were excluded on this basis.

In-Depth Review of Population-Based Health Information Systems

As a first step, key aspects of each identified health information system were identified and summarized. This involved outlining major objectives, summarizing major areas of data presentation and emphasis, and identifying sponsoring agencies and sources of funding. Finally, information was obtained on the extent to which each information system has been used in planning and evaluation processes. Where systems were very new and, therefore, not likely to have yet been used (or if they were not Canadian), the latter step was not undertaken.

Initiatives were then reviewed in terms of how they met explicit criteria related to content, comparative focus, and reporting mechanism. These criteria were initially identified in consultation with the "Evidence-Based Decision Making" working group in a conference call on January 12, 1996. Subsequently, they were modified and expanded to amplify differences between initiatives identified for in-depth review.

The first set of criteria focused on assessing population-based health information systems in terms of "content domains" relevant to a population health perspective. The list of domains used was derived from published population health frameworks, including those of Evans and Stoddart (1990), Roos et al. (1996), and Frank (1995). Within each content domain, major categories of indicators were also identified.

Major content domains and categories of indicators are described below.

1. Regional and demographic information – Key attributes of the identified population, including population size, age and sex distribution, fertility rates, and other characteristics.

2. Determinants of population health external to the health care system – Areas that are identified as important contributors to population health, but are outside the traditional perspective of the health care system. They include factors such as biologic influences, which are not generally considered amenable to intervention, as well as other factors that form the background for approaches to improving population health such as social environment, economic environment, physical environment, health knowledge and beliefs, and health behaviours.

3. Health status – Including several broad categories that define general approaches to measuring population health. Health status can be considered as either an "outcome" of factors that are known to influence it (consistent with a population health approach), or as a factor that contributes to the "need" of a population for interventions (both internal and external to the health care system).

4. Use and cost of health care services – Comprising several major categories of health care services. The category of preventive services was defined to include primary and secondary preventive services, such as public health and screening services. The category of community services was defined to include services such as home care, community mental health services, and others. Other identified categories included physician services, allied professional services, hospital services, personal home care services, drugs, and ambulance services.

5. Supply and capacity of the health care system – An area identified as relevant for consideration because of potential links between supply/capacity and use, and costs of health care, although not important from the perspective of population health.

6. Health outcomes – An area also considered because in some cases, health status measures are used explicitly as indicators of end results in a population health framework. While it was not always clear whether indicators of health status were being used as need or outcome variables, the presence of certain key variables (such as proportion of babies born with low birthweight, and avoidable mortality) was interpreted as an indicator that there was a focus on health outcomes.

7. Health care outcomes – Included because, theoretically, it may be possible to differentiate outcomes that are amenable to medical intervention.

Each population-based information system was reviewed against the set of content domains and indicators, and decisions were made as to whether it contained indicators within each category. If the answer was yes, a decision was made about whether there was a major or minor emphasis in a given category. In general, systems that included two or more indicators within a given category were considered as having a major emphasis in a particular area, but consideration was also given to the extent to which a particular set of indicators received emphasis within each system.

Each initiative was assessed according to several additional criteria. First, systems were reviewed to determine whether they explored linkages across content domains, especially those relevant to a population health focus. For example, were the systems exploring the relationship between indicators in the "determinants of health" and "health status" domains? From an evidence-based perspective, were they exploring the relationship between the "health status" and "use and cost" domains? Systems were also reviewed to assess comparative focus: which questions do they address, as identified by their measurement approaches and the comparative analyses on which they focus? Aspects of the reporting mechanism used by the different population-based health information systems were also reviewed. Finally, summary analyses were conducted to assess the relative strengths and weaknesses of various approaches to arrive at an understanding of critical characteristics useful for defining a national approach to conducting comparative population-based analyses.

RESULTS

Identification and Screening of Initiatives

Contacts made with key sources across the country identified 52 potential initiatives for consideration.[1] Screening revealed that many initiatives were not health information systems as defined for this report. Some simply provided lists of indicators or were in very preliminary stages of planning; others presented health goals; others represented reports about health information or allocation formulae for regional funding; still others were

---

1. A list of contacts made as part of this process is provided in appendix 1. A complete listing of initiatives identified for consideration appears in appendix 2.

provincial health surveys. A few initiatives, while health information systems, were not population based. For example, Alberta's Psychiatry Database: An Integrated Information System and the Hartford Foundation's Community Health Management Information System were excluded on this basis. Eighteen of the 52 initiatives met both criteria and were identified for further analysis, including general review, content, comparative focus, and reporting mechanisms (table 2).

General Review of Information Systems

The Geography of Death: Mortality Atlas of British Columbia 1985– 1989

- Main objective is to describe and disseminate relevant community-level health information to the public and to local health service providers, planners, and educators so communities can identify and address their own specific health challenges. These efforts are expected to lead to the identification of local health priorities and more appropriate decision making.
- The atlas presents mortality patterns in British Columbia, for selected and leading causes of death, over the five-year period from 1985 to 1989 (based on vital statistics death registrations). The general physical and socioeconomic characteristics of British Columbia, a brief overview of the health services network in the province, and a descriptive summary of the physical, economic, and social milieu of the geographical units, which are used for mapping, are presented. Each map is accompanied by a brief description of major geographical patterns and data relating to the mortality trend for the period. Three additional volumes in the geographical series have been published: *Community, Environment and Health*, volume 27; *Determinants of Population Health: A Critical Assessment*, volume 29; and *A Persistent Spirit Toward Understanding Aboriginal Health in British Columbia*, volume 31.
- Published 1992, University of Victoria. Supported by the Leon and Thea Koerner Foundation, the Social Science Federation of Canada, the National Centre for Atmospheric Research, the International Geographical Union Congress, the University of Victoria, the Natural Sciences Engineering Research Council of Canada, the Institute of the North American West, and the British Columbia Ministry of Health and Ministry Responsible for Seniors.
- The editor for the book states he has been contacted by various groups involved in health promotion initiatives for British Columbia; however, the specifics of use for these projects is unknown. The document was used by the federal government at international cartography/geographical conferences as representative of Canadian work in this area.

Table 2

Initial screen: Is the initiative a population-based health information system?

Province	Initiative	Information system?	Population based?	For further analysis?
BRITISH COLUMBIA	*The Geography of Death: Mortality Atlas of British Columbia 1985–1989*	Yes	Yes	Yes
	User's Guide—Operational Indicators for Community Health Programs 1993	No	No	No
	A Report on the Health of British Columbians—Provincial Health Officer's Annual Report 1994 (1995 report forthcoming)	Yes	Yes	Yes
	Mortality and Health Status in Vancouver: An Analysis by Neighbourhood Areas 1995 (update of *Vancouver Health Atlas 1991*)	Yes	Yes	Yes
ALBERTA	*Healthy Edmonton 2000—Goals Project 1992*	No	Yes	No
	Health of Calgarians 1995	Yes	Yes	Yes
	Alberta Health Survey 1995	No	Yes	No
	Psychiatry Database: An Integrated Information System 1996	Yes	No	No
SASKATCHEWAN	*Needs-Based Allocation of Resources to Saskatchewan Health Districts 1994–1995*	No	Yes	No
	Community Profile System— Saskatchewan Health System Project 1995	Yes	Yes	Yes
MANITOBA	*Populis—The Manitoba Centre for Health Policy and Evaluation (MCHPE) 1995*	Yes	Yes	Yes
	Manitoba Population Health Assessment Template 1995	No (proposal only)	Yes	No
ONTARIO	*Ontario Health Survey 1990*	No	Yes	No
	Information Products and Tools —Information to District Health Councils 1993–1995	No	Yes	No

Table 2 (cont.)

Province	Initiative	Information system?	Population based?	For further analysis?
ONTARIO (cont.)	Patterns of Health Care in Ontario—ICES Practice Atlas 1994	Yes	Yes	Yes
	POHEM Project—work in progress	No	Yes	No
	McMaster Comprehensive Health Status Measurement System (Mark III)/Proposed Population Health Index 1995	No	Can be (depends on application)	No
	A Model for Community Health Profiles—Ontario Public Health 1995 (draft report)	Yes	Yes	Yes
	HELPS Initiative—pilot project	No	Yes	No
	Geographic Information Management System—work in progress	Yes	Yes	Yes*
	SE Toronto Health Profiles Project 1994	Yes	Yes	Yes
QUEBEC	Quebecers in the Quebec Health and Social Survey 1992	No	Yes	No
	Politique de la santé et du bien-être 1992	Not available for review		
	Policy on Health and Well-Being 1992	No	Yes	No
	User's Guide to 40 Community Health Indicators, 1992 (CHIS indicators)	Yes	Yes (in part)	Yes
	Les coûts relatifs de production et l'équité interrégionale—cadre conceptuel et révision méthodologique 1994	No	Yes	No
	L'équité dans l'allocation inter-régionale des ressources du champ de la santé physique 1994	No	Yes	No
	Des indicateurs de besoins pour l'allocation interrégionale des ressources 1995	No	Yes	No
	Les indicateurs de la politique québécoise de la santé et du bien-être 1995	Yes	Yes	Yes
	Le Québec comparé: indicateurs sanitaires, démographiques et socioéconomiques 1995	Yes	Yes	Yes

Table 2 (cont.)

Province	Initiative	Information system?	Population based?	For further analysis?
NEW BRUNSWICK	*Health Status Reports 1988 and 1994* (1996 mandated by deputy minister)	Not available for review		
	Resource Allocation Model for Family Community and Social Services 1995	No (proposal only)	Yes	No
NOVA SCOTIA	*Report Card on Health 1995*	No	No	No
	NS Health Survey 1995	Initiatives in different stages of development.Communication with George Kephart and Dan Rice/Brenda Ryan: no population-based information systems at present.		
	Health Information Technology Initiative 1995			
PRINCE EDWARD ISLAND	*Island Health Information System 1993–1996*	No	No	No
	Health Indicator Resource Project 1995—presented to Atlantic Regional Health Indicators Conference	Yes (framework only)	Yes (framework only)	No
NEWFOUNDLAND	Requested information on systems	Communication with Jorge Segovia: unique identifier for health insurance—not always valid due to deaths, migration, update irregularity; Ministry of Health maintains computerized databases for hospital separations and physicians' claims—good quality; research projects related to health issues, i.e., health survey; referral to chair, Health System Information Task Force.		
	Improved Health for Newfoundland and Labrador through Improved Health Information 1995	No (proposal only)	No (proposal only)	No
	The Way Forward—Health Information Systems Vision 1995	No (proposal only)	No (proposal only)	No

Table 2 (cont.)

Province	Initiative	Information system?	Population based?	For further analysis?
ATLANTIC REGION	*Atlantic Regional Health Indicators Conference 1995*	No	No	No
		(summary of information re Atlantic Province initiatives)		
OTHER CANADIAN	*Health Information for Canada: Report of the National Task Force on Health Information 1991*	No	Yes	No
	Canadian Centre for Health Information (CCHI) Indicators 1993	Yes	Yes	Yes**
	Comparative Analysis of the CCHI Health Indicators and CHIS Health Indicator Guidelines 1993	No	No	No
		(summary of Analysis of CCHI Health Indicators and CHIS Indicator Guidelines)		
	Health Statistics Division (formerly CCHI) *Health Indicators 1994* (update of CCHI Indicators 1993; further update for release in 1996)	Yes	Yes	Yes***
	Community Health Indicators: Definitions and Interpretations 1995 (also titled *Health Status Indicators;* update of *User's Guide to 40 Community Health Indicators 1992;* CHIS indicators)	Yes	Yes	Yes
	Canadian Child Health Atlas 1995	Yes	Yes	Yes
	Use and Impact of Information Technologies in Health (External Version)—A Report to Health Programs and Promotions Branch 1995	No	No	No
		(summary of information about patient-oriented service management systems)		
	Report Card on the Health of Canadians: Technical Version October 1995—draft (planned release September 1996)	Yes	Yes	Yes
UNITED STATES	*The Truth about Where You Live —An Atlas for Action on Toxins and Mortality 1991*	Yes	Yes	Yes
	Healthy People 2000—National Health Promotion and Disease Prevention Objectives 1991	No	Yes	No

Table 2 (cont.)

Province	Initiative	Information system?	Population based?	For further analysis?
UNITED STATES (cont.)	*Community Health Management Information System 1992*	Yes	No	No
	Oregon Benchmarks 1994	Yes	Yes	Yes

* Report not available for further analysis.

** The CCHI Indicators 1993 were updated as Health Statistics Division Health Indicators 1994.

*** The Health Statistics Division Health Indicators 1994 is an update of CCHI Indicators 1993.

Mortality and Health Status in Vancouver: An Analysis by Neighbourhood Areas 1995

- Main objective is to provide information to a wide audience of potential users involved in the process of health policy reform. Although the focus is Vancouver, the intent was to develop methods that are applicable to other urban areas (census metropolitan areas) of the province.
- This report is an update of the 1991 document, *Vancouver Atlas,* and provides a descriptive analysis of variations in mortality and selected health status indicators among 13 neighbourhood areas within Vancouver. The 13 areas were defined so as to maintain some degree of homogeneity with respect to the social characteristics of the residents in order to link observed variations in mortality to social influences on health. The analysis combines mortality information, obtained from the province's vital statistics data with census population estimates provided by Statistics Canada. Two three-year time periods are analyzed (1985–87 and 1990–92).
- Produced by the British Columbia Ministry of Health and Ministry Responsible for Seniors.
- According to one of the developers of the document, the information has been reviewed by policymakers; however, he believes it has had little input into decision making. One of the problems with the information produced is that the boundaries used for mapping and graphing the data have been changed with the introduction of the regional health authorities and, therefore, does not accurately represent the current health divisions of the city.

A Report on the Health of British Columbians: Provincial Health Officer's Annual Report 1994 (1995 Report Forthcoming)

- Main objective is to produce an annual report on the health of British Columbians "as measured against population health targets." These have not yet been established. The purpose of the current report, which is required by the Health Act, is to serve as a starting point for discussions on provincial health goals, objectives, and targets.

- Health status indicators (e.g., life expectancy, infant mortality, teen pregnancy, etc.) and the major determinants which influence health (i.e., socioeconomic environment, physical environment, biological influences, health knowledge and beliefs, and health services) are discussed. Recommendations for action to improve the identified health problems and issues facing British Columbians are presented.

- Produced by British Columbia Ministry of Health and Ministry Responsible for Seniors.

- The report has been used at the regional health unit level as a framework for determining indicators for a needs assessment profile of the unit, local planning and project proposals for local programs. Socioeconomic indicators, which demonstrated disparities in health status, have been used for building the funding formula for health regions. In addition, the report was used for background information by the Northern and Rural Task Force to assess and identify gaps in health and health care in northern British Columbia. Recommendations for injury prevention and tobacco reduction have contributed to action on strategies in these areas. The report has also been used to provide a policy framework for designated populations (e.g., Aboriginal peoples' health, women, etc.). The data on indicators have become the de facto standard for tracking indicators at the health unit level and have provided a basis for discussion on health goals for the population.

Health of Calgarians 1995

- Main objective is to provide a key component of the Regional Needs Assessment by reporting on the health status of Calgarians. Ultimately, it is expected that reporting of health status will provide information to measure the progress being made toward the achievement of health goals for Region 4 (Calgary and surrounding communities).

- Information is presented on the state of health of Calgarians through the use of health status indicators (e.g., physical, social, mental, and spiritual state of people) and on factors that determine, or are strongly correlated with, health (i.e., changes in the social, economic and cultural environment; the physical environment; health behaviour and skills; and health service). A public health focus, with major emphasis on types of morbidity, trend data and benchmarks, is presented. Issues and recommendations for action at the individual, community, and government levels are outlined in each section.

- Produced by the Calgary Regional Health Authority.

- Several requests have been received for further information on the data and statistics within the report. It is anticipated the information will be used in the development of business plans for the public health sectors of the different regions. As a result of working together on the project, members of the public health sector have developed a more cohesive identity.

Community Profile System—Saskatchewan Health System Project 1995

- Main objective is to provide an integrated and accessible source of information to support district planning, needs assessment, and the ongoing management of services at district and provincial levels. The emphasis is on building a database, together with easier-to-use tools to access the data, so that evaluators and planners can find the data themselves. In the interim, the Community Profile System has been developed to summarize data at community and district levels.
- The Community Profile System summarizes information for 850 communities and 30 health districts in the province. Data have been analyzed by five-year age categories to provide comprehensive community health profiles for planning. The profiles contain population and demographic information, a complete set of variables from both the 1986 and 1991 census, and five years of administrative data. The administrative data include hospital, physician, home care, mental health, addiction treatment, and ambulance information. These community profiles have been provided for storage in electronic format (e.g., personal computer hard drives) so users can get access to the information directly. Developers are currently working with education and justice information to incorporate other variables of importance to developing community profiles.
- Developed by Saskatchewan Health, Corporate Information and Technology Branch.
- The Community Profile System has been used in a number of ways, including creating districts and defining boundaries, developing a new regional funding formula, and conducting needs assessments and planning at the district level.

Populis—the Manitoba Centre for Health Policy and Evaluation (MCHPE) 1995

- Main objective is to report on the health of the population and on the relationship between health and the use of health care services. The information is provided to the provincial government for planning and decision making on policies and programs related to health and health care.
- The information system is designed around administrative data collected as part of the provincial health insurance system; for this program,

every contact the population makes with hospitals, nursing homes and physician visits is documented. Vital statistics data documenting date and cause of death and public use census information have also been integrated into the information system. Health status indicators provide the base for assessing both inequalities across regions of the province and the prevalence of specific health-related problems in a particular region. A socioeconomic risk index is used as a measure of health needs. A major focus is on understanding linkages among health status, socio-economic status, and usage of health care. Both cross-sectional and longitudinal analyses have been conducted.

- Produced by the Manitoba Centre for Health Policy and Evaluation (MCHPE), a research unit based in the Department of Community Health Sciences, Faculty of Medicine, University of Manitoba. MCHPE is active in health services research, evaluation and policy analysis, concentrating on using the Manitoba health database to describe and explain patterns of care and profiles of health and illness. The Manitoba Department of Health provides funding for ongoing operational and infrastructure costs.

- Populis has been used in applied analyses around specific questions related to health reform. Numerous requests have been received for information tailored to specific jurisdictions. It is anticipated that arrangements will be made to provide data to regional health authorities as part of an MCHPE deliverable to Manitoba Health.

Patterns of Health Care in Ontario—ICES Practice Atlas 1994[2]

- Main objective is to offer information on health indicators and patterns of health care to clinicians, administrators, planners, and policymakers working to maintain and improve medical care delivery. A secondary purpose is to provide information that may be useful in the broader debate about how Canada's health care system should be adapted to meet the financial demands of the future.

- Data for most analyses are derived from administrative data (e.g., hospital discharge data), which provide general information on temporal and regional patterns of medical care use. The atlas identifies counties, cities, and regions and shows population-based rates of utilization for different types of health care services. The report also includes an overview of the health status of Ontario residents derived from a combination of the Ontario Health Survey, Hospital Medical Records Institute (HMRI) (now the Canadian Institute for Health Information) data, and mortality data.

---

2. Since this review was conducted, a second edition of the report has been released.

- Produced by the Institute for Clinical Evaluative Sciences (ICES), a nonprofit research corporation established in 1992 and sponsored by the Ontario Ministry of Health and the Ontario Medical Association. The mandate of ICES is to examine how Ontario's health system works and how health care services can be improved. Research is undertaken to address the quality, efficiency, and accessibility of medical and allied professional services in Ontario.
- The atlas has been used at three levels: by hospitals for quality audit processes, by district health councils at the community level for activities and planning, and by the Ministry of Health for assessment of hospitals (e.g., efficiency, etc.). It also resulted in the establishment of a hysterectomy task force to assess differences between rates in northern and southern Ontario.

A Model for Community Health Profiles—Ontario Public Health 1995 (Draft Report)

- Main objective is to provide an assessment of the health of a population, through the analysis and interpretation of a variety of data. The resulting health data and information can then be used for planning by both public health units and district health councils, as well as other community agencies.
- The model focuses on the assessment of community health (encompassing health and wellness and measures of disease burden) and not on the provision of health services. Indicators are drawn from a number of sources to provide measures of the broader determinants of health and to capture aspects of the economic, physical, and social environment. Indicators were either included, modified, or excluded in the model based on the availability of data valid at various levels, with the objective of providing a sampling of indicators across the broad spectrum of health.
- Produced as part of the Community Health Framework Project by the Ontario Ministry of Health.
- It is anticipated the document will be used at the health intelligence unit level as a basis for developing regional status reports. Additional indicators (e.g., those related to crime, etc.) will be added to provide a broad picture of each region.

SE Toronto Health Profiles Project 1994

- Main objective is to produce understandable, useful, and timely information on the health of the population of southeast Toronto. A series of working papers has been designed as the basis of an ongoing discussion with users of health information.

- The diverse population groups living in southeast Toronto are profiled in a series of working papers which examine patterns of hospitalization by census tract (*Working Report No.1, Patterns of Morbidity*), demographic and socioeconomic factors (*Working Report No. 2, Sociodemographic Profiles*), and health care needs in relation to demographic and socioeconomic factors (*Working Report No. 3, Sociodemographic Factors Associated with Hospitalization*). Additional papers are being developed. Differences among the 28 census tracts in southeast Toronto are investigated using 1991 Canadian census data and the Canadian Institute for Health Information data for hospital usage (HMRI data in first report).

- Produced by the Wellesley Hospital Research Institute. Support and assistance provided by the city of Toronto Department of Public Health and the administration of the Wellesley Hospital. Funding provided by grants from the Pan American Health Organization and the Wellesley Hospital Urban Health Initiative.

- The working papers have been used by the health and social agencies of southeast Toronto and Wellesley Hospital to determine the needs of the population in the area. Wellesley Hospital has used the information to indicate to government the importance of inpatient services for the community as opposed to a transfer of hospital services to ambulatory care as recommended by the District Health Council. In addition, links have been established with the University of Toronto to use the data in the development of an advanced geographic information system.

User's Guide to 40 Community Health Indicators 1992
(Also Referred to as CHIS Indicators)

- Main objective is to promote the development of community health information systems and improve decision making on health services and programs by providing accurate information and appropriate guidelines to assist in the interpretation of indicators commonly used in community health. The document is intended to establish standards for future publications on indicators.

- Health indicators are described and presented in a reference framework in which conceptual, methodological, and practical aspects are clearly defined. The indicators cover various dimensions of health, which assist in the development of a health profile of a population. Summary information is divided into sections (i.e., determinants of health, health status, and consequences of health problems), providing definitions, interpretations, limitations and possible uses of, and references for, each indicator. Sources of data, the method of calculation, and the observed values for Quebec and Canada for selected years (where data are available) are included.

- Produced by workers in a number of community health departments in Quebec and published by Health Canada's Health Services and Promotion Branch in collaboration with the National Health Information Council and the Health Information Division of the Policy, Planning and Information Branch of Health Canada. The Community Health Division of the Health Services and Promotion Branch of the former Health and Welfare Canada provided technical and financial assistance.
- The document has been used by several health and social agencies and organizations, both within Quebec and across Canada, to assist in program planning and decisions related to health and social issues.

Les indicateurs de la politique québécoise de la santé et du bien-être 1995

- Major objective is to track Quebec's progress in meeting 19 objectives identified in the document, *Policy on Health and Well-Being*, published in 1992.
- Forty-five indicators pertaining to social adjustment, physical health, public health, mental health, and social integration are presented. The document includes both trend data and projections to the year 2002. Where data are available, comparative analyses across health and social regions are also presented. Graphs and tables are accompanied by interpretive comments in relation to the specific objective which the given indicators are addressing.
- Produced by the Direction générale de la planification et de l'évaluation, Ministère de la Santé et des Services sociaux, Gouvernement du Québec.

Le Québec comparé: indicateurs sanitaires, démographiques et socioéconomiques 1995

- Main objective is to present a broad picture of Quebec's health, demographic and socioeconomic status over time and in relation to other settings. It is intended to serve as a tool and reference for people working in, or involved with, the health care sector. In particular, it is intended to help policymakers make decisions about the best measures to improve the health of the population and the efficiency of the health care system.
- This work builds on the direction profiled in the 1992 document, *Policy on Health and Well-Being*; however, it is not directly tied to the 19 objectives outlined in that report. Instead, it presents a broader picture of the demographic and socioeconomic context, mortality, and resource use related to health, using recognized and accepted indicators. It focuses on addressing two perspectives: first, presenting data about how circumstances have changed over time and where Quebec now stands

and second, how Quebec compares to other Canadian provinces and regions as well as to other industrialized countries. The document contains tables and graphs with related interpretive text as well as conclusions that identify similarities and differences between Quebec and other jurisdictions.

- Produced by the Ministère de la Santé et des Services sociaux, Gouvernement du Québec.

Health Statistics Division (Formerly CCHI) Health Indicators 1994

- Main objective is to calculate, publish, and disseminate those indicators for which data are available to assist in decision making related to health planning, policies, and programs. It is intended that, as the indicator program evolves, it will prove useful in establishing health goals for the population and offer objective measures of their success.
- This work is an update of the *Canadian Centre for Health Information (CCHI) Indicators 1993*, which lists indicators together with their availability periods, quantifiers, and disaggregations. Both the 1993 and 1994 databases group indicators into four categories: health determinants, health status, health resources, and health resources utilization. The 1994 data are provided in three formats: hard-copy tables and graphs, a personal computer diskette database and the CANSIM database. In the hard-copy format each indicator is presented in a one-page summary, consisting of a table of figures for Canada, the provinces, and territories for the latest available year, a time series graph for Canada, and a detailed description of the indicator. For both computer retrieval options, a detailed data dictionary specifying disaggregation and category information has been provided. The 1996 update, which uses IVISION software and includes indicators derived from the National Population Health Survey, is planned for release in April 1996.
- Produced by the Health Statistics Division of Statistics Canada (formerly the Canadian Centre for Health Information [CCHI]).
- A representative from the Health Statistics Division of Statistics Canada reported that it is difficult to state how the indicators have been used; however, some market research has recently been completed to determine how to update and present the 1996 indicators for better use in health planning and program decisions.

Community Health Indicators: Definitions and Interpretations 1995 (Also Titled Health Status Indicators; Update of User's Guide to 40 Community Health Indicators [CHIS] 1992)

- Main objective is to provide theoretical and functional information on a broad range of population health indicators available at the national, provincial, and intraprovincial levels. It is designed to promote the use of common concepts, definitions, procedures, and standards in public health, as well as a core set of data/indicators for interjurisdictional comparison.

- This work is an extension of the *User's Guide to 40 Community Health Indicators 1992*. The number of indicators has been expanded from 40 to 60. Indicators relating to the environment, organization of health care, and the use of services have been added. The first section describes the conceptual and operational aspects of the indicators as well as the classification model and selection process. The second section consists of summary information about each indicator, including definitions, possible interpretations, limitations, and references. In addition, it contains the sources of data and method of calculation, and it updates observed values for Quebec and Canada with the most recent data (where available).
- Produced by the Working Group on Community Health Information Systems (CHIS) and Directions de la santé publique, Quebec. The Canadian Institute for Health Information (CIHI) provided financial support for the study and for distribution of the document.

Canadian Child Health Atlas 1995

- Main objective is to provide information on children's hospitalization patterns to health care providers, parents, caregivers, and policymakers. Investigating the determinants of morbidity and the use of health services should lead to improved interventions and policies to reduce identified differences and, in so doing, improve the health of all Canada's children.
- The leading causes of hospitalization among children (i.e., four hospital diagnostic groupings: all causes of hospitalization, respiratory illness, injuries, and gastrointestinal illness) are selected for mapping. In each province, a record is attributed to the census division in which the child lives. Each census division is categorized as to whether or not its observed hospitalization experience was significantly different from what would be expected if the all-Canada rate were applied to the census division. The maps then depict census divisions of each province coded in one of three ways: significantly lower than expected, not significantly different than expected, or significantly higher than expected.
- Produced by the Canadian Institute of Child Health (CICH), a national nonprofit organization dedicated to improving the overall health and well-being of children in Canada. Funding was provided by Health Canada.

Report Card on Health of Canadians: Technical Version October 1995
(Draft)

- Main objective is to report, for policymakers and the public, information on the current health status of Canadians within a health determinants framework. By strengthening public understanding about the broad determinants of health and increasing support for the population health approach, policymakers can subsequently develop comprehensive population health initiatives for a few key priorities that have the potential to improve the health of the overall population significantly.
- The report card incorporates 87 topics organized into two major sections: determinants of health (i.e., social and economic environment, physical environment, health services, individual coping strategies, knowledge and attitude, and lifestyle behaviours) and health status (i.e., well-being and function, disease and conditions, including mental health, and mortality and potential years of life lost). The data sources are derived from a range of statistics published in the 1990s, including the *National Population Health Survey*. The detailed technical report will provide health policymakers and program planners with a broad overview of health status, including temporal trends and provincial and international comparisons. A less-detailed, user-friendly report will be produced for distribution to the public, using a selection of key indicators from the technical report. The public version of the report was released in the fall of 1996.
- The Conference of Deputy Ministers of Health approved the work plan for the *Report Card on the Health of Canadians* as part of the business plan for the Advisory Committee on Population Health (ACPH). An ACPH subcommittee, with representatives from British Columbia, Ontario, Manitoba, Alberta, Health Canada, the Canadian Institute of Health Information and Statistics Canada, was formed to direct the Report Card project. Thomas Stephens and Associates was contracted to carry out the project, and Health Canada provided project management support.

The Truth about Where You Live—An Atlas for Action on Toxins and Mortality 1991

- Main objective is to transform complex and highly technical data on toxins and mortality into information that can be easily accessed, understood, and used for determining the extent of local environmental contamination and potential health effects. The maps and data are a starting place to assist local efforts to prevent toxic hazards and to minimize the health impact on the population.
- *The Truth about Where You Live* provides a comprehensive picture of communities across the United States that are suffering from dispro-

portionate shares of environmental contamination and death. Using computer mapping techniques, the book synthesizes over a hundred million pieces of data culled from government files. Each map displays geographic, pollution and mortality data, enabling the reader to see at a glance, where people are dying at rates significantly above national norms and where toxins may pose particular problems for the environment and human health.

- The atlas represents the culmination of five years of work at Public Data Access, Inc. (PDA), which was established to make government information more easily available to the general public. The work was funded by the contributions of the Deer Creek Foundation, Environmental Research Foundation, Grassroots Leadership, and a number of individual supporters of PDA. Various aspects of the database were developed as a result of work for the Association on American Indian Affairs, Inc., Clean Water Action Project, Commission for Racial Justice of the United Church of Christ, Council on Economic Priorities, Greenpeace USA, National Toxics Campaign, Michigan Public Interest Research Group, and the Radiation and Public Health Project.

Oregon Benchmarks 1994

- Main objective is to provide measurable indicators that can be used statewide to assess, guide, and monitor Oregon's progress toward broad strategic goals. Trends and problems are analyzed to facilitate the identification of priorities and policy decisions that will ensure a better future for Oregonians.
- The 1994 report (made to the 1995 state legislature) summarizes the need for a long-range vision, while focusing on acute and growing problems; reviews Oregon's strategic vision and core benchmarks that measure progress (core benchmark summary: promote family stability and capable people, enhance quality of life and the environment, and promote a strong, diverse economy); describes critical trends shaping Oregon; and identifies urgent benchmarks that require immediate work to stay focused on the long-term vision. There are 259 benchmark measures, divided and labelled as historical and target indicators. A description of the data sources for each benchmark is also included. The Oregon Progress Board reviews each indicator every two years. Based on the review and on substantial public comment, additions, deletions, and modifications to existing benchmarks are made.
- Produced by the Oregon Progress Board. Funding is provided by the State of Oregon Economic Development Department.

Review of Content Domains

In summarizing content areas covered by the set of information systems, it is clear that most provide information about regions and their associated demographic features (table 3). Where this information is provided, it receives major emphasis (i.e., several indicators were included), reflecting both an orientation toward regional comparisons and the relative ease of obtaining information for these indicators from Statistics Canada census data and provincial vital statistics registry information. Several systems did not contain such indicators, however, consistent with their major focus on issues other than regional comparisons. For instance, the British Columbia *Provincial Health Officer's Annual Report* and the Quebec report, *Les indicateurs de la politique québécoise de la santé et du bien-être*, can be characterized as emphasizing health goals rather than regional comparisons, while the 1994 *ICES Practice Atlas* is oriented toward issue-specific regional comparisons.

It is clear from reviewing table 3 that many systems provide information in content areas related to determinants of population health that are external to the health care system. Almost every health information system reviewed provides some emphasis on the social and economic environment that influences health, reflecting an emerging understanding of the importance of these issues, as well as data availability from Statistics Canada sources and provincial social services agencies. A smaller number of information systems contain indicators about the physical environment. Many of the systems reviewed derive indicators about health behaviours from population health survey information that is becoming increasingly available (e.g., the British Columbia *Provincial Health Officer's Annual Report*, the Ontario *Model for Community Health Profiles*, the Health Statistics Division Health Indicators and the CHIS *Community Health Indicators*). In addition, the draft *Report Card on the Health of Canadians* provides information about health knowledge and beliefs. The *Health of Calgarians* report is noteworthy in that it makes good use of both provincial and local surveys to provide a comprehensive set of indicators relating to the determinants of health that are external to the medical care system.

Health status is an area that also receives major emphasis in many of the information systems reviewed for this report. Across systems, the most consistently reported set of indicators is based on mortality data, reflecting

Key to initiatives for tables 3 and 4

Key	Initiative
A	*The Geography of Death: Mortality Atlas of British Columbia 1985–1989*
B	*A Report on the Health of British Columbians: Provincial Health Officer's Annual Report 1994*
C	*Mortality and Health Status in Vancouver: An Analysis by Neighbourhood Areas 1995**
D	*Health of Calgarians 1995*
E	*Community Profile System—Saskatchewan Health System Project 1995*
F	*Populis—The Manitoba Centre for Health Policy and Evaluation 1995*
G	*Patterns of Health Care in Ontario—ICES Practice Atlas 1994*
H	*A Model for Community Health Profiles—Ontario Public Health 1995*
I	*SE Toronto Health Profiles Project 1994*
J	*User's Guide to 40 Community Health (CHIS) Indicators, 1992*
K	*Les indicateurs de la politique québécoise de la santé et du bien-être 1995*
L	*Le Québec comparé : indicateurs sanitaires, démographiques et socioéconomiques 1995*
M	*Health Statistics Division Health Indicators 1994***
N	*Community Health Indicators: Definitions and Interpretations 1995**** (also titled *Health Status Indicators*)
O	*Canadian Child Health Atlas 1995*
P	*Report Card on the Health of Canadians: Technical Version* October 1995, draft
Q	*The Truth about Where You Live—An Atlas for Action on Toxins and Mortality 1991*
R	*Oregon Benchmarks 1994*

* Update of *Health Atlas*—Vancouver Health Department 1991. Relevant information from both reports included.

** Update of *CCHI Indicators 1993*. Relevant information from both reports included.

*** Update of *User's Guide to 40 Community Health (CHIS) Indicators, 1992* (J).

Table 3

Comparison of initiatives—Domains: On which of the following domains does the initiative focus?

DOMAINS	A	B	C	D	E	F	G	H	I
Regional and demographic information *(e.g., population size, population characteristics, land area)*	●			●	●	●		●	●
Determinants of population health external to the health care system									
Biological influences		*							
Social environment	O	●	●	●	●	●	O	●	●
Economic environment	O	●	●	●	●	●	O	●	●
Physical environment		●		●				●	
Health knowledge and beliefs				●					
Health behaviours		●		●				●	
Health status									
Self-assessed health status		O		O			O	●	
Functional status		O		O			O	●	
Morbidity		●		●		●	O		●
Mortality	●	●	●	●	●	●	●	●	
Use and cost of health care services									
Preventive		O		O		O			
Community				O	●				
Physician		O		O	●	●	O		
Allied professional									
Hospital		O		O	●	●	●	●	●
Personal care home					●	●			
Drugs					●	**	O		
Ambulance					●	O			
Supply and capacity of the health care system	●				●	●			
Health outcomes *(e.g., low birthweight, avoidable mortality)*	●	●	●	O	O	●		O	
Health care outcomes *(e.g., diabetic coma, diabetic limb amputation)*						**			

* Mentioned, no data. ** In development.
● Major emphasis   O Minor emphasis

Table 3 (cont.)

DOMAINS	INITIATIVES								
	J	K	L	M	N	O	P	Q	R
Regional and demographic information *(e.g., population size, population characteristics, land area)*	●		●	●	●		●	●	
Determinants of population health external to the health care system									
Biological influences									
Social environment	●	●	○	●	●		●	●	●
Economic environment	●		●	●	●		●	●	●
Physical environment					●		●	●	●
Health knowledge and beliefs							●		
Health behaviours	●	●	●	●	●		●		●
Health status									
Self-assessed health status	●			●	●		●		○
Functional status	●	●		●	●		●		
Morbidity	●	●	●	●	●	●	●		●
Mortality	●	●	●	●	●		●	●	●
Use and cost of health care services									
Preventive			○	○	●		●		●
Community								○	○
Physician				○	○		○		
Allied professional									
Hospital	●	○	●	●	●	●	●		
Personal care home									○
Drugs			○	○	●				
Ambulance									
Supply and capacity of the health care system			●	●	●			●	
Health outcomes *(e.g., low birthweight, avoidable mortality)*	○	○	○	○	○	○	○	●	
Health care outcomes *(e.g., diabetic coma, diabetic limb amputation)*									

● Major emphasis   ○ Minor emphasis

the relative availability of such information from provincial vital statistics registries. The second most frequently used set of health status indicators is based on measures of morbidity. Some of these are derived from survey sources and others from hospitalization data. Some information systems contain morbidity indicators derived from only the former source (e.g., the 1994 *ICES Practice Atlas*), some contain those derived from only the latter source (e.g., Populis, the Manitoba Centre for Health Policy and Evaluation system), while others contain indicators derived from both sources (e.g., the Ontario *Model for Community Health Profiles*, the CHIS *Community Health Indicators*, and the draft *Report Card on the Health of Canadians*). A number of health information systems also include self-assessed and functional measures of health status, which are based largely on survey data sources.

Across most of the systems reviewed for this report, there was relatively minor emphasis on the utilization content domain, in comparison to the determinants of health and health status domains. The only exception was in the area of hospital use, for which some systems have access to provincial administrative data systems and others have access to the summary information provided by provinces to Statistics Canada. Several information systems include indicators on the use of preventive services (such as mammography and pap smears), most of which are derived from population surveys. In contrast, very few systems compile indicators about use of community services (such as home care and community mental health services), largely related to problems with availability of data. Only a few systems report on the use of physicians, personal care homes, drugs, and ambulance services. Two systems, the Saskatchewan Community Profile System and Populis, the Manitoba Centre for Health Policy and Evaluation system, are notable for the comprehensiveness of use indicators that they contain. However, even these systems are missing indicators in important areas. Only two systems, the Manitoba system and the Health Statistics Division Health Indicators system contain data on costs. Finally, very few information systems contain information on supply and capacity of the health care system.

Relatively few reports explicitly consider health status indicators as an outcome of the determinants of population health. Several recent initiatives (e.g., the Ontario *Model for Community Health Profiles*, the 1995 CHIS *Community Health Indicators*, and the *Report Card on the Health of Canadians*) tend to group health status indicators in a section that follows an earlier one on determinants of health. While the frameworks used in these systems imply that health status is being considered as an outcome, there is little consideration given to which indicators within the health status domain provide the most meaningful information in this regard. Systems that focus on comparative mortality (i.e., the British Columbia *Mortality Atlas*, the Vancouver report on *Mortality and Health Status*, and the U.S. *Atlas for Action on Toxins and Mortality*) are much more explicit in their presentation of mortality as an outcome. Two other information systems place strong emphasis on links between determinants of health and various measures of health status: the British Columbia *Provincial Health Officer's Annual Report* and reports from the Manitoba Centre for Health Policy and Evaluation. The former focuses on broad determinants in relation to a number of health outcomes, while the latter focuses on measures of health status (and primarily mortality) as outcomes of socioeconomic and health care determinants. No systems currently provide indicators of outcomes that can be more directly related to medical care.

Linkages across Domains

Six of the 18 systems reviewed contain explicit analyses that compare indicators across two or more domains (table 4). Several of these systems conduct such analyses for only a subset of indicators derived from survey data (i.e., the *ICES Practice Atlas* and the Health Statistics Division Health Indicators). Others present such analyses across many of their indicators, based on having data that contain relevant indicators at the level of the individual- or ecological-level data that can be attributed to persons and used in population-based analyses (i.e., the Manitoba Centre for Health Policy and Evaluation system, the Vancouver *Mortality and Health Status* report and the *SE Toronto Health Profiles Project*). It is not clear whether some of the systems that focus primarily on describing indicators have been developed with the intention of emphasizing this aspect of analysis.

Comparative Focus

Some of the health information systems provide counts of events (table 3). All use rates, but surprisingly, not all use age- and sex-adjusted rates for comparative analysis. In particular, the Health Statistics Division Health Indicators are developed from aggregate counts of events provided at the provincial level; while mortality rates are standardized, utilization rates are not.

Table 4

Comparison of initiatives—Parameters

Parameters	Initiatives		
	A	B	C
LINKAGES ACROSS DOMAINS Are there linkages across major domains? If yes, across which ones?	No	SES x mortality Income x health behaviours and preventive use Education x self-assessed health status and activity limit	SES x mortality
COMPARATIVE FOCUS What measurement approaches does the initiative use?			
Counts		√	
Rates	√	√	√
Does the initiative highlight differences and similarities across populations?	Yes	Yes	Yes
Does it include comparative analysis of groups at risk? (*e.g., Aboriginal peoples, women, low SES*)	No	Yes	No
Does it provide comparisons at different levels?			
National		√	
Provincial	√	√	
Regional	√	√	√
Other small areas	√		√
Does it highlight trends over time?	No	Yes	Yes
Does it provide benchmarks?	No	No	No
REPORTING MECHANISM Does the initiative have a comprehensive reporting mechanism?	Yes	Yes	Yes
What type of reporting mechanism is used?			
Print	√	√	√
Electronic			

Table 4 (cont.)

Parameters	Initiatives		
	A	**B**	**C**
What type of reporting format is used?			
Tables	√	√	√
Figures, graphs	√	√	
Maps	√	√	√
How frequently are reports updated?			
One time only	√		
Serial updates		√	√

Parameters	Initiatives		
	D	**E**	**F**
LINKAGES ACROSS DOMAINS Are there linkages across major domains? If yes, across which ones?	No	No	Health need variables x use Sociodemographic factors x use
COMPARATIVE FOCUS What measurement approaches does the initiative use?			
Counts	√	√	
Rates	√	√	√
Does the initiative highlight differences and similarities across populations?	No	Yes	Yes
Does it include comparative analysis of groups at risk? (*e.g., Aboriginal peoples, women, low SES*)	No	No	No, but possible
Does it provide comparisons at different levels?			
National			
Provincial		√	√
Regional	√	√	√
Other small areas		√	√
Does it highlight trends over time?	Yes	Yes	Yes
Does it provide benchmarks?	No	No	No
REPORTING MECHANISM Does the initiative have a comprehensive reporting mechanism?	Yes	Yes	Yes

Table 4 (cont.)

Parameters	Initiatives		
	D	**E**	**F**
What type of reporting mechanism is used?			
Print	√		√
Electronic		√	√
What type of reporting format is used?			
Tables	√	√	√
Figures, graphs	√	√	√
Maps		√	√
How frequently are reports updated?			
One time only			
Serial updates	√	√	√

Parameters	Initiatives		
	G	**H**	**I**
LINKAGES ACROSS DOMAINS Are there linkages across major domains? If yes, across which ones?	Need variables x use Sociodemographic factors x use, need, age. Others.	No	Sociodemographic factors x hospitalization
COMPARATIVE FOCUS What measurement approaches does the initiative use?			
Counts			√
Rates	√	√	√
Does the initiative highlight differences and similarities across populations?	Yes	Not currently	Yes
Does it include comparative analysis of groups at risk? (*e.g., Aboriginal peoples, women, low SES*)	No	No	No
Does it provide comparisons at different levels?			
National			√
Provincial	√	√	√
Regional	√	√	√
Other small areas	√	√	
Does it highlight trends over time?	Minor emphasis	Yes	No
Does it provide benchmarks?	No	No	No

Table 4 (cont.)

Parameters	Initiatives		
	G	H	I
REPORTING MECHANISM Does the initiative have a comprehensive reporting mechanism?	Yes	Yes (main focus is describing indicators)	Yes (related series of reports)
What type of reporting mechanism is used?			
Print	√		√
Electronic		√	
What type of reporting format is used?			
Tables	√		√
Figures, graphs	√	√	√
Maps	√	√	√
How frequently are reports updated?			
One time only	√	√	√
Serial updates	Proposed	Proposed	Proposed

Parameters	Initiatives		
	J	K	L
LINKAGES ACROSS DOMAINS Are there linkages across major domains? If yes, across which ones?	No	No	No
COMPARATIVE FOCUS What measurement approaches does the initiative use?			
Counts			
Rates	√	√	√
Does the initiative highlight differences and similarities across populations?	Yes	Yes	Yes
Does it include comparative analysis of groups at risk? (e.g. Aboriginal peoples, women, low SES)	No	No	No

Table 4 (cont.)

Parameters	Initiatives		
	J	**K**	**L**
Does it provide comparisons at different levels?			
National	√		√
Provincial	√	√	√
Regional		√	
Other small areas			
Does it highlight trends over time?	Yes (for some indicators)	Yes	Yes
Does it provide benchmarks?	No	Yes	No
REPORTING MECHANISM Does the initiative have a comprehensive reporting mechanism?	Yes	Yes	Yes
What type of reporting mechanism is used?			
Print	√	√	√
Electronic			
What type of reporting format is used?			
Tables	√	√	√
Figures, graphs		√	√
Maps			
How frequently are reports updated?	Periodic reports with changes in indicators and format		
One time only		√	√
Serial updates		Proposed	

Parameters	Initiatives		
	M	**N**	**O**
LINKAGES ACROSS DOMAINS Are there linkages across major domains? If yes, across which ones?	Health behaviour x education Demographics x income (minor emphasis)	No	No
COMPARATIVE FOCUS What measurement approaches does the initiative use?			
Counts	√		
Rates	√	√	√
Does the initiative highlight differences and similarities across populations?	Yes	Yes	Yes

Table 4 (cont.)

Parameters	Initiatives		
	M	**N**	**O**
Does it include comparative analysis of groups at risk? (*e.g., Aboriginal peoples, women, low SES*)	No	No	Yes (children)
Does it provide comparisons at different levels?			
National	√	√	
Provincial	√	√	√
Regional		Possible	
Other small areas		Possible	√
Does it highlight trends over time?	Yes	Yes	No, but possible
Does it provide benchmarks?	No	No	No
REPORTING MECHANISM Does the initiative have a comprehensive reporting mechanism?	Yes	Yes	Yes
What type of reporting mechanism is used?			
Print	√	√	√
Electronic	√		
What type of reporting format is used?			
Tables	√	√	√
Figures, graphs	√		
Maps			√
How frequently are reports updated?			
One time only			√
Serial updates	√	√	

Parameters	Initiatives		
	P	**Q**	**R**
LINKAGES ACROSS DOMAINS Are there linkages across major domains? If yes, across which ones?	No	No	No
COMPARATIVE FOCUS What measurement approaches does the initiative use?			
Counts			
Rates	√	√	√

Table 4 (cont.)

Parameters	Initiatives		
	P	Q	R
Does the initiative highlight differences and similarities across populations?	Yes	Yes	No
Does it include comparative analysis of groups at risk? (*e.g., Aboriginal peoples, women, low SES*)	No	Yes	Yes
Does it provide comparisons at different levels?			
National	√		√
Provincial	√		√
Regional	Possible		Possible
Other small areas	Possible	√	
Does it highlight trends over time?	Yes	No	Yes
Does it provide benchmarks?	No	No	Yes
REPORTING MECHANISM Does the initiative have a comprehensive reporting mechanism?	Yes	Yes	Yes
What type of reporting mechanism is used?			
Print	√	√	√
Electronic			
What type of reporting format is used?			
Tables	√		√
Figures, graphs	√		
Maps		√	
How frequently are reports updated?			
One time only	√	√	
Serial updates			√

Most initiatives highlight differences and similarities across populations. Two of the information systems (*Health of Calgarians* and *Oregon Benchmarks*) focus on providing information for the area of interest and, hence, do not contain comparative observations. The third system that does not include comparative observations is the *Model for Community Health Profiles*, which focuses on describing indicators rather than providing information itself. Within systems that provide comparisons, a relatively small number provide comparative information for population groups considered to be at high risk. Some provide comparisons for only a few regions, while others focus on providing comparative indicators across many regions. Depending on information sources, systems have different capabilities in terms of reporting information at smaller levels of aggregation. Some systems clearly are only capable of providing comparative information at national and provincial levels. For instance, the data compiled by the Health Statistics Division are based on aggregate provincial-level data and cannot be broken down for smaller analyses. Systems that derive many of their indicators from survey data, such as the *Model for Community Health Indicators* and the *Community Health Indicators* system, are dependent on the adequacy of the sample for small area analysis. In national surveys, samples are usually drawn at a level adequate to support estimates at the provincial level, but not to provide stable estimates for smaller areas within provinces. Collecting survey data to support small area analysis is very expensive. Many systems include analyses of trend data over time. Only a few systems provide benchmarks or standards for measuring progress and performance.

Reporting Mechanism

All the systems reviewed have a comprehensive reporting mechanism. Only one system, the Saskatchewan Community Health Profile System, relies solely on an electronic format: summary tables are provided for storage on hard drives of users' personal computers. A second, the Health Statistics Division Health Indicators system, provides both print and electronic format reporting mechanisms. Most systems use a combination of tables, figures, and graphs to present information. Others have found mapping approaches to be useful. Many systems plan to provide updated reports and several have already produced multiple versions of reported information.

Role in Providing Evidence for Decision Making

An important aspect of the performance of these health information systems relates to the extent to which they have been found to play a useful role in the policy process. For many, such an assessment is premature, since they have had little experience "in the field." This includes the draft *Report Card on the Health of Canadians* which has not yet been released and the 1995 *Model for Community Health Profiles* project which provides information about indicators that can be used to develop community profiles and which contains no comparative information. It also includes the 1995 *Community Health Indicators* report, as well as the 1992 *User's Guide to 40 Community Health Indicators* (on which the 1995 report was based). These two reports both contain little comparative data and focus primarily on providing theoretical and functional information on a broad range of indicators. Their utility in contributing to the policy process has, therefore, not been well established. Many of the other information systems that have been available for a longer time have been received enthusiastically by decision makers. Subsequently, however, they have fallen short of expectations in terms of identifying appropriate levers for the policy process. Notable exceptions include the information systems and reports that have been developed in Quebec, in which information has been tightly linked to funding and service delivery perspectives, and the Populis system of the Manitoba Centre for Health Policy and Evaluation, which has been used to produce answers in response to specific policy questions.

Major Strengths and Weaknesses across Information Systems

All the information systems reviewed for this report have important strengths, many of which deserve consideration for implementation at a national level. Clearly, most have incorporated a population health focus. Several initiatives, notably the 1992 *User's Guide to 40 Community Health Indicators*, the 1995 *Community Health Indicators* report and the Ontario *Model for Community Health Profiles*, outline comprehensive sets of indicators for community health assessment. These initiatives have made great progress in expanding measurement of various dimensions of health and in enabling development of community health profiles. While there is substantial overlap in the content of these lists, there are also many differences. Nonetheless, these initiatives represent an important achievement in defining common approaches to measurement of determinants of health and health status indicators within a population health focus.

The draft *Report Card on the Health of Canadians* goes well beyond discussions of indicators. It contains provincial comparisons for a comprehensive set of indicators using recent data (i.e., 1990 to 1995). The *Health of Calgarians* report has demonstrated that individual regions can draw on local health surveys and obtain information from municipal and provincial agencies to develop comprehensive local community health profiles.

In spite of the progress made in comparative approaches to measuring health and the determinants of health, there has been little progress in measuring utilization of health care in most comprehensive frameworks. Indeed, the draft *Report Card on the Health of Canadians* (October 1995) acknowledges that, despite taking a deliberately broad and comprehensive approach to the selection of indicators, the report contains relatively few indicators that describe the resources and costs of the health care delivery system, because "these fall under close and continuous scrutiny in other programs." In fact, the provincial comparisons that are compiled for the Health Statistics Division Health Indicator system (and incorporated into the Report Card) are not useful for comparative analysis because they have not been age- and sex-adjusted. However, while usage and costs, as well as supply and capacity issues, have received little emphasis in the new comprehensive frameworks, information systems that focus on using administrative data, such as the Manitoba Centre for Health Policy and Evaluation system and the *ICES Practice Atlas*, have developed expanded capabilities to conduct small area analyses of important aspects of usage.

Mortality atlas approaches, such as the British Columbia *Mortality Atlas*, the Vancouver *Mortality and Health Status Atlas*, and the U.S. *Atlas for Action on Toxins* show the power of mortality data to highlight large differences in health outcomes across populations at the subprovincial level. Similarly, the Manitoba Centre for Health Policy and Analysis system found premature mortality to be one of the most powerful measures of health status for demonstrating regional differences. Because of the compelling nature of death as an outcome measure, all of these systems have found mortality differences to be extremely useful for raising questions about the determinants of observed differences.

Several systems have demonstrated the power of conducting explicit analyses that compare indicators across two or more domains, especially those involving health status. The Vancouver *Mortality and Health Status Atlas* has demonstrated powerful relationships between socioeconomic circumstances and mortality outcomes within the city. Using only data from the Ontario Health Survey sample, the *ICES Practice Atlas* demonstrated strong relationships between health status and reported usage of health services. The SE Toronto Health Profiles Project has used information about socioeconomic risk to address issues related to needs for inpatient care during an era of hospital bed closures. By virtue of compiling comparative data at the level of eight regions, the Manitoba Centre for Health Policy and Evaluation has been able to look at important questions about the relationship of social and economic circumstances to health and the relationship between socioeconomic risk and use of health care services. The British Columbia *Provincial Health Officer's Annual Report* also contains many compelling analyses across domains, with a focus on analyzing and understanding indicators in the context of a population health framework.

The Saskatchewan Community Profile System has demonstrated that useful profiles can be developed across multiple subprovincial regions and, more important, that the boundaries for areas covered can be configured to be relevant to regional health authorities that are assuming responsibility for resource allocation. The *Canadian Child Health Atlas* has demonstrated that it is possible to develop small area comparative analyses of hospital-based morbidity at a national level.

Other systems have demonstrated the strengths of measuring trends over time (*Le Québec comparé*) and of measuring progress towards goals (*Les indicateurs de la politique québécoise de la santé et du bien-être*, and the *Oregon Benchmarks* project). The U.S. *Atlas for Action on Toxins and Mortality* shows that there is much that can be done to further our understanding of the impact of the physical environment as an important determinant of population health. The *Canadian Child Health Atlas* suggests that there is potential for developing comprehensive comparative national information systems that focus on vulnerable populations. Reports such as *Le Québec comparé* and the British Columbia *Provincial Health Officer's Annual Report* demonstrate the usefulness of integrating regional and provincial comparisons with relevant national and international references.

Finally, some systems have stronger track records than others in providing information that can be useful to the policy process. These include initiatives from Quebec and Manitoba.

DISCUSSION

This report has reviewed a number of health information systems to describe their characteristics and to identify their strengths and weaknesses, with particular emphasis on determining their potential to contribute to the policy process. There are some limitations to the review, since the 18 health information systems identified do not necessarily represent a comprehensive set of Canadian initiatives currently under way. Some important initiatives may have been overlooked. Moreover, by focusing only on systems that are up and running and currently providing information, this report has not been able to consider systems and approaches that are at an even more preliminary stage of development. Several of these, especially the data systems being developed to manage provincial health care systems, have the potential to contribute vastly more powerful data sets to underpin future health information systems. In spite of these limitations, the initiatives reviewed represent a relevant sample in terms of the lessons to be learned and the implications for approaches that could prove useful for wider implementation.

Findings in Relation to Objectives

Objective 1

In addition to the specific findings of this report, summarized in the previous section, one very important finding was the discovery that a great deal of activity is being spent in the development and implementation of information systems across the country. A total of 52 initiatives were identified, of which 18 were classified as population-based information systems, representing a tremendous investment of national energy and resources.

Detailed analysis of the 18 health information systems revealed that they have very different "personalities." While all have adopted a population health framework for presentation of indicators, each uses this framework in a somewhat different manner. Furthermore, there are also many differences in the way indicators are used within these frameworks. Some of these differences relate to selection of indicators (e.g., which of the many measures of income available from census data are used for describing income distribution) and others relate to selection of cut-points for creating indicators. This has resulted in a set of approaches that use slightly different frameworks composed of slightly different indicators across different Canadian settings. The emerging patchwork of information does not support understanding of population health from a national perspective. The draft *Report Card on the Health of Canadians* scheduled for release in the fall of 1996 will address some of these issues, but has additional weaknesses (see below).

An additional summary observation from the review is that in adopting a population health framework, most of the information systems have focused more directly on measuring health status and the determinants of health that fall outside of the medical care system than has previously been possible. One result of this emphasis is that aspects of use of medical care and elaboration of the contribution of medical care to population health remain underdeveloped in all but a few of the initiatives. This has implications for policy relevance (see below).

Objective 2

During this review, it became apparent that most of the 18 initiatives were at a very early stage in developing links to support decision making. In particular, the usefulness of information systems to inform policy decision making around population health initiatives could not be assessed because many of the systems have not had adequate time to demonstrate it. Many of the current initiatives are clearly able to provide an increasing focus on important health outcomes, but there has been concern among policymakers that they may fall short in terms of identifying appropriate policy levers. Several do not include information about health services use and resource consumption, which are clearly very important issues to policymakers. Where health information systems do include indicators of usage, these are often not presented in a format that supports consideration of policy options. Furthermore, elaboration of the relative contributions of nonmedical and medical care factors in influencing health status have not been clearly laid out. Only two of the initiatives stand out in terms of how they link to and support policy and planning processes. These are the information systems and reports that have been developed in Quebec, in which information has been tightly linked to funding and service delivery perspectives, and the Populis system of the Manitoba Centre for Health Policy and Evaluation, which has been used to produce answers in response to specific policy questions.

It is clear that much remains to be learned about how to make health information systems relevant to the policy process. It appears that several characteristics are central to a system's ability to support the decision-making process. These include a focus on comparative analysis across planning areas, with analyses to highlight an understanding of the relative contributions of nonmedical and medical care inputs to health, and the linkage of information to current funding and delivery perspectives. Finally, flexibility to provide focused responses to well-articulated policy questions enhances a system's capability to contribute meaningful information from the perspective of policymakers. Over time, different types of evidence will likely be required from health information systems to support policy decision making. These will probably include pre- and postevaluations of policy changes as well as comparisons of effects across jurisdictions that have made fundamentally different choices in implementing initiatives to improve health. Models based on current information systems clearly will not be able to provide all the answers. Additional information will be required from more rigorous study of the determinants of health based on different methods and data. However, this review has highlighted the importance of encouraging continued and future development of information systems that can support policy decision making. As members of the "Evidence-Based Decision Making" working group are aware, we are clearly only beginning to provide robust evidence to the policy process.

Objective 3

This review strongly supports the need for a national initiative to permit assessment of population health and to provide information to support important policy decisions that face a country trying to maximize the health of its population. Such an initiative should clearly draw on the strengths of various systems that have been reviewed for this report and to some extent, build on work already done. Such an initiative should be national in scope, with a major focus on providing information to support decision making at national, provincial, and regional jurisdictional levels. It should provide population-based information within a comprehensive population health framework, meaning that emphasis should be placed on providing information about determinants of health that fall both within and outside of the health care system. Initially, there should be a focus on conducting comparative analyses of indicators to highlight differences and similarities across populations, using relevant policy and program (i.e., geographic) jurisdictions. Because provinces have different capabilities in terms of available data, the initiative should be flexible enough to accommodate different strengths and weaknesses. Finally, it should link information to funding and service delivery perspectives to provide information about policy directions that arise from a population health perspective.

The draft *Report Card on the Health of Canadians* has taken an important step in this direction. It has compiled cross-provincial comparative data for a comprehensive set of indicators using a framework of population health, thereby elaborating a more comprehensive set of provincial profiles than has previously been available. However, in emphasizing population health, the draft Report Card has highlighted comparisons of health states and health determinants that fall outside the health care system, with less development of indicators of usage of health care. The relative weakness of this area means that this initiative, in its current format, will not support important linkage questions about what relationship there is, if any, between various measures of health status and use at the provincial level. This is, potentially, an area in which provinces that have greater data availability and analytic capability could provide a more robust set of comparative provincial utilization indicators. At a minimum, comparative indicators of use in the draft Report Card could be age- and sex-standardized, even if only indirect methods were to be used. The review of information systems conducted for this report suggests that many additional useful indicators of comparative hospital usage could be developed: all the information systems reviewed incorporated measures of hospital utilization, and the *Canadian Child Health Atlas* (and Statistics Canada) conducted a national comparative analysis using a combination of discharge summaries from the Canadian Institute for Health Information and the Quebec Medécho system. Similar work could be done to provide more robust hospital usage data as a companion to the comprehensive set of indicators in other areas of the Report Card. This more comprehensive set of measures (i.e., that includes use) could address important questions about linkages between social and economic circumstances, health status and use of hospital services at the provincial level, using the approach taken in the Manitoba Centre for Health Policy and Evaluation Populis system as a model. Provinces that have capabilities to refine comparative indicators of other aspects of use (e.g., physician and personal care home services) and of supply, capacity, and costs could be supported to develop these indicators for similar comparative analyses.

One of the most important areas in which there is a need for national capability is the development of community profiles congruent with boundaries used by regional decision-making bodies. While the jury is still out as to how comprehensive community profiles must be to provide information that is useful for managing the system, it is clear from this review that the ingredients are present to develop powerful regional profiles across the nation. Existing data sources such as the census, provincial vital statistics registries, and hospital usage data from the Canadian Institute for Health Information and the Quebec Medécho system, provide data that can be configured at the levels of both provincial and regional health authorities. Many important indicators pertaining to social, economic, and physical environment factors that are important determinants of health can be put into operation across the nation using existing data. Premature mortality, life expectancy, and potential years of life lost can be developed using a combination of vital statistics and census data. Finally, comparative and standardized measures of hospital usage data can be developed to highlight many different aspects.

Experience with the Manitoba Centre for Health Policy and Evaluation system has suggested that configurations of regional data provide powerful information for managing the system, even if only hospital data are used. If more comprehensive profiles are ultimately required for regional health planning, putting in place a set of comparative indicators across the nation would provide a powerful tool for interim planning. Since experience in this area has been developed using comparisons from a few areas, expanding the scope to include all regional authorities across the country would likely strengthen or challenge conclusions drawn in the series of reports from the Manitoba Centre.

In terms of presentation, the availability of a comprehensive reporting mechanism in electronic as well as print format is likely to be useful and to decrease distribution costs. A large number of summary tables can be made available through electronic means of distribution with no threat to the privacy of confidential information. As well, mapping techniques provide useful approaches to conveying complex information about regional variation.

In structuring the information system, emphasis should be placed on analytic comparisons and interpretation of comparative data. It is clear that much work has gone into developing individual health information systems. On the other hand, the systems that appear to be having an influence are those that present comparative data in an integrated format that raises issues from the perspective of population health. Integrated and comparative analysis across the nation would likely be beneficial to advancing concepts of using evidence to support decision making in a manner that is congruent with a population health framework.

Over the longer term, other approaches deserve emphasis. These encompass measuring trends over time, measuring progress toward goals, and including international comparative data. In addition, emphasis deserves to be placed on developing comprehensive, comparative national information systems that focus on vulnerable populations such as children, Aboriginal peoples, and persons living in poverty. Other analyses that could be conducted include pre- and postevaluations of major reforms and comparisons of effects across jurisdictions that have chosen different policy options to address population health. Finally, experience regarding which approaches provide the most useful information for the decision-making process to support improvements in population health at various levels of jurisdiction (i.e., federal, provincial, and regional authority) should be assessed.

Objective 4

The differing personalities of the 18 health information systems reviewed for this report reflect different data capabilities, conceptual models, and perceived requirements for information. While it is possible to identify general approaches that might consolidate and build on some of these systems for implementation of a national initiative, cooperation and partnerships will be required to move such an agenda forward.

RECOMMENDATIONS

As discussed, there is a very high level of activity being invested in the development of information systems. Much of the focus is on data collection and the development of indicators, while paying less attention to understanding the needs of decision makers for information to manage the health system. The importance of tailoring information in a manner that is responsive to important policy questions is an important direction for development. Moreover, it is fitting that the "Evidence-Based Decision Making" working group should be actively encouraging such a direction.

Recommendation 1

It is recommended that the National Forum on Health champion investment in information systems that go beyond data warehousing and are designed to provide evidence to support policy and health services decision making within the context of a population health perspective.

This review strongly supports the need for a national initiative to permit assessment of population health and to provide information to support important policy decisions that face a country trying to maximize the health of its population. Such an initiative should clearly draw on the strengths of various systems that have been reviewed for this report and, to some extent, build on work already done. Such an initiative should be national in scope, with a major focus on providing information to support decision making at national, provincial, and regional jurisdictional levels. It should provide population-based information within a comprehensive population health framework, meaning that emphasis should be placed on providing information about determinants of health that fall both within and outside the health care system. Initially, there should be a focus on conducting comparative analyses of indicators to highlight differences and similarities across populations, using relevant policy and program (i.e., geographic) jurisdictions. Because provinces have different capabilities in terms of available data, the initiative should be flexible enough to accommodate different strengths and weaknesses. Finally, it should link information to funding and service delivery perspectives in order to provide information about policy directions that arise from a population health perspective. The National Forum on Health has the capability to argue for a national approach to enhance understanding of population health and identification of the policy options that are available to address differences in the health of Canadians and to contribute to overall improvements in population health.

Recommendation 2

It is recommended that the National Forum on Health encourage and support the development of a national population-based health policy information network.

Such an initiative should draw on the best aspects of systems that have been developed and have proven useful in the policy process, but should be flexible enough to incorporate strengths from emerging initiatives. A modular approach, as outlined in table 5, would permit development of a core set of analyses for all jurisdictions at both the provincial and regional authority levels, but would also support development of more in-depth comparative analyses, depending on data availability and interests. After production of an initial report, information should be updated and a new report produced on a regular basis, possibly every two or three years, to monitor change over time.

Table 5

Modular approach to development of a national population-based health policy information network

Data source and comparative focus	Level of analysis	
	Province	Regional authority
Survey-based measures	Core (from Report Card)	Optional
Vital statistics–derived measures	Core (from Report Card)	Core
Census-based measures	Core (from Report Card)	Core
Measures derived from provincial administrative data:		
Hospital services	Core	Core
Personal care home services	Optional	Optional
Physician services	Optional	Optional
Drug use	Optional	Optional
Physician supply	Optional	Optional

Clearly, cooperation and partnerships will be required to launch such an initiative. Consideration must be given to the interests of groups that have been involved in developing information systems, as well as those of decision makers at regional, provincial, and federal levels. Ideally, a national initiative should be developed in a manner that is cognizant of the priorities and specificities of different jurisdictions, but also coordinated to maximize usefulness in terms of comparability and to minimize duplication.

In this review, four options were identified in considering who should assume responsibility for conducting and supporting such a project. First, Statistics Canada may have the resources to undertake initiatives in this area but, arguably, this project may not sit well within its mandate. The Canadian Institute for Health Information (CIHI) clearly has a mandate that is more congruent with this activity, but concerns have been expressed about its ability to be responsive to provincial policy needs for information. A third potential option would be to support cooperative work among some of the applied health services research units across the country (Centre for Health Services and Policy Research at the University of British Columbia, the Manitoba Centre for Health Policy and Evaluation at the University of Manitoba, the Institute for Clinical and Evaluative Sciences and the Health Intelligence Units in Ontario, the Interdisciplinary Research Group on Health and researchers from Laval University, Quebec City and the Population Health Research Unit at Dalhousie University), and ministries of health in remaining provinces. This option is likely to be difficult to launch unless one group were to take leadership and obtain some specific funding to undertake the initial project. As a fourth option, the Federal/Provincial/ Territorial Conference of Deputy Ministers of Health could be encouraged to support such an initiative, modelled on the approach used to support the development of the draft *Report Card on the Health of Canadians*. For this report, the Conference of Deputy Ministers approved the work plan as part of the business plan for the Advisory Committee on Population Health (ACPH), which is advisory to the former. An ACPH subcommittee, with representatives from British Columbia, Ontario, Manitoba, Alberta, Health Canada, the Canadian Institute for Health Information (CIHI), and Statistics Canada was formed to direct the project. An independent consulting group was contracted to carry out the project, with Health Canada providing project management support. A similar process led by the Conference of Deputy Ministers might provide a strong mechanism to support the partnerships required to launch such a project as well as to ensure its policy relevance. In this case, the National Forum on Health could petition to make a representation to the Conference of Deputy Ministers to outline the need for, and possibilities associated with, a national population-based health policy information network. Development of a first report through this mechanism would likely benefit from input of both the ACPH as well as the Advisory Committee on Health Services, both of which are advisory to the Federal/Provincial/Territorial Conference of Deputy Ministers of Health.

Charlyn Black, *M.D., Sc.D., is an associate professor in the Department of Community Health Sciences, Faculty of Medicine, University of Manitoba. She is a senior researcher and codirector of the Manitoba Centre for Health Policy and Evaluation. Her current research interests focus on applications of population-based information systems, the use of administrative data to assess and monitor quality, effectiveness and outcomes of medical interventions, and the development of data-driven information tools to inform and improve physician practice.*

Acknowledgements

The author wishes to thank the National Forum on Health for financial support to this project as well as the thoughtful direction and comments provided by the "Evidence-Based Decision Making" working group.

Many individuals and organizations took the time to respond to questions about the initiatives in which they are involved. Their contribution in time, energy, and ideas is much appreciated.

In particular, the author wishes to acknowledge the tremendous contribution of Mary Thliveris to this report. As project manager, she made numerous contacts with individuals, facilitated my understanding of 52 initiatives, organized information, wrote descriptions of several information systems, and orchestrated production of the final report.

Finally, advice about policy considerations from Ulrich Wendt, senior policy advisor to Manitoba Health is greatly appreciated.

BIBLIOGRAPHY

EVANS R. G., and G. L. STODDART. 1990. Producing health, consuming health care. *Social Science Medicine* 31(12): 1347–1363.

FRANK, J. W. 1995. The determinants of health: A new synthesis. *Current Issues in Public Health* 1: 233–240.

ROOS, N. P., C. M. BLACK, N. FROHLICH, C. DECOSTER, M. COHEN, D. J. TATARYN C. A. MUSTARD, L. L. ROOS, F. TOLL, K. C. CARRIERE, C. A. BURCHILL, L. MACWILLIAM, and B. BOGDANOVIC. 1996. Population health and health care use : An information system for policy makers. *Millbank Quarterly* 74(1): 3–31.

APPENDICES

APPENDIX 1

Key Contacts for Initiatives

BRITISH COLUMBIA

Guy Costanzo
Research Officer
Vancouver Health Department

Harold Foster
Geography Department
University of Victoria

John Millar
Provincial Health Officer
Province of British Columbia

SASKATCHEWAN

Neil Gardner
Executive Director
Corporate Information and
Technology Branch
Saskatchewan Health

Valerie Phillips
Senior Analyst
Strategic Programs Branch
Saskatchewan Health

ALBERTA

Brent Friesen
Medical Officer of Health
Calgary Public Health Unit

Heather Holly
Department of Community Health
Sciences
University of Calgary

James Howell
Medical Officer of Health and
Vice-President, Public Health
Services
Edmonton

Mamoru Watanabe
Health Sciences Centre
Faculty of Medicine
University of Calgary

MANITOBA

Joel Kettner
Department of Community Health
Sciences
Faculty of Medicine, University of
Manitoba

Cam Mustard
Manitoba Centre for Health Policy
and Evaluation
Department of Community Health
Sciences
Faculty of Medicine, University of
Manitoba

Noralou Roos
Director
Manitoba Centre for Health Policy
and Evaluation
Department of Community Health
Sciences
Faculty of Medicine, University of
Manitoba

Evelyn Shapiro
Manitoba Centre for Health Policy
and Evaluation
Department of Community Health
Sciences
Faculty of Medicine, University of
Manitoba

ONTARIO

Lawrence Chambers
Department of Epidemiology and
Biostatistics
McMaster University

Richard Glazier
Clinical Epidemiology Division
Wellesley Hospital Research Institute

John Hoey
Public Director (interim)
Health Intelligence Unit for Eastern

Neil Johnston
Faculty of Health Sciences
McMaster University

David Naylor
Institute for Clinical Evaluative
Sciences

George Pasut
Ontario Public Health Unit
Ontario Ministry of Health

Anne Premi
Manager, Community Health
Frame Work Project
Ontario Ministry of Health

Mark Speechley
London and Western Ontario
Health Intelligence Unit
University of Western Ontario
Medical School

Pat Stuckless
Information, Planning and
Evaluation Branch
Ontario Ministry of Health

George Torrance
Centre for Health Economics
and Policy Analysis
McMaster University

Evelyn Vingilis
Department of Population
and Community Health
University of Western Ontario
Medical School

QUEBEC
Francois Béland
Professor
Département d´administration de la
santé
Université de Montréal, GRIS
Faculté de médecine

Lorraine Bernier
Régie régionale de la santé et des
services sociaux de Montréal-Centre

Pierre Cliche
Directeur général par intérim de la
planification et de l'évaluation
Gouvernement du Québec
Ministère de la Santé et des Services
sociaux

Jean-Pierre Duplantie
Director General
Régie régionale de la santé et des
services sociaux de l'Estrie

NEW BRUNSWICK
Jean-Claude Hache
Director of Information Systems
Ministry of Health

PRINCE EDWARD ISLAND
Wayne Hooper
CIHI Representative, PEI

NOVA SCOTIA
George Kephart
Department of Community Health
and Epidemiology
Dalhousie University

Dan Rice
Policy Planning
Nova Scotia Department of Health

Brenda Ryan
Director
Research, Statistics and Evaluation
Nova Scotia Department of Health

NEWFOUNDLAND
Elizabeth Davis
Health System Information Task
Force, Chair

Jorge Segovia
Division of Community Medicine
Memorial University of
Newfoundland

Other Canadian

Canadian Institute of Health
Information
Ottawa, Ontario

Robert Evans
Director of Population Health
Canadian Institute for Advanced
Research

Deirdre Gillieson/Lorna Bailie
Health Statistics Division of
Statistics Canada

Matthew J. Hodge
Child Health Atlas

Francine Leduc
Seniors Independent Research
Program
Division of Aging and Seniors
Health Canada

Cecilie Lord, Chair
National Advisory Committee on
Population Health

Ivan Pless
Child Health Atlas

Michael Wolfson
Director General
Statistics Canada

U.S.A.

John A. Hartford Foundation
CHMIS

Benjamin Goldman
Atlas for Action

James Mason
Healthy People 2000

Duncan Wyse
Oregon Benchmarks

APPENDIX 2

Initiatives Considered for Review

Province	Initiative	Contact person	Report status
BRITISH COLUMBIA	The Geography of Death: Mortality Atlas of British Columbia 1985–1989	Harold Foster	Book received
	User's Guide—Operational Indicators for Community Health Programs 1993	CHIS NHIC	Report received
	A Report on the Health of British Columbians—Provincial Health Officer's Annual Report 1994 (1995 report forthcoming)	John Millar	Report received
	Mortality and Health Status in Vancouver: An Analysis by Neighbourhood Areas 1995 (update of Vancouver Health Atlas 1991	Guy Costanzo	Report received
ALBERTA	Healthy Edmonton 2000—Goals Project 1992	James Howell	Report received
	Health of Calgarians 1995	Brent Friesen	Report received
	Alberta Health Survey 1995	Mamoru Watanabe	Information received
	Psychiatry Database: An Integrated Information System 1996	Heather Holly	Report received
SASKATCHEWAN	Needs-Based Allocation of Resources to Saskatchewan Health Districts 1994–1995	Valerie Phillips	Report received
	Community Profile System—Saskatchewan Health System Project 1995	Neil Gardner	Report received
MANITOBA	Populis—The Manitoba Centre for Health Policy and Evaluation 1995	Noralou Roos	Book received
	Manitoba Population Health Assessment Template 1995	Joel Kettner	Report received
ONTARIO	Ontario Health Survey 1990	Ontario Ministry	Information received
	Information Products and Tools—Information to District Health Councils 1993–1995	Pat Stuckless	Report received

Appendix 2 (cont.)

Province	Initiative	Contact person	Report status
ONTARIO (cont.)	*Patterns of Health Care in Ontario—ICES Practice Atlas 1994*	David Naylor	Report received
	POHEM Project—work in progress	Michael Wolfson	Information received
	McMaster Comprehensive Health Status Measurement System (Mark III)/Proposed Population Health Index 1995	George Torrance Michael Wolfson	Information received
	A Model for Community Health Profiles—Ontario Public Health 1995 (draft report)	Anne Premi	Draft report received
	HELPS Initiative—pilot project	George Pasut	Information received
	Geographic Information Management System—work in progress	Neil Johnston	Information received
	SE Toronto Health Profiles Project 1994	Richard Glazier	Report received
QUEBEC	*Quebecers in the Quebec Health and Social Survey 1992*	Santé Québec	Information received
	Politique de la santé et du bien-être 1992	Report not available for review	
	Policy on Health and Well-Being 1992	Ministère de la Santé et des Services sociaux	Report received
	User's Guide to 40 Community Health 1992 (CHIS Indicators)	Lorraine Bernier	Report received
	Les coûts relatifs de production et l'équité interrégionale – cadre conceptuel et révision méthodologique 1994	Jean-Pierre Duplantie	Report received
	L'équité dans l'allocation interrégionale des ressources du champ de la santé physique 1994	Jean-Pierre Duplantie	Report received
	Des indicateurs de besoins pour l'allocation interrégionale des ressources 1995	Jean-Pierre Duplantie	Report received
	Les indicateurs de la politique québécoise de la santé et du bien-être 1995	Lorraine Bernier	Report received

Appendix 2 (cont.)

Province	Initiative	Contact person	Report status
QUEBEC (cont.)	Le Québec comparé: indicateurs sanitaires, démographiques et socioéconomiques 1995	Pierre Cliche	Report received
NEW BRUNSWICK	Health Status Reports 1988 and 1994 (1996 mandated by deputy minister)	Jean-Claude Hache	Information requested
	Resource Allocation Model for Family Community and Social Services 1995	Chris Robinson	Report received
NOVA SCOTIA	Report Card on Health 1995	George Kephart Dan Rice Brenda Ryan	Information received
	NS Health Survey 1995		
	Health Information Technology Initiative 1995		
PRINCE EDWARD ISLAND	Island Health Information System 1993–1996	Wayne Hooper	Information received
	Health Indicator Resource Project 1995—presented to Atlantic Regional Health Indicators Conference	Information received from Kayla Estrin	Report received
NEWFOUNDLAND	Requested information on systems	Jorge Segovia	Information received
	Improved Health for Newfoundland and Labrador through Improved Health Information 1995	Elizabeth Davis	Report received
	The Way Forward—Health Information Systems Vision 1995	Elizabeth Davis	Report received
ATLANTIC REGION	Atlantic Regional Health Indicators Conference 1995	Informatiom received from Kayla Estrin	Report received
OTHER CANADIAN	Health Information for Canada: Report of the National Task Force on Health Information 1991	Martin Wilk NHIC	Report received
	Canadian Centre for Health Information (CCHI) Indicators 1993	Deirdre Gillieson M.C. Ryan	Information received

Appendix 2 (cont.)

Province	Initiative	Contact person	Report status
OTHER CANADIAN (cont.)	*Comparative Analysis of the CCHI Health Indicators and CHIS Health Indicator Guidelines 1993*	M.C. Ryan	Report received
	Health Statistics Division (formerly CCHI) *Health Indicators 1994* (update of CCHI Indicators 1993; further update for release in 1996)	Deirdre Gillieson Statistics Canada	Report received
	Community Health Indicators: Definitions and Interpretations 1995 (also titled *Health Status Indicators*; update of *User's guide to 40 Community Health Indicators 1992*; CHIS Indicators)	CIHI CHIS	Report received
	Canadian Child Health Atlas 1995	Matthew J. Hodge/Ivan Pless	Report received
	Use and Impact of Information Technologies in Health (External Version)—A Report to Health Programs and Promotions Branch 1995	Health Canada	Report received
	Report Card on the Health of Canadians: Technical Version October 1995—draft (planned release September 1996)	Cecilie Lord John Millar	Draft report received
U.S.A.	*The Truth about Where You Live—An Atlas for Action on Toxins and Mortality 1991*	Benjamin Goldman	Book received
	Healthy People 2000— National Health Promotion and Disease Prevention Objectives 1991	James Mason	Report received
	Community Health Management Information System 1992	John A. Hartford Foundation	Report received
	Oregon Benchmarks 1994	Duncan Wyse	Report received

Foundations for Evidence-Based Decision Making

ROBERT B. BUTCHER, PH.D.

Professor
University of Western Ontario

SUMMARY

Evidence is the information used in making a decision or judgement or in solving a problem. The nature of evidence is as varied as the situations in which it is used. Beyond the well-known and readily accepted rules of deductive and inductive logic, what counts as good evidence varies by decision type, academic discipline, the values and objectives of the decision maker, the context, and so on.

In the field of health care, almost all decisions have a values component. Where resources are scarce, every decision to do one thing has a corresponding consequence of not doing something else, implying that the action chosen is valued more highly than the option rejected. Not to make a decision at all also reflects certain values.

Evidence used in supporting values decisions is quite different to that used in finding the solution to a problem. Before making a decision, evidence of the validity of a proposal, or of its fairness, may be required. Limited resources drive the need to strike a balance and make trade-offs and, as such, there will always be some people left unsatisfied.

In problem solving, the goal or end-state of affairs is specified and what is sought is the most efficient means to that end. In decision making, the very goal of action is itself up for discussion. Health care consumers may be keen to play a role in decision making, but they are less interested in problem solving.

The nature, role, type, and use of evidence, as well as evaluation of that use must all be considered. It is also very important to examine the interests and objectives involved in any decision and the impact these have on the relevance of evidence. Decisions must be analyzed by level as well as through the perspective of the decision makers. Finally, any analysis of the impact of evidence must take into account its context.

Evidence is not always strong or clear; methods are therefore required to evaluate its validity. Decisions may affect the interests of more than just the individual or a group, and sometimes conflicting values must be taken into account in the decision-making process. Use of evidence in decision making requires a careful partnership between decision makers and those who produce and evaluate the information.

The conclusion that can be drawn from these observations is that each decision at every level, from policy to the bedside, should be justified by reference to evidence and good reasoning. Projects, treatments, or interventions should not be undertaken without first establishing a method of evaluating their chances of success or failure. Evidence must be examined with impartiality and account taken of its diversity. In a whole-person, whole-life concept of health, evidence must be sought that can be brought to bear in evaluating social interventions. Finally, evidence must be made accessible to decision makers, even if this means setting up a nationally sanctioned bridging agency.

TABLE OF CONTENTS

INTRODUCTION

The Nature of Evidence

A piece of evidence is a fact or datum which is used, or could be used, in making a decision or judgment or in solving a problem. The evidence, when used with the canons of good reasoning and principles of valuation, answers the question why, when asked of a judgment, decision, or action. As such, the nature of what can count as evidence in the justification of a decision or judgment is as varied as the types of possible judgments themselves.

The elements common to all decision making are the rules of deductive and inductive logic. These are well known, readily accepted, and provide the framework for making inferences and deductions. But beyond this framework what counts as good evidence will vary by decision type, academic discipline, the values and objectives of the decision maker, the context of the decision, and so on. Thus, what can be done in this brief paper is to provide a framework for understanding decision making in health that points out the varied roles evidence might play. A much larger project would be required to map and evaluate all the types of information that may be proffered as evidence in the making of a health-related decision.

At some level, almost all decisions in and around health have a values component. Sometimes those values, and the role they play, are obvious, sometimes less so. Where resources are scarce, every decision to do one thing has a corresponding consequence of not doing something else. In each case this implies that the action chosen is valued more highly than the option rejected. Not to make a decision at all also reflects certain values; it is not value neutral. The role and nature of evidence supporting values decisions is quite different from its role and nature in finding the solution to a problem. In a decision, evidence of the justice of a proposal may well be required, or of its fairness to all the stakeholders.

Limited resources also drive the need to strike a balance and make trade-offs. Because everything cannot be done, some things will be left undone and some people left unsatisfied. Justification of such decisions requires evidence—but once again, the evidence will be quite different from that required to defend the solution of a problem.

The Structure of This Paper

This introduction first draws a distinction between decision making and problem solving and then lays out the components of good or justified decision making. The section "Evidence" looks at the nature, roles, types, evaluation, and uses of evidence. The section "Interests and Objectives" examines the interests and objectives involved in any decision in health and analyzes the impact these have on the type and relevance of evidence. This issue is approached from two angles: by an analysis of decisions by level and through the perspective of the decision makers themselves. The section "Situation—Decision Context" looks briefly at the situation or context of decision making and, once again, analyzes the impact it may have on what would count as valid evidence and good reasoning. The section "Short Literature Review" presents a brief overview of the relevant medical literature. The conclusions in the final section move from the varieties of decision making to the processes of providing relevant, usable, and reliable evidence.

Distinction between Problem Solving and Decision Making

Professor Raisa Deber (National Forum on Health 1995), in her presentation to the "Evidence-Based Decision Making" (EBDM) working group's Consumer Dialogue in June 1995, made a distinction between problem solving and decision making and suggested that health care consumers are keen to play a role in decision making but are less interested in problem solving. That distinction permeates the discussion of evidence-based decision making.

In problem solving, the goal or end-state of affairs is specified, or agreed to, in advance. What is sought is the most efficient means to that end. (Problem solving can be thought of as "means-end" reasoning.) What will count as "efficient" may well be subject to debate, but the goal is not. In problem solving, the values are known and assumed to be agreed on by the problem solver (or the person or people for whom the problem is being solved).

By contrast, in decision making, the very goal of action is itself up for discussion and debate. In decision making, the first step is to establish the values, and hence the goals, that are being sought. The second step is to find means for achieving those goals.

The distinction is important for this debate because lack of clarity about whether one is problem solving or decision making may mask the need for decisions rather than solutions.

For example, the Health Information Dialogue, sponsored by the EBDM working group, in May 1995, presented two Quebec examples of studies and solutions to problems. The first concerned the use of low-osmolar contrast media (LOM) and routine preoperative chest X rays (RPCX). In both cases, current practices were more costly than the alternatives and did not improve health. Both are excellent examples of problem solving. The health goals are agreed on, as is the assumption that more-efficient rather than less-efficient means should be used to achieve those goals. Current practices are less efficient, so they should be changed. In cases like this, the encouragement of improvements through evidence-based decision making is itself a matter of problem solving—how to make the information available most efficiently, and how to encourage those who face the problems to use it.

In decision making, the situation is more complex. Before the process of finding the most efficient means to a desired outcome can begin, the desired outcome must be determined. For example, in a situation of limited resources, is it better to work toward saving a small number of lives at a relatively high cost per life, or to improve the quality of life of many people at a relatively low cost per person?

Basing decisions on, and solving problems through, evidence is a cornerstone of rationality and, as such, is opposed only with great difficulty. But agreement with the principle masks a series of vital questions which include: what are the goals to be achieved, what are the acceptable means of achieving those goals, what is the type and level of the decision, by whom is the decision being made, what is the nature of the evidence and, indeed, what would even count as evidence and how is that evidence related to a decision?

"Good" or Justified Decisions

A "good" decision, or one that is justified, can be seen as a combination of three elements: evidence, interests, and situation.

Evidence can be weak or strong, clear or murky, and so on. It can come from a variety of sources—science, personal experience, theory. Methods are required for evaluating evidence—for determining how much credence should be given any particular piece of information.

Interests often (though not always) enter the decision-making process through the identity of the decision maker. A rational patient/client would make a decision in his interests, given his values, desires, etc. A patient's decision may well not be the same as a policymaker's decision, given that the policymaker has to make decisions in the interests of a group or community. It is in the analysis of interests that values most clearly play their role in decision making.

Situation (or context) must be taken into account. It may be stating the obvious, but a justified decision must be sensitive to its context. In the medical context, it may well be rational for a dying person to try treatments that have great risks, or are untested and untried. While jumping out of a third-floor window is not generally a good idea, it might be if the building was burning. A good decision will take into account the situation and other possible courses of action.

In problem solving, one of those elements (interests) is already agreed on or assumed. In decision making, all three elements come into play. The first of those three elements is analyzed in more detail.

EVIDENCE

In general terms, "evidence" is the information provided, in the form of reasons, to justify decisions, judgments, or conclusions. Evidence is the facts or data used as premises in arguments in support of conclusions. How a fact can be used to play an evidential role depends on the type of decision that is being made. For instance, Sherlock Holmes concludes that the perpetrator was known to the household of the victim, because on the night of the crime the dog did not bark. The Red Wings may be predicted to win the Stanley Cup on the basis of the evidence of their record over the season. (A prediction which neatly illustrates the way in which many judgments based on evidence will be at best probable rather than certain.) Treatment X for illness Y for patient Z may be prescribed because in a clinical trial the treatment was shown to be effective for similar people in a similar situation.

The Sherlock Holmes example can also be used to illustrate two further points. First, the fact that the dog did not bark was a piece of information available not only to Holmes but also to the inspector from Scotland Yard. The inspector failed to recognize its importance and relevance. This can happen, too, for any other piece of evidence (or potential piece of evidence). Relevant information, information that could feature as evidence, may be missed, unavailable, or suppressed. Second, Holmes recognized the non-barking dog as evidence by incorporating it into a theory, a theory that says that dogs bark at strangers. The information becomes evidence and, hence, can play its role in an argument designed to support a conclusion only by being incorporated into a theory.

Evidence, therefore, can be questioned or disputed in a variety of ways. First, its accuracy may be disputed. Here the question concerns the facts of the case. Second, and more problematic, the relevance of the evidence may be questioned. For instance, it is widely reported that Nancy Reagan consulted horoscopes during her husband's presidency. There could be no disputing the fact that Mars really was in Cancer on any particular day. However, there would be a great deal of dispute about whether that piece of information was relevant as evidence for any decisions that might be made. This is clearly an extreme example, but even within science what should be taken as relevant information, and how that evidence may feature in a decision, may well be a matter for dispute and discussion.

The Roles of Evidence

Confidence

The purpose of considering evidence is to be able to make judgments. Sometimes these judgments are about the future, or about what will happen in new situations. In other cases, the judgments are about the past—the butler did it, or the universe started with a big bang.

But evidence is used in a wide range of situations and across the entire spectrum of decision making. What will count as evidence will vary according to the situation and the type of decision. For instance, consider what would count as the evidence in the following situations: in the deliberations of a Papal Court considering canonization, that a miracle had truly occurred; in determining whether or not he really does *love* her; in determining whether Wayne Gretzky is the greatest hockey player that has ever lived; or in determining whether or not treatment X should be used for illness Y for person Z.

The purpose of these examples is twofold. First, evidence comes in many forms, and what is counted as evidence in one situation for one type of decision may not count elsewhere. Second, sometimes what would count as evidence is itself contested.

Even within the field of health care, the notion of evidence has many facets. Evidence-based decision making in medicine tends to refer strictly to decisions based on the results of clinical trials. But, in a sense, medical decision making has always been based on evidence, sometimes in the form of theories of disease and pathology, sometimes as personal experience of what seemed to work.

Wherever evidence is used, its role is to support a judgment. The evidence provides confidence that what is concluded, or judged, is indeed the case. The better the evidence, the more confidence there can be that the judgments are correct.

Description and the Inference to Causality (Observation and Experimentation)

Description (Observation)

Some of the information required for making informed decisions in health is straightforwardly descriptive. Knowledge is required of the incidence rates of diseases, the prevalence of ailments, the frequency of certain behaviours, and so on. Sometimes this information can simply be collected by keeping appropriate records. In other cases, distribution in the general population is inferred from distribution in a representative sample. For instance, the number and type of admissions to an emergency ward can be ascertained by keeping and reviewing relevant records. However, the incidence of smoking among the population of teenage girls is inferred from a sample taken to be representative. In the former case, accuracy (and hence confidence) is dependent on the state of record keeping. In the latter case, confidence is dependent on the representative nature of the sample (assuming that the statistician's methods of evaluating the representative nature of a sample do not need discussion here).

In scientific terms, this sort of data is often called descriptive or observational. While descriptive information may include inferences (for instance from sample to population) it does not, in contrast with what follows, involve manipulation of the variables.

Inferring Causality (Experimentation)

In the quest to understand (and in Skinner's phrase—"predict and control") the world around them, people often wish to know not merely what is the case, but why it is the case. That is, they wish to know the causes of the observed effects. It is often unhelpful to try to infer causation merely from observation of a correlation. For instance, if height is correlated with intelligence in children, it would be found that tall children tend to be smarter: obviously true, because tall children tend to be older. In this case, both elements of the correlation are caused by a third factor, age, which was not incorporated in the original data.

In an experiment, a deliberate and conscious attempt is made to isolate the variables under examination so inferences about causation can be made.

J. S. Mill (1843) formulated several methods of establishing causation: agreement, difference, concomitant variation, and residues. These methods form the basis of the rules of scientific induction.

- Agreement: the search for a common factor whenever the given effect occurs.
- Difference: remove a factor, hold everything else constant, and see if the effect still occurs.
- Concomitant variation: similar to the method of difference, only operating quantitatively rather than qualitatively. One varies the intensity of a factor and looks for variations in the effect.
- Residues: a slightly more complex method. It is used when part of an effect, E, observed in the presence of factors A, B, C, is attributable to factors known to be causes, A and B. The residue is then attributable to C (providing A, B, and C are the only causal factors at play.) For example, Marie and Pierre Curie noticed that the radioactivity of pitchblende (an ore of uranium) was higher than could be explained by the uranium it contained. The residual radioactivity had to be caused by something else—it was—radium.

These methods form the basis of contemporary experimental design. The attempt in experimental design is to isolate the relationship of causality between the independent variable, that is, the manipulated variable (the cause) and the dependent variable (the effect). The better designed the experiment, the more confident the researcher can be that effect E really is caused by factor A.

The principle limitation of observational evidence, when compared with experimental evidence, is that the former is of limited use for inferring causation. At heart, this is the basis of the preference for the evidence provided by clinical trials. Because these trials are carefully designed and controlled experiments, they allow one to speak with far greater confidence about the causal factors at play.

Types of Decisions, Types of Evidence

As indicated above, the nature of what would count as evidence depends on the type of reasoning that is being conducted. Evidence in a trial is different from evidence in a religious or scientific debate. However, even within the field of science, what counts as evidence, and what counts as good reasoning, varies from discipline to discipline. To take an obvious example, the reasoning, and the evidence, brought forward to support a Freudian psychoanalytic diagnosis are quite different from the type of evidence produced to support a neurological explanation of the same behaviour.

Similarly, the sort of epidemiological evidence that supports conclusions, for instance about cancer rates at the community level, is quite unlike the evidence produced to support a diagnosis of cancer for some particular individual.

The point is that debates about the quality and cogency of evidence are conducted within the disciplines of science using the criteria established by the standards of good practice in each discipline. Other than the broad canons of logic—which apply to any type of reasoning—what counts as evidence and what counts as a good explanation is decided within each discipline. Other than these broad canons of logic (such as the law of non-contradiction, A and not A cannot both be true), there is no overarching template which can be applied to evaluate all and any form of reasoning.

In the section "Interests and Objectives," we examine decisions in health by level: macro, meso, and micro. In each of these cases, we look at the type of decision being made and the relevant requirements for evidence. (The table in the appendix lays out type of decision, decision maker and evidence, etc., schematically.)

To a certain extent this is unsatisfying. We need not go very far into the history of medicine itself to find examples of all sorts of, to our current standards, bizarre forms of reasoning. Phrenology is perhaps the classic example, but warnings about the physiological consequences of masturbation or women's sport make precisely the same point. The practice of science is continually self-correcting. Because scientific theories and scientific evidence continually expose themselves to the facts, eventually, when a sufficient body of contradictory evidence has built up, the theories themselves give way (what Kuhn [1962] called a "paradigm shift"). The outcome is that the standards of good reasoning in any discipline constitute a moving target.

There is no substitute for taking the best available advice in any field—where "best available" is established by the practitioners themselves.

This general point, however, requires a caution. As noted, even assuming goodwill and a commitment to seeking the truth, there is sometimes contradictory evidence, and experts can disagree on the relevance or meaning of the data. In addition, scientists are as human as everyone else and so operate with their own vested interests and biases. The process of seeking advice from experts is one which requires acknowledging the limitations of particular perspectives and seeking appropriately broad-based consultation.

Scientific Evidence and a Bias toward Traditional Medicine

We need to be sensitive to the possibility that scientific approaches to evidence add a bias toward traditional over alternative medicine. However, the other extreme, where we abandon any rigorous sense of evidence for the benefit of inclusivity is just as problematic. Standards of evidence must permit the evaluation of alternative therapies—and the therapies themselves must be amenable to such evaluation.

One of the major challenges posed by alternative therapies is that they tend to treat the whole person, rather than operating on the model of treating the disease that is the standard approach in traditional health care. This treatment of the person tends to result in personal treatment—where the client feels closer to the practitioner. This closeness not only results in positive feelings for the client, it may also feature in the creation of positive outcomes.

The challenge of treatment of the person should be viewed as positive. One of the failings of traditional health care may well be its impersonality and its concentration on diseases rather than people. However, this approach leads to problems of evaluation. The effectiveness of alternative therapies may depend on the complete relationship between client and practitioner, a relationship that does not lend itself readily to the atomization into elements required by standard evaluation processes and clinical trials.

It was noted above that the process of seeking expert advice needs to be sensitive to vested interests and the parochial nature of certain viewpoints. This is a case in point. Alternative therapies cannot be dismissed because they do not fit traditional models. Nor can they be accepted merely because of a desire to be open and nondiscriminatory. What is required is an open-minded willingness to seek appropriate methods of evaluation and to develop theories which integrate the different approaches to health and well-being.

In some respects, alternative therapies face tougher entry conditions than were faced by current medical practices. Many current procedures and therapies are conducted without having had the benefit of thorough review and evaluation. That is unfortunate, but it is changing. Many groups around the world are looking at standards of evidence for medical practice and working toward subjecting as many current procedures as possible to critical reevaluation. The same standards of scrutiny should be applied to alternative therapies.

Alternative therapies need validation as much as any other type of therapy. What is required is that the therapies are shown to be effective, where "shown to be effective" requires both that the therapies are correlated with the desired result and integrated into a theoretical account of how that effect is brought about.

Evaluating Evidence

As has been seen, evidence can arise from a variety of different sources, but even when the evidence is pretty standard (as in scientific evidence found in academic journals) a number of questions still arise regarding the design of the intervention, the transferability of the data to other populations, the exact nature of the questions asked, and so on. Also, given that there are often conflicting and changing research results, a method is required for evaluating scientific studies before applying their results in treatments.

The task of systematic evaluation of research results, and their consequent synthesis and promulgation, has to be assigned to experts in the fields concerned. The careful review of research design and methods in any discipline can only be conducted by the experts in that discipline itself. This is the process of expert peer review and analysis. In practical terms, this means that the practice of evidence-based health care requires a careful partnership between decision makers—policymakers, administrators, physicians and users who need to articulate the sort of information they require—and expert peer reviewers to evaluate the evidence and make it available in a form that is useful. This process operates at many levels. Expert peer review can assess the reliability of any specific scientific study. The users of that information, for example policymakers, must then integrate that information with evidence of the effectiveness of alternative therapies or other means of achieving the social goals of health and personal well-being. Finally, all the relevant information, in the form of practice guidelines, research reports and so on, must be made available in an accessible form to physicians, practitioners, and clients.

But evidence can also come from other sources, including anecdotes, personal experience, social mores, and so on. Such evidence cannot be discounted, nor should its effects on decision makers be underestimated.

If we restrict ourselves to discussions of the effectiveness of any proposed intervention, it is possible, in broad terms, to produce a rough and ready priority ordering based on the confidence that each type of evidence provides reliable causal explanations.

Experimental Evidence

Clinical trials tend to be favoured as the standard of medical evidence because they have been specifically designed to search for causal explanations that can be transferred to new situations and other subjects. This is true in general for other, specifically designed, experimental manipulations. Experiments are designed to isolate the relevant variable and control extraneous and confounding factors.

The case-by-case evaluation of experimental evidence should be left to the experts in the field.

The general difficulty with the application of experimental results is the extent to which the field use of the relevant treatment or procedure will correspond to the conditions of the trial or test. *Again, there is no substitute for careful case-by-case evaluation.*

Observation

Detailed observation is the foundation of evidence in many scientific disciplines. (In many cases, experimental manipulation of the variables is simply not possible.) The general problem is in inferring causation to observed correlations. Correlations can be inferred more reliably as causes if both, other corroborating evidence, and a theoretical explanation of the connection exist. For instance, correlation of high cancer rates with smoking does not by itself show a causal connection. However, when that correlation is coupled with laboratory studies of the effects of smoking on other animals and theoretical models which show how smoking can cause the effects it does, the evidence of a causal connection becomes overwhelming.

Theory

In the first place, theory provides a framework for placing and evaluating evidence. A piece of data is only evidence within the framework of a theory which shows how the data can be used in an explanation. So theory brings together disparate pieces of data and unifies them within a coherent structure. As such, theory is also used to evaluate data. Experimental results may be discarded on the basis that they do not fit with extant theory in the field concerned. (The interplay between theory and evidence is complex and nuanced. While theory arranges and evaluates data, data can also bring a theory down. This process is the stuff of scientific advance and revolution. Kuhn [1962] argued that there are no extrascientific or superrational processes available for evaluating just when the weight of evidence is such that the theory should be changed; or when such evidence is available, that we should maintain theory anyway and discount contrary evidence.) It should also be pointed out that theories operate within traditions. Alternative therapies, for instance, may not fit easily with current medical traditions. The task of theory review and development requires an openness to alternative methods of viewing things.

A course of action may also be justified solely on the basis that it fits a theory of human biology or functioning. This should only be done in the absence of direct evidence.

Authority

Although in the canons of informal logic an appeal to authority is a standard fallacy, it is a useful way of cutting down the time and energy one spends on one's own research. What one must do, however, is evaluate the authority. If the authority is generally reliable and is pronouncing on his area of expertise, it may well make sense to accept the judgment of the authority. If that judgment contradicts other evidence, the judgment must rest with how well the authority deals with the conflicting evidence or counter-examples.

Personal Experience

While the claims of personal experience are hard to ignore, such experiences are notoriously unreliable as predictors of transferability to new cases or different situations. *Although it may be difficult, direct evidence should be favoured over personal experience.*

This five-category approach is similar to that adopted for grading evidence by the Canadian Task Force (CTF) on Periodic Health Examination.[1]

---

1. Its grades of evidence are: I Randomized controlled trial, IIi Controlled trial without randomization, IIii Cohort or case-control study, IIiii Comparison of times or places, III Opinions of respected authorities, case report, or case series. CTF category I corresponds (in a restricted form) to our category 1 Experimental evidence. Category II (all three subsections) are forms of observation, our category 2. Opinions of respected authorities III corresponds to our category 4. Our category 3 Theory, pervades the assessment of all the other categories.

   It should be noted that the CTF guidelines have limitations. They only evaluate the type of research design and do not probe more deeply to look at the actual conduct of the research (for example, sample size). They cannot deal with contradictory randomized controlled trial results. While a simple formula is useful for superficial comparisons, the detailed work of evaluating particular pieces of research requires a great deal of expertise in the areas concerned.

Using Evidence

As we have seen, a piece of data or a fact only becomes evidence when it is used. A piece of evidence is a premise in an argument, an argument which leads to a judgment, a conclusion, or an action. To return to the example from Sherlock Holmes, the fact that the dog did not bark on the night of the crime is evidence for the conclusion: the perpetrator was known to the household. To complete the argument we also need the premise that dogs bark (or this dog would have barked) at strangers. The point is, that *the notion of evidence is empty without an understanding of the decision type and the context in which the evidence is being used.*

This also points to the need to provide information in ways and forms which are accessible, and thus useful, to decision makers. We turn now to an analysis of the interests and objectives of decision makers and the role those interests play in shaping the nature of evidence and in decision making.

INTERESTS AND OBJECTIVES

Introduction

Decision Makers, Levels of Decision, and Interests

Decision making is done by a decision maker. The appropriate relationship of evidence to decision depends on the interests and objectives of the decision maker and the context of the decision.

In broad terms, decisions made in health can be divided into three levels and interests, and objectives identified at each level. That is done in the section on levels of decision making in health. In the section on decision makers, we look more closely at the decision makers themselves and the roles they play.

The concept of "locus of responsibility" refers to the person or group toward whom the decision maker is responsible. In some cases, the decision maker and his locus of responsibility coincide. This is so for a patient or

---

(Continued)

It should also be apparent that using the grading criteria appropriate to one type of evidence may well be disastrous when applied to another. For instance, while the standards listed are useful for evaluating claims of causality, they are inapplicable when evaluating evidence of attitudes or values. In the latter case, one would need to look at the nature and order of the questions asked, the alternatives offered, the sample size and distribution, and so on. It would also be erroneous to argue that the only sort of evidence of any use in medical decision making is evidence of causality. As shown more clearly in the discussion of types of decision, evidence from quite different sources and of quite different types is often needed (Canadian Task Force on Periodic Health Examination 1994).

client. He will make decisions based on his own interests and preferences. (These interests may include concern for the interests of others, but they need not.) The physician, however, makes decisions in the interests of the patient/client, so while the physician is the decision maker, the locus of responsibility is the patient/client. Finally, policymakers or administrators make decisions on behalf of a group or community. In such cases, the interests of the decision maker ought not to play a role. The decision should be dominated by the interests of the group concerned.

Constraints on, and Biases in, Decision Making

The Ethical Principle of Efficient Use of Resources

The decisions made in a situation of unlimited resources are not likely to be the same as those made in a situation where every choice entails a corresponding decision not to do, or not to fund, something else. No assumptions are made about the absolute level of funding required for health care, but it is assumed that each decision has financial consequences, both within and outside of health care. *Because resources are finite, there is an ethical obligation to ensure that the methods used to achieve any agreed-on goal are the most efficient available.*

It might sound odd to talk of fiscal efficiency as an ethical obligation, but it is. Even if we leave aside the notion of public service as stewardship— which imposes its own obligations—if it is assumed the resources available for health are fixed, because each choice leaves something else undone, we have a prima facie obligation to make the choices that bring about the most good. For example, if $100,000 spent on procedure X could have been spent to better effect on prevention program Y, there is an obligation to opt for Y. (The obligation is prima facie because it may be defeated by other moral obligations, such as justice or a prior commitment, and the notion of "better effect" is as yet unanalyzed, but the obligation exists nonetheless.)

This principle reinforces the point made earlier that all health practices should be open for review and evaluation. Even if there is no alternative to current practices, there are other actions that could be taken to promote health and well-being, so each procedure requires justification.

Opportunity Cost

In addition to financial costs to any decisions, there are also opportunity costs. The decision to use treatment X is a decision to treat rather than not treat and may also be a decision to forego alternative treatment. This means that all aspects of the status quo are candidates for review. To put this another way, the mere fact that there is not a currently viable alternative treatment does not mean that current practice should be immune from review (for example, RPCX). *There is always an alternative to treatment (no treatment), and there is always a cost in terms of foregone opportunities.*

The "Do Something" Principle

In the face of uncertainty or danger, people tend to feel better if they are doing something rather than waiting to see what happens. This general fact of human life applies in health care. When a patient/client has a problem, both the patient/client and the physician are likely to feel better if action is taken to try to remedy the situation. This means that treatments are apt to be implemented in the absence of good evidence, just because acting is more comfortable than waiting. (This may in itself be therapeutic as it may act as a form of placebo effect, but if that is what is desired we ought at least to be explicit about what is being done.) However, *the therapeutic effects of a placebo may not justify the unthinking adoption of the "do something" principle.*

The "Better Safe Than Sorry" Principle

In medicine, there are many situations where, if action is not taken now, an opportunity is missed which will never be repeated. Cesarean sections offer an obvious example. The inclination is to act in the presence of worrying signs in order to prevent possible serious damage or death. The inclination is perfectly understandable, but it leads to very high rates of cesarean sections in medical jurisdictions that monitor and treat childbirth in a particular way. *The outcome of following the "better safe than sorry" principle is that interventions may be conducted too often and too soon.*

In addition, physicians and other health care professionals may well feel potential legal or malpractice pressures to act, even in the absence of good evidence, rather than not act. Both physician and patient are likely to *feel* better if they believe they "did all that they could."

Levels of Decision Making in Health

Broader Determinants of Health

The promotion of health and well-being is a far broader enterprise than the mere provision of health care. The health of a community is determined by more than its medical infrastructure. One dominant theme of the summaries collected as *What Determines Health?* (National Forum on Health 1996) is that feelings of personal empowerment, control, and autonomy are prime determinants of health and well-being. This theme of personal empowerment—an empowerment that is created by healthy communities and supportive families—was seen for all ages, from infants to seniors, and for conditions as diverse as preschool development, suicide, and drug misuse by elderly persons.

But the recognition that health and well-being are determined by far more than medical care entails that the promotion of health must encompass far more than treatment of diseases after they occur. This, in turn, means that a wide range of social interventions requires evaluation as alternative methods of promoting health and well-being. This is notoriously difficult. A second recurring theme in the summaries contained in *What Determines Health?* was that many of the interventions cited had not undergone formal evaluations of effectiveness. The evidence of their efficacy and relative effectiveness against other approaches to promoting health is, in many cases, simply unavailable.

Consider, for example, the difficulty of assessing the effectiveness of a program to prevent suicide in a teenage Aboriginal population. First, one must determine what would count as an appropriate measurement. This could range from actual or attempted suicides, to a measurement of attitudes to self-determination and autonomy. Second, the time frame for measurement needs to be determined. Could the program be counted as a success after one year? Or when the participants reached age 18 or 25, and so on? Third, what relation would the measured variable need to have to the baseline measurement for the program to be counted a success? Suicide rates may fluctuate wildly from year to year. Similarly, if the rate was on an upward trend, merely holding it constant over a number of years may count as success. But the difficulties of measurement cannot be allowed to preclude the attempt. To justify social interventions designed to promote health, we need the best reasons and evidence available. In the case of such interventions, it is unlikely that the type of evidence available will resemble the evidence that is generated by experiments. What will be found are arguments that lead to conclusions— this intervention will have the desired and intended effect because.... Evaluating evidence when examining social interventions and programs requires an acceptance of arguments that work from theory and analogy.

For our purposes at the moment, we will consider all health decisions as resource allocation decisions. That is, we are viewing each decision as an opportunity to take (or forego) an action, and each action is taken as having costs (financial and other)—both directly and indirectly through other opportunities foregone.

Macroallocation Decisions

These are high-level, political, allocation and policy decisions, which could include, for instance, the percentage of the budget allocated to health, social, and educational programs and the percentages of those budgets allocated to research, prevention, hospital, home care, drugs, and so on as well as standards of care, permissible (or funded) treatments, etc. Decisions made at this level are systemwide and objectives are determined by reference to the interests of the entire community.

The first key step in deciding what would count as evidence in a decision of this type is to look at the objectives of the decision. Assume for a moment that the objective is for a province to achieve the best standards of health for its citizens compared with any other province in Canada. The first task is to define what would count as the best standards of health.

The World Health Organization's definition of health, "Health is a state of complete physical, mental and social well-being and not merely the absence of disease or infirmity," is extremely broad and very difficult to measure. The very choice of measurement standards will presuppose value choices which will, in turn, influence the way the goal can be pursued. For instance, we could survey people's subjective accounts of their health and well-being, or we could count the services provided by hospitals and physicians, or we could look at the amounts spent per capita on health care (and so on and so on). Each piece of data could feature as evidence in an argument designed to support the conclusion: "so our province has the best standards of health in the country." Yet each measurement method would lead to different steps to gain an improvement.

These are not insurmountable difficulties, but they do indicate the need for decisions and agreement. Only when the idea of "health benefit" has been decided, defined, and agreed on is it possible to measure means of achieving it. However, even this does not answer the question of what would count as evidence for making the decision.

Riegelman (1995), in *The Measures of Medicine: Benefits, Harms and Costs*, took what he called a quantitative approach to making medical decisions at each of the three levels (macro, meso, and micro) discussed here. He contrasted this with what he called a rule-based approach. In effect, he adopted a problem-solving rather than a decision-making approach with the objective already determined as the maximization of benefit. He assumed that the goal is the maximization of benefit and all that is sought is a method for calculating relative benefits, harms, and costs. On this account, the action which brings the greatest net benefit is calculated—and his book is full of examples and methods for making those calculations—and then that action is performed. Following this method, the evidence needed for making good decisions is evidence of the relative effectiveness, harms, and costs of alternative treatments or approaches.

But this is far from the complete story.

Churchill (1987), in *Rationing Health Care in America: Perceptions and Principles of Justice*, while discussing allocation decisions for specific services (renal dialysis, comprehensive prenatal health program, expansion of neonatal intensive care, artificial heart research, health insurance for the uninsured, cancer research, health care coverage for the elderly, and support for persons in persistent vegetative states), listed eight possible principles of allocation:

- pure egalitarianism: give the same amount to each;
- equitable egalitarianism: give same proportion of request to each;
- help neediest or most ill first;
- seek the greatest good for the greatest number;
- choose in accordance with long-range efficiency and effectiveness;
- act on principle of restorative justice—give greater aid to those whose maladies were caused or exacerbated by past injustices;
- honour long-standing commitments; and
- choose by lottery.

Of these eight, only four and five can be directly related to Riegelman's methods. The point, of course, is to illustrate that decisions about the macro-allocation of resources may feature evidence not merely of effectiveness, cost, etc., but also of justice or prior obligation.

It is also worth pointing out that it is assumed the interests of the population we are trying to serve can be assessed. Take, for example, the contrast between preventive and restorative medicine. In terms of general measures of population health, an intervention that saves a life by vaccination is equivalent to one that saves a life through surgery. The difference is that the individual that gains the benefit of surgery can be identified, but it is not possible to know which individual gained the benefit from the vaccination program. (Such a person is sometimes called a "statistical beneficiary.") This tends to militate against prevention programs and in favour of dealing with identified victims. But, in terms of the impact on population health, this bias could well be counterproductive.

A further difficulty with prevention, in the traditional model of health care, is that the people who receive the intervention are otherwise healthy. They do not appear at the physician's office seeking treatment for an ailment that troubles them. On the other hand, a person who is seeking treatment does so because he is suffering. The pressure of compassion to relieve that identified individual's suffering is felt far more keenly than the desire to save the life of someone who is nameless, faceless, and unidentified. This fact makes us feel less like supporting prevention over treatment.

In practical terms, this means that actions which may bring the greatest benefit to a community as a whole—and which are thus in its best interests— are not seen as most beneficial to the individuals in that community. We can identify our friends and relatives who did not get the best possible health care, but we cannot identify those people who benefitted from prevention. This makes decision making even more difficult in what are, after all, political decisions.

A further type of decision at both this macro- and the mesolevel, concerns limitations on the services offered by individual physicians and caregivers. These limitations come in two ways. In the first, the service may simply not be funded by the community or the institution concerned. A second type of limitation is where there are systemic constraints on treatment options for specified conditions. In both cases, the requirement for good decision making will be evidence that the treatments or programs concerned either do not bring benefits, or obtain the benefits only at far too great a cost. In the latter case, the idea of "too great a cost" has ethical support from the requirement that we spend scarce resources in the most efficient way possible. "Too great a cost" means that there are other ways of bringing about greater good with the same allocation of resources.

Decision making at the macrolevel will thus require three, quite different, sets of evidence. The first concerns the health goals and objectives of the system or program under consideration. This type of evidence is derived from the values of the people to be served. The research would need to be conducted through surveys, focus groups, and the like. The second type of evidence concerns the relative efficacy of proposed programs, treatments, or procedures in reaching those goals. This sort of information may come from epidemiological and other research sources (for instance, randomized clinical trials). Finally, the decision makers need information about costs, not only the actual and opportunity cost of the measures under consideration, but also evidence of the costs the payer (government and then taxpayer) is willing to bear. With evidence derived from each of those three sources, the decision maker is in a position to make a judgment that can be justified.

Decision making may be further biased (and this applies at all three levels) by the "do something" and the "better safe than sorry" action principles. In the desire to do all that is possible, especially when the situation is desperate, we may engage in practices that are, statistically, almost futile. While this may offer hope to the patient and comfort to the practitioner, we all pay the price in other opportunities foregone.

Mesoallocation Decisions

These are institutional-level decisions, which include funding levels for particular services and programs, and institutional priorities and practices.

Whereas macroallocation decisions looked to the interests of the entire community, mesolevel decisions have a restricted constituency. Individual institutions may well have competitive goals vis-à-vis other similar institutions within the same system. While rationalization of services may well make excellent sense from a system perspective, this may not be the case at the level of each institution.

Similarly, the streamlining of services at one institution (e.g., early discharge of surgical patients) may result in repercussions elsewhere in the system: increased use of home care services, or even higher probability of relapse.

Having said that, many of the principles that operated at the macrolevel also operate here. The cost-benefit-harm approach can still be used to great effect—subject, however, to the constraints of justice and prior commitment.

The requirements of evidence are also similar.

Microallocation Decisions

Whereas macro- and mesodecisions were about allocations to programs, microdecisions allocate resources within a program to a client. The principal difference between this type of decision and the previous two, concerns the decision maker and the interests he is required to take into account.

If the microallocation decision is made by the patient/client and his physician, generally, the financial cost aspect of the decision falls out of consideration entirely. As shown in the next section, in a microdecision, if the locus of responsibility is the patient/client, then in a publicly funded system, financial costs play no part in the calculation.

It is worth reiterating the influence of the action principles at this level of decision. Because costs tend not to be considered and because the interests of the patient/client are taken to be paramount, there is great pressure, especially in desperate situations, to try almost anything. If we wish to prevent this type of next-to-futile intervention, the decision to limit physician freedom must be made elsewhere in the system.

Decision Makers

Clients or Users

Interests and Preferences

An individual's interests are dependent on his values, desires, way of life, and so on. Even for people with a very similar health status, individual interests may dictate quite different treatment choices. Risks and benefits of a treatment are assessed relative to the client's interests.

It is generally accepted that a person has privileged knowledge of his own preferences and interests. In the case of a treatment decision being made jointly by a patient/client and his physician, each supplies different information. The patient brings information about interests and preferences, the physician brings knowledge about treatments and consequences. The dual information roles bring dual responsibilities. In this model of decision making, the patient/client is responsible for knowing and articulating his interests and preferences, and the physician is responsible for presenting treatment information in a way that the patient/client can use.

Costs and Benefits

A rational patient/client (and there are many issues surrounding the quality of patients' decisions given their state of health, unfamiliarity with the concepts, traditional relationship with physicians, and so on) would probably undertake some form of cost-benefit analysis as he decides what to do.

However, given the locus of the responsibility of the patient/client, that cost-benefit analysis may well be somewhat limited.

- *Unconsidered costs: health of others* – It may be rational (self-interested) for me, as an individual, to forego a vaccination, to avoid the small but potentially fatal, effects of an adverse reaction. If sufficient numbers of other people have the vaccination, my risk of contracting the disease itself may be relatively remote. However, if other people follow my self-interested reasoning, vaccination as a practice loses its effectiveness. My decision not to have the vaccination freeloads on a system where most people do have vaccinations.

  Education may work to encourage individuals to take the long-term interests of others into account as they make their own health decisions. But while the option for self-interested action is open, many are likely to take it, whatever the health consequences to others. The solution may be to limit the choices that are available in certain situations.

- *Unconsidered costs: financial* – In decision making about medical treatment, the patient/client is not required to take the financial costs into consideration. So, for example, if two treatments are available, one of which carries a risk of minor side effects, while the other, which is far more expensive, does not, the rational self-interested patient would chose the more expensive treatment.

  Similar considerations apply regarding demands for expensive diagnostic tests for low-probability illnesses.

  The patient/client is not generally required to have the good of the medical system—or Canadian society, or the national debt—in mind as he makes a decision and is not really responsible to any one else for that decision. While the physical costs and benefits of a procedure are borne by the patient/client, the financial costs are not.

Risks

Part of the assessment of costs and benefits includes an assessment of risk. Here, sensitivity to differential assessments of risk is required. It is generally accepted that experts tend to accept higher levels of risk than nonexperts. Individuals can be classified as risk takers or risk avoiders by the characteristics they exhibit across a range of decisions. Is there a level of risk that is objectively reasonable? Or is it the sort of decision that should be left to individuals on a case-by-case basis?

Care Providers

One part of the role of the care provider is in straightforward problem solving. The care provider should present to the patient/client the options for treatment and an assessment of relative efficacy and effects. The physician therefore needs access to information that he can use in this way. It is unrealistic to expect individual practitioners to have the time or the expertise to perform literature searches and reviews and to evaluate all of the sometimes conflicting information that is available. This is the role for expert review committees. The physician needs access to sources that are known to be reliable. The patient, with knowledge of his own preferences and values, should then be in a position to make an informed choice.

The care provider is in a difficult position, because he acts in the best interests of the client and also plays the role of gatekeeper to the medical system. In effect, caregivers are asked implicitly to think both about the interests of their individual patients and about the medical system and medical costs, but this is done within the rhetoric of physicians and care providers acting in the interests of the patient.

These dual roles place physicians and others in an intolerable position. On the one hand, they are explicitly assumed to be acting in their patients' interests (which means, presumably they would be supporting their patients' decisions) yet, on the other hand, they are often looked to for cost containment within the health care system.

In terms of locus of responsibility they have two—one explicit and acknowledged (the patient), the other not explicit and not acknowledged (the medical system, and by extension, the taxpayer).

It is not clear what a care provider should do when confronted with situations where these dual responsibilities come into conflict. To preserve the relationship between patient and physician it may be necessary to limit the range of options a physician might recommend to a patient. That is, permissible treatments might need to be delimited by some individual, or group, other than the physician. The physician could then be seen to act on behalf of the patient, but within the confines of generally accepted limits. This decision to impose systemic constraints on practice would have to be made at the meso- or macrolevel.

Administrators

In the cases of both the patient or client and the caregiver, the perspective is generally that of the interests of the individual, and the physical benefits or costs are borne by that person. For administrators the situation is very different. The physical costs and benefits of a decision are borne by others, as are the financial costs. (Unless remuneration is tied to cost control.) Both administrators and policymakers are responsible to a broader constituency—their institutions and the clients they serve, rather than individuals—for their decisions.

Policymakers

Given the assumption of finite resources for health care, the decision to employ any procedure entails a corresponding decision not to do something else. Those decisions all have costs which will be borne by individuals who are often not the ones to receive the corresponding benefit. The task of the policymaker is to develop policies and priorities that reasonable people would accept as fair, whatever their current health status.

This requires, as noted above, information—evidence—of three quite different types. The policymaker needs evidence of the values and interests of the constituency concerned (for these form the objectives of any decision), of the relative efficacy of treatments or procedures, and of the actual costs and the costs the constituency is willing to bear. Each piece of information offered as evidence will need to be assessed by the standards of the discipline concerned.

SITUATION—DECISION CONTEXT

It is very clear that any decision needs to take into account its context, which will often be discussed in an analysis of the interests involved. Naming this element separately introduces the requirement that context be formally considered.

Evidence and Risk

High standards of evidence for high-risk, low-benefit procedures and lower standards for low-risk, high-benefit ones are required, but there are complicating factors. This paradigm works in the ideal case of a healthy decision maker deciding between a series of possible options. In the case of someone who is desperate, where there is no available and recognized therapy, almost any treatment might rationally be seen as better than nothing. (This common response gives rise to the expression that a drowning man clutches at straws.) Similar pressures apply for the administrator or policymaker. It may be rational to stop a clinical trial and make the treatment broadly available in cases where the data are not complete, but where the preliminary evidence indicates that the treatment may save lives. (Both of these problems have arisen in treatment of persons with AIDS.)

Other Options

There is always at least one other option (do nothing) so rational decision making needs to evaluate each possible course of action in the light of the alternatives. The context of the decision is framed by other treatment or program options.

Evidence for Change

There is a conservative principle that better evidence for a change is required than that to maintain the status quo. That seems right, but how much better must the evidence be to warrant a change? This conservative principle is itself undermined in the case of treatments or actions for which there is no good evidence of efficacy.

Scarcity of Resources

Scarcity of resources is assumed to be behind all decision making in health. It reappears in the context of each decision. For the individual, the scarcity of resources shows itself in terms of a lack of energy and time. For the policymaker and the administrator, the constraints are financial as well. There is interesting evidence that national and provincial levels of health care expenditure are politically optional, that is they can be chosen, at least within certain limits, by policymakers. This means that general economic factors, such as the health of the economy, will form part of the context of macrolevel decision making.

SHORT LITERATURE REVIEW

General

In Canada, most of the work on the theory and practice of evidence-based medicine has been conducted by the McMaster Evidence-Based Medicine Working Group. The series of articles in the *Journal of the American Medical Association (JAMA)* (see below) lays out quite clearly the rationale for, and practical problems of, implementation of evidence-based practices.

In the United States, D. M. Eddy is the grandfather of evidence-based medicine. He has numerous articles in *JAMA*, from the early '90s onward, once again laying out the rationale and implications of evidence-based practice. One consistent theme is the role that cost considerations should play in the evaluation of possible treatments. Because Eddy writes from a U.S. perspective, his recommendations are often unhelpful. For instance, he recommended (Eddy 1992) that interventions designated "investigational" (where outcomes are not known or uncertain) should be offered as options but not covered by insurance, with the patient left with the bill.

While this specific approach is not useful, the general issue of the role of cost considerations is of vital importance. Discussion of costs (indeed whether such discussion even occurs) varies widely depending on the discipline of the writer concerned. Writers with backgrounds in the practice of medicine, tend to view the issues as problems to be solved, i.e., what is the most efficient way of dealing with a disease or condition. Health economists tend to write almost solely from the standpoint of cost-effectiveness, thus leaving out consideration of social values other than the maximization of benefit. As we have repeatedly seen, a justified decision at the macrolevel will need to include evidence of efficacy, costs, and values.

Evidence-Based Medicine as a Practical Problem of Implementation

Much of the currently available literature concentrates on the practical difficulties of encouraging a culture of evidence-based decision making. For example, the series of articles produced by Dr. Oxman and colleagues from McMaster (Oxman et al. 1994) dealt with the problems of setting priorities and guidelines, and measuring and reviewing performance. It is taken for granted that the introduction of evidence-based decision making is a good thing and that what needs to be determined is the means (Evidence-Based Medicine Working Group 1994). This approach sees the introduction of evidence-based medicine as a problem to be solved.

Reviewing Medical Evidence

A second practical problem is the assimilation and review of information available in the medical literature. The task here is to synthesize and evaluate data from a variety of sources and develop guidelines for practice that can readily be used by practitioners. The normal point of departure is the randomized clinical trial where a treatment or procedure is evaluated, in a controlled way, against other treatments, and its effectiveness is assessed on the basis of whether the observed results are consistent with normal distributions in the population. If the observed results are sufficiently unlikely (often a one-in-20 chance or less), it is concluded that the treatment is having the observed effect.

Given the explosion of randomized clinical trials, there are vast amounts of data available in all sorts of areas of medicine. Often, the results of these studies appear (or indeed are) contradictory. The end user of the information is not in a position, either through lack of time or training, to evaluate the data and apply them to a specific situation.

There appear to be two basic approaches to evaluating and synthesizing the medical data to transfer them into a usable form.

Review by Expert Advisory Groups

Perhaps the best-known international effort to review and synthesize medical literature is that undertaken by the Cochrane Collaboration (The Cochrane Centre 1996). The process establishes working collaborations of experts and information users with particular interests who review the evidence in their area of interest. The method is one of continuous peer review, criticism, and revision. The end product is a database of systematic reviews (Oxman and Guyatt 1988; Mann 1994).

Metanalysis

A second general approach is to use the statistical tool of metanalysis. In this process, a large number of clinical trials are aggregated and, in effect, their results pooled. This allows the detection of smaller effects than would otherwise be seen in individual studies (Mann 1994).

CONCLUSION AND POLICY IMPLICATIONS

Conclusion

The issues raised by evidence-based decision making in health care range from the overtly practical to the deeply theoretical. By distinguishing between problem solving and decision making, we can clarify our conceptualization of the issues. For practical problems, practical solutions are needed. Decisions require discussion, debate, and a willingness to share and defend values. In both cases, evidence is needed that will act as the reasons and justifications for judgments and solutions.

A recurrent theme has been the variety of situations in which evidence is required and, hence, the variety of evidence itself. Use of evidence in decision making requires a careful partnership between decision makers and those who produce and evaluate the information.

Physicians require evidence of efficacy that is accessible, authoritative, and reliable. This means mechanisms are required to review, evaluate, and synthesize carefully the mass of clinical data that is currently available. This work is painstaking and laborious and can only be carried out by experts in the relevant fields.

Policymakers, whether operating at the macro- or mesolevels, need this kind of information, but they also have additional requirements. They need to know the values, attitudes, and preferences of their constituents. Further, they need to know the relative costs of the available alternatives. Each type of evidence must be evaluated for reliability by the experts in each field. No single type of data nor of evidence has priority in policy decisions. A justified decision will carefully, and defensibly, blend elements of all three.

At one level, evidence-based decision making in health care cannot be opposed. It is impossible to object to decisions based on good reasons. However, "evidence-based" cannot merely mean based on randomized clinical trial, nor is it a complete description of the means of making medical (or for that matter, any other) decisions. There is no substitute for case-by-case careful evaluation and thoughtful judgment.

Policy Implications

The Culture of Evidence and Good Reason

Canadian health promotion should commit itself to a culture of best practices for evidence and reasoning. This means that each decision at every level, from policy to the bedside, should be justified by reference to the best available evidence and reasoning. For any decision or solution to a problem there should be a clearly articulated answer to the question "why is this course of action better than the alternatives?"

The Culture of Evaluation

A commitment to evidence brings a commitment to evaluation. Projects, treatments, or interventions should not be undertaken without first establishing a method of evaluating their success or failure. Project funding should be contingent on ongoing evaluation.

The Diversity of Evidence

A commitment to evidence and good reason is not a commitment to one specific model of health or medicine. Sometimes the best available evidence will come from clinical trials; in many other cases it cannot and could not. A commitment to evidence requires openness and sensitivity to different types and forms of treatment and therapy and, consequently, to different types and forms of evidence.

A Whole-Person, Whole-Life Concept of Health

The goal of health promotion and care in Canada is the creation of communities and individuals who are healthy across their lifetimes. People are not made healthy merely by the removal of disease. The goal of health requires a commitment to the creation of the conditions of health and that, in turn, requires a sensitivity to the types of evidence that can be brought to bear in evaluating social interventions.

Using Evidence

All too often, evidence or potential evidence is available but not accessible to the people making the decisions. This happens in the policy arena where, for example, the social determinants of health may be studied in the academic setting, but where the data are not readily accessible to policymakers. It is similar at the treatment level, where best practices may have been established but the information is not accessible to the practitioner.

Canadian health care and promotion requires a nationally sanctioned, bridging agency to collect, review and analyze the mass of available evidence, make recommendations, and formulate guidelines for practice. Practitioners, policymakers, and others would then be able to turn to a single source for expert and authoritative evidence and advice.

Robert B. Butcher *completed his Ph.D. in philosophy at the University of Western Ontario in the Bioethics Program. He currently teaches at the University of Western Ontario and is a researcher in the area of philosophy, in particular ethics and its application to the health sciences. Dr. Butcher also works as a private consultant on ethics and values through his company Foundations. Some of his clients have been the Canadian Centre for Ethics and Sport, Fitness and Amateur Sport, the Canadian Olympic Association, and Health Canada. His most recent interests lie in analyzing the concept of "wellness" and its application in the health sciences with particular emphasis on the moral point of view.*

BIBLIOGRAPHY

BERO, L., and R. DRUMMOND. 1995. The Cochrane Collaboration: Preparing, maintaining, and disseminating systematic reviews of the effects of health care. *JAMA, Journal of the American Medical Association* 274(24): 1935–1938.

CANADIAN TASK FORCE ON PERIODIC HEALTH EXAMINATION. 1994. *The Canadian Guide to Clinical Preventive Health Care.* Ottawa (ON): Health Canada.

CHURCHILL, L. 1987. *Rationing Health Care in America: Perceptions and Principles of Justice.* Notre Dame: Notre Dame Press. pp. 147–150.

EDDY, D. M. 1992. *A Manual for Assessing Health Practices and Designing Practice Policies: The Explicit Approach.* Philadelphia (PA): American College of Physicians. p. 55.

EVIDENCE-BASED MEDICINE WORKING GROUP. 1994. "Evidence-based medicine: A new approach to the practice of medicine. *JAMA, Journal of the American Medical Association* 268(17).

KUHN, T. S. 1962. *The Structure of Scientific Revolutions.* Chicago (IL): University of Chicago Press.

MANN, C. 1994. Can meta-analysis make policy? *Science* 266, November.

MILL, J. S. 1843. *A System Of Logic.*

NATIONAL FORUM ON HEALTH. 1995. *Summary Report: Changing the Health Care System—A Consumer Perspective.* Government of Canada, June, p. 13.

_____. 1996. *What Determines Health?* Ottawa (ON): Government of Canada.

OXMAN, A., and G. GUYATT. 1988. Guidelines for reading literature reviews. *CMAJ, Canadian Medical Association Journal* 138: 697–703.

OXMAN, A., D. A. DAVIS, J. W. FEIGHTNER, N. V. FINNIE, B. G. HUTCHISON, S. LUSK, P. S. MACDONALD, R. G. MCAVLEY, and J. W. SELLORS. 1994. Evidence-based care: 1. Setting priorities: How important is that problem? *CMAJ, Canadian Medical Association Journal* 150(8): 1249–1254.

_____. 1994. Evidence-based care: 2. Setting guidelines: How should we manage this problem? *CMAJ, Canadian Medical Association Journal* 150(9): 1417–1423.

_____. 1994. Evidence-based care: 3. Measuring performance: How have we managing this problem? *CMAJ, Canadian Medical Association Journal* 150(10): 1575–1579.

_____. 1994. Evidence-based care: 4. Improving performance: How can we improve the way we manage this problem? *CMAJ, Canadian Medical Association Journal* 150(11): 1793–1796.

_____. 1994. Evidence-based care: 5. Lifelong learning: How can we learn to be more effective? *CMAJ, Canadian Medical Association Journal* 150(12): 1971–1973.

RIEGELMAN, R. 1995. *The Measures of Medicine: Benefits, Harms and Costs.* Cambridge (MA): Blackwell Science.

THE COCHRANE CENTRE. 1996. *The Cochrane Centre Handbook.* Oxford (U.K.): The Cochrane Centre, Summertown Pavilion, Middle Way.

APPENDIX

APPENDIX

Decision/Evidence

Decision level	Decision maker	Locus of responsibility	Decision	Evidence	Problem	Evidence
Macro	Politician Bureaucrat Policymaker	Community	Community objectives, definitions, values, principles, services/ programs, policies	Measures of population health (need), community values, justice/ fairness, resources	Most efficient means (in accordance with community values)	Measures of relative program costs and effectiveness, values
Meso	Administrator	Institution Clients	Institutional priorities, objectives, values, services/programs, policies	Community needs, resources, institutional expertise	Most efficient means (in accordance with institutional/ community values)	Measures of program costs and effectiveness, values
Micro	Patient Physician	Patient	Patient values Objectives	Interests, values, options, benefits/ harms	Means available, (in accordance with personal values)	Harms/benefits, values

Civic Lessons: Strategies to Increase Consumer Involvement in Health Policy Development

CAROL KUSHNER AND MICHAEL RACHLIS, M.D.

SUMMARY

The purpose of the paper is to identify strategies for broadening the role of consumers in health care management and policy making, including how they might influence the research agenda, standards of practice (including clinical guidelines), and other relevant health care policies. It concludes that consumers can be a potent voice in advocating for and effecting change within the health care system. However, it also observes that consumers are often poorly informed and have limited access to organized resources. Therefore, extraordinary effort by government is required to enable them to play an effective advocacy function.

The Rationale for Consumer Involvement

While Canadians are continually told that our health care system is one of the best, this rhetoric masks serious problems stemming largely from the structure of health care delivery itself. These problems include documented shortcomings in the quality of care and services. Other problems are apparent in the persistent failure of health care systems to translate promising directions from the research literature into desirable policies and programs, where this translation calls for fundamental system restructuring. To many consumers, the system is a "non-system"—a bewildering maze of seemingly unconnected providers who focus only on one part of a person's care.

Some solutions including the need for reform have been known for at least 25 years, yet few changes and little progress have been made. Even now, as provinces restructure, there is relatively little action in changing how services are delivered. Most policy development has focused on accommodating budget cuts and on changing governance and administration.

What Consumers Bring to the Reform Process

Most system reviews and provincial reports on health reform call for more public participation, and many reform proposals have specific measures aimed at increasing consumer control over health care delivery. Consumers can facilitate government reform processes and may, in fact, be essential to overcoming the predictable resistance to change that will come from those who work in the system. Consumers have unique information, which improves decision making by ensuring that services are better tailored to consumer expectations and preferences. They also bring balance and fresh perspectives to the traditional debates that occur between funders and service providers. This balancing function can moderate or bolster resource demands or influence reallocation decisions. Finally, consumer involvement can contribute to a society's "civic sense" by strengthening the public's sense of ownership over public institutions and processes.

However, consumer involvement—and specifically, information—is not the primary influence in the policy development process. Other factors that are typically more significant include the environment external to the health policy process (e.g., how debt and deficits are perceived), the decision-making process within the health policy system, and the values, beliefs, and interests of stakeholders and the public.

Analytical Frameworks

In developing the case for more consumer involvement, the paper presents several analytical frameworks:

- *The first and most important looks at* interest groups *within the health care system and the tensions between dominant and repressed interests. These frameworks build on the imbalances in the strengths both within and between groups. Consumers, unlike physicians and drug companies, are poorly served by current arrangements and would gain greatly from a differently organized system. They have enormous difficulty organizing for change.*
- *The second framework builds on* policy-oriented learning. *This approach looks at why and how coalitions form and work to alter policy, and how creating opportunities for public debate among coalitions can change beliefs, foster learning, and affect change.*
- *Several frameworks focus on* levels of consumer participation. *One suggests that consumers have different levels of experience and expertise and that processes to involve them need to take this into consideration. Another develops a "ladder of participation" where different kinds of processes are equated with differing levels and expectations of decision making.*

- *A final framework illustrates different assumptions associated with* how consumer involvement is perceived. *Differing orientations (scientific, market, legal, and democratic) dictate different methods for approaching issues, different roles for the consumer, and different strategies of participation.*

Current and Emerging Opportunities for Consumer Involvement

The last five years have seen several new opportunities for increased consumer involvement in health care decision making. Regionalization was at least partly envisioned to facilitate greater local community participation and better decision making. The Cochrane Collaboration is an international attempt to review the research literature on the effectiveness of health care interventions in order to derive policy directions. Ontario's new law governing health professionals requires that lay representatives comprise up to 49 percent of the governing councils. While some of these initiatives appear to promise more consumer control, the authors' analysis casts doubt on whether these new governance mechanisms actually do foster consumer participation, given the extent to which providers tend to dominate boards or otherwise influence their decisions.

Case Studies

Three case studies are used to illustrate the potential and limitations of increased consumer participation. The studies were selected because they demonstrate the benefits of consumer input and because health care policies have changed as a result of consumer involvement. However, each study also contains cautionary tales about some of the limitations and barriers that can impede consumer participation.
- Case no.1: Consumers and long-term care in Ontario. *This study examines the impact of the Senior Citizen Consumer Alliance for Long-Term Care Reform. This coalition of three large consumer organizations representing most seniors in the province was established in 1990 to bring the influence of senior citizens to bear on government policy proposals to change long-term care in Ontario. Using their own project funding, the Alliance conducted a variety of successful initiatives related to long-term care reform, including a policy proposal to create a network of nonprofit, neighbourhood-level, multiservice agencies.*
- Case no. 2: The influence of consumers on breast cancer policy. *This study examines the efforts of breast cancer survivors to influence public policy. At the National Breast Cancer Forum held in Montreal in 1993, for the first time, 150 breast cancer survivors and their families were able to challenge the research and treatment community and direct attention to a series of issues that were important to them. Additional indicators of survivor influence include the National Breast Cancer Network (which permits survivor groups*

to link up across the country), the Canadian Breast Cancer Research Initiative, and survivor involvement in advising the Canadian Breast Cancer Initiative on clinical guidelines for care and treatment.

- Case no. 3: The Consumers' Health Forum of Australia, Inc. (CHF). *This study examines the influence of the CHF which was established in 1987. The CHF promotes the role and importance of consumer perspectives on health policy and practice, supports a network of consumer and community groups that pools knowledge, resources and efforts on health issues (at national, state, and local levels), and develops and pursues research and policies of concern to consumers. The CHF speaks for all of its members on broad issues (e.g., doctors' fees and pharmaceuticals) while providing access to government decision makers on matters specific to member groups' interests.*

Lessons from the Case Studies

A number of lessons can be drawn from these case studies:
- *Meaningful changes to the structure of health care delivery are unlikely unless extraordinary efforts are made to organize the consumer sector and to make adequate resources available.*
- *Consumers treasure their independence and fear being co-opted, regardless of whether their funding comes from government or business. It is important, therefore, that funders recognize that advocacy has a legitimate policy-making role and that criticism not affect funding support.*
- *People who sit on policy-making bodies must be accountable to those they represent. Groups need to have democratic processes for selecting representatives and strong mechanisms for seeking input and feedback as policies develop.*
- *Creating more boards or consumer positions on boards will not likely increase consumer influence, as governance mechanisms appear to provide relatively weak levels of accountability.*
- *People with direct experience in the health care system (e.g., patients) may be in the best position to judge its quality of service and care. However, their illness or condition may impede their participation or there may be issues that survivors do not wish to address directly (e.g., palliative care).*
- *Certain specific measures might increase and strengthen consumer participation in Canada, including helping consumers to become more knowledgeable about the policy process, creating more opportunities for public debate, and helping consumer groups to network and share information, analyses, and resources.*
- *Bringing small, single-issue groups and large groups together in a broad-based coalition and encouraging them to develop a united position on specific health reform proposals could dramatically change the political balance of some debates.*

What Governments Can Do

- *Clarify the goals of consumer participation. The consumer organizations in the case studies were very clear about their goals and objectives, but government processes involving consumer input have not always been quite so explicit.*
- *Ensure funding for consumer interest groups. Most industrial and professional interest groups can pay their own way. Many disease-specific groups established primarily to raise funds for research (e.g., Heart and Stroke Foundation, Canadian Cancer Society) are also in a position to be self-financing. However, consumer interest groups with a major focus on advocacy are different. They need stable core funding to be involved in the policy process in a meaningful way. To help advocacy groups raise funds in the private sector, government should change the current rules for charitable giving to permit these groups to retain their charitable status even though more than 20 percent of their resources are spent on advocacy activities.*
- *Support and mandate more consumer participation in decision making. Governments are in charge of designing processes that can either include or exclude consumer participation. They can further the opportunities for consumer impact by explicitly mandating consumer participation.*
- *Develop and fund a national consumer health forum. The Consumers' Health Forum of Australia provides an excellent organizational template for strengthening consumer participation in health policy development. Many officials in the Australian government acknowledge the useful role consumers can play in moving the health policy agenda forward.*
- *Sponsor a national consumers' health conference. A developmental step to explore the potential of these recommendations would be for the federal government to host a national consumers' health conference in 1997. The conference could encourage consumer advocacy organizations from across the country to review their current perspectives on health reform and could promote their willingness to work together on a joint agenda.*

TABLE OF CONTENTS

INTRODUCTION

This paper identifies strategies for broadening the role of consumers[1] in the health care management and policy-making process including an examination of consumers' influence on the research agenda, standards of practice (including clinical guidelines), and other relevant health care policies such as resource allocation. Three case studies illustrate the potential and limitations of more participation.

To flesh out the case studies, interviews were conducted with a number of key informants including consumers, health policy and communications consultants, current and former government officials, policymakers, and researchers. Most interviews were by telephone, but most of the Australian case study interviews were conducted in person during one author's (CK) recent trip to that country. A complete list of those contacted is provided in the appendix. Information from these sources and selected articles from the literature have guided the analysis of this report.

The rationale for more public participation in decision making is outlined first. Next the analytical frameworks are described. They reveal some limitations and barriers which can interfere with consumers' meaningful input, as well as some opportunities. A brief review of current and emerging opportunities for consumer involvement in health care, including regionalization, the Cochrane Collaboration and the new law governing health professions in Ontario, follows.

Three case studies highlighting consumer involvement in health care decision making are then considered in light of the analytical frameworks. This is followed by a discussion of whether they can be applied to the broader Canadian context and possible lessons for the future. Finally, the paper ends with some specific recommendations regarding support for more consumer involvement in health care decision making.

RATIONALE FOR INCREASED CONSUMER INVOLVEMENT

Various government reports document serious problems with our health care system. For example, a review of Ontario's system reported: "Evidence

---

1. The use of the term "consumer" incorporates both currently active and potential recipients of care from the system (although in the breast cancer case study, the term "survivor" is used for those with the disease). While most non–health care providers seem to prefer "consumer" over "patient" or "client," some analysts argue that the word belies the uneven power relationship between providers and patients, and that it suggests "the right to buy the services they want... as opposed to simply those they need" (Deber 1995). Another alternative term—"user"—is almost universally rejected, on the basis that in common parlance it means those who take IV drugs or those who operate computers.

on inappropriate care can be found throughout the Province's health care system, from inappropriate institutional admissions to overuse of medications among the elderly" (Ontario Health Review 1987).

Some physicians, such as Dr. Adam Linton (1988), former president of the Ontario Medical Association, have also been outspoken about these problems: "Evidence exists to suggest that laboratory tests are overused, ineffective drugs and technologies continue to be used, new technology is inadequately evaluated before introduction, and we do not as yet have any reliable system to monitor our spending and minimize waste."

And yet, Canadians are continually told that our health care system is the best, or one of the best. This rhetoric masks very serious quality problems stemming largely from the structure of health care delivery itself. It is our hypothesis that improvements in the quality of care and service require greater consumer participation in both the development of health policy and the restructuring of health care delivery. In fact, consumer involvement may be essential to overcome the predictable resistance to change from those who work in the system.

There is substantial evidence about problems with quality in Canada's health care system. Here are just a few examples.

- A recent study from Quebec showed that half of all elderly patients were given at least one questionable drug prescription in 1990 (Tamblyn et al. 1994).

- Dr. Ronald Grossman (*Toronto Star* 1996), chief of respirology at Mount Sinai Hospital in Toronto, recently deplored the increasing deaths from asthma. "It is clear the deaths are largely preventable. We see asthmatics in the emergency ward every day. And it's so unnecessary. If they managed their asthma properly... they wouldn't have to endure such severe attacks."

- A Harvard University study on hospital quality in New York State in the analysis of 30,000 randomly selected discharge records from 1984, found among other things that nearly 7,000 people died and a further 1,700 were permanently disabled because of negligent hospital care (Brennan et al. 1991). Even assuming an injury rate from hospital care in Canada of only half that found in this U.S. study, it would mean 5,000 deaths a year due to negligent hospital care and over 1,300 cases of permanent disability every year in this country.[2]

- A study conducted in the Montreal suburb of Laval found that less than one-third of people with high blood pressure had their hypertension controlled. Untreated hypertension confers a greatly increased risk for

2. Assuming a New York State population in 1984 of 17.7 million, and a Canadian population in 1994 of 28 million, a rate of death due to negligence of 0.00039 and a rate of permanent disability of 0.000099 (Brennan et al. 1991, 373).

heart attack and stroke. Pica et al. (1988) commented: "The study suggests that follow-up and counselling on modifiable risk factors in borderline and mild hypertensives might not be up to recent Canadian and American guidelines."

In addition, it is noted that health care systems often fail to translate promising directions from the research literature into programs or policies if doing so requires fundamental system restructuring. For example, few changes to our system have occurred as a result of these "prescriptions" for change.

- Many studies (Hall et al. 1992; Vetter, Jones, and Victor 1984; Pathy et al. 1992; Stuck et al. 1995; Rich et al. 1995; Hendriksen, Lund, and Stromgard 1984; Cupples and McKnight 1994) indicate that better organized primary care for people with chronic illness can reduce their need for specialist and hospital care and reduce short-term mortality rates by 25 percent or more. In one such experiment (Hall et al. 1992) conducted in New Westminster, British Columbia, people applying for long-term care were randomly assigned to a control group (who received the standard package of services depending on eligibility), or the experimental group which received individually tailored health promotion from a visiting nurse. After 36 months, patients in the health promotion program were 39 percent less likely to have died or to have been placed in a long-term care institution.

Recent critiques show consumers have considerable difficulty with the system's failure to integrate services and coordinate care. A number of reports document the consumers' perspective that the system is a "nonsystem," a bewildering maze of seemingly unconnected providers who focus only on one part of a person's care. Quebec's Rochon Commission (1988), for example, noted:

> Services are at present fragmented, with the establishments centred narrowly upon their respective missions and practically ignoring each other. In the course of the consultations carried out by the Commission, this state of affairs resulted in many complaints about impersonal care and a complete absence of any global approach to problems of the individual.

The Ontario Health Review Panel (1987) concluded its executive summary with this:

> There is a remarkable consistency and repetition in the findings and recommendations of improvements in all the information we reviewed. Current submissions and earlier reports highlight the need to place greater emphasis on primary care, to integrate and co-ordinate services, to achieve a community focus for health and to increase the emphasis on health

promotion and disease prevention. The panel notes with concern that well-founded recommendations made by credible groups over fifteen years have rarely been translated into action.

This suggests that we have known how to reform our health care system for at least 25 years but have been unable to make much progress with appropriate reforms. Even now as provinces restructure their systems and refocus on quality, there is relatively little action on changing how services are actually delivered. Most policy development has focused on budget cuts and changes to governance and administration. Consumers—particularly those with chronic illness—still face an uncoordinated system.

At the same time, it must be acknowledged that, in general, information is the weakest factor affecting any policy development process (Lomas 1990). Other more significant factors typically include the environment external to the health policy process (e.g. how deficits and debt are perceived), the decision-making process within the health policy system (e.g., centralized or decentralized, top down or bottom up), and the values, beliefs, and interests of stakeholders and the public (that is, those who derive incomes from the health system as providers, public officials, manufacturers of drugs and durable medical equipment, as well as those who currently, or may in future, need to rely on its services).

WHAT CONSUMERS COULD BRING TO THE REFORM PROCESS

There are at least three justifications for involving consumers in the development of public policy.

- Consumers have unique information relevant to the decisions being considered by policymakers. The implication is that better decisions will result if consumer input is tapped to tailor services to consumer expectations and preferences.
- Consumers bring balance and fresh perspectives to the traditional debates that predictably occur between funders and service providers. This balancing function can often be used to moderate or bolster resource demands, or to influence reallocation decisions.
- Consumer involvement in policy development can contribute to society's "civic sense." Democracy provides either for citizens to be represented in decision making via clear lines of accountability (usually elections) or for citizens to be directly involved in decision making themselves. The latter is seen as a way to strengthen the public's sense of ownership over public institutions and processes.

Most provincial reports on health reform and system reviews call for more public participation, and many reform proposals have specific measures aimed at increasing consumer control over health care delivery, a subject discussed in more detail in the section on regionalization.

ANALYTICAL FRAMEWORKS

In developing the case for more consumer involvement, this report relies on a number of analytical frameworks. The first, and arguably the most important, deals with the very powerful interest groups which dominate our health care system and are greatly threatened by reform. For example, the British Columbia Royal Commission on Health Care and Costs (1991) made the following pointed observation: "Too often creative and cost-effective solutions to health care problems—particularly problems in the delivery of services—are opposed by a fortress mentality that equates change with threat, shifts in priorities or reallocation of funds with cutbacks, and integration and accountability with loss of control."

The term "interest group" is often used quite loosely, usually to describe some association complaining to government. However, there are clear differences in the "bench strength" of various types of interest groups. Some represent individuals or organizations—for example, physicians or drug companies have enormous resources, can autonomously make many policy decisions themselves and are automatically included in consultations about new health policies. Others, including most consumer health groups, have few resources, little decision-making authority, and are rarely included in meaningful consultation.

Of course, some so-called "disease groups" (for example, the Heart and Stroke Foundation or the Canadian Cancer Society) have quite good resources. Their main function is to raise funds for research and to provide specific member services, with advocacy playing only a minor role in their overall activity. Such organizations are not generally considered true "consumer" groups. On the other hand, many women's groups, much of the environmental movement, activist groups from the disabled community, and some groups with a disease-specific focus (people with AIDS, breast cancer action groups, etc.) do focus much of their energy on advocacy.

Consumers who are ill have a direct stake in how well the health care system operates—what's called a "concentrated" interest—as distinct from the majority in the population whose interests in health care are far more diffuse (Marmor and Morone 1980) By contrast, people who work in the system also have a concentrated interest and are, in general, far more powerful in exerting influence over policy. When those with chronic illnesses join forces to effect change, they may experience great difficulty obtaining access to and influencing the relevant policy tables—reflecting a fundamental imbalance between different types of concentrated interests.

Robert Alford (1975) outlined his insights on interest group politics in the health care system in his classic book *Health Care Politics: Ideological and Interest Group Barriers to Reform*.

He began by making a distinction between those who have a direct stake in the present health care system, which he called "structural interests," and those who merely stand to benefit from a differently organized system, which he called "potential interests."

He noted that among the various structural interests in the health care system, some are well served by the current arrangements (e.g., physicians, drug companies). These he called the "dominant structural interests" noting that typically they had no need to organize for change since the system as currently set up serves their members very well. Although Alford categorized medicine's professional monopoly as the dominant structural interest in health care, he noted that there is always conflict *within* interest groups as well as conflict *among* groups. The result is that, although private fee-for-service practitioners, specialists, family doctors, academic physicians, and salaried practitioners do not have identical interests in the system, they all "share an interest in maintaining physician autonomy and control over the conditions of their work."

In contrast to the dominant structural interests, Alford identified the second category as "repressed structural interests." These interests are characterized as being poorly served by current arrangements. In addition, they have enormous difficulty organizing for change "unless extraordinary political energies are mobilized." Alford said that most other health care workers, (nurses, lab technicians, ambulance attendants, physiotherapists, etc.) are "repressed structural interests."

Alford also proposed a third category, "challenging structural interests," and pointed to the "corporate rationalizers"—the planners, administrators, public health agencies, medical schools, hospitals, government departments, and researchers who are increasingly contesting medicine's professional monopoly. Alford said that challenging structural interests emerge when major developments in the structure of society occur—for example, when new technologies, shifts in the division of labour, or new incentives create pressure for "a new way of doing things around here."

Alford considered consumers to be both repressed structural interests and potential interests, noting that they have little in the way of resources or authority from present system relationships but that they would gain greater interests from system restructuring.

The second framework used for analysis was developed by the political scientist, Paul Sabatier (1987), who identified two key factors to achieve what he called "policy-oriented learning." The first is the need to create coalitions for change—bringing individuals and groups together to work on an issue or reform idea. Sabatier noted that shared ideology is a more powerful glue than common financial interests over the long term and that this should be considered in developing effective coalitions. The second factor is to ensure public policy forums where at least two coalitions can openly debate their beliefs and present their evidence. Sabatier warned against debating core values and ideologies which are not amenable to change.

However, he pointed out that learning can occur when the coalitions debate beliefs, and that beliefs can change in the face of compelling evidence.

The implication from Alford is that governments trying to restructure the health care system will benefit if they develop a coalition of repressed groups to take on the dominant interests. From Sabatier, we learn more about the details of how coalitions work to alter policy and how opportunities for public debate can change beliefs and foster learning.

This paper also uses several frameworks to examine levels of consumer participation. Consumers have different levels of experience and expertise. Processes intended to involve them need to take this into consideration. Charlotte Williamson (1995) proposed three categories: patients and carers,[3] consumer groups, and consumerists. The first two are self-explanatory but the third refers to people with a level of understanding that is "wider and more abstract than that of any single consumer group or patient care-group." She noted (Williamson 1995) that consumerists tend to focus on general principles such as "access, information, choice, advocacy, equity, safety and redress— with the additional health care principles of autonomy, respect, support, control and decision making and co-ordination and continuity of care."

Another framework useful in approaching levels of consumer involvement is the "ladder of participation" (Charles and DeMaio 1993) where the higher the rung, the greater the decision-making authority (Church et al. 1995).

Lowest level: Processes that are mainly consultative comprise the lowest rungs on the ladder. Examples include royal commissions, advisory committees, focus groups. This level involves no real power transfer, only the right to have concerns heard.

Middle level: Processes that provide for consumers and providers to share decision-making responsibility. Examples include joint policy boards and planning committees. Some transfer of power from traditional decision makers is required.

Top level: Processes that put the power over decision making entirely in consumers' hands. Examples include health boards that exclude providers. This requires a substantial transfer of decision-making authority from providers, government officials, etc.

Finally, Mary Draper and Sophie Hill (1995) from the Royal Melbourne Institute of Technology developed the following table to illustrate some of the different assumptions at work in involving consumers.

---

3. The term carers refers to informal (usually unpaid) providers of services.

Table 1

Approaches to consumer empowerment

Scientific approaches	Market solutions	Legal approaches	Democratic participation
Rely on objective measurement and statistics	Rely on either market information as a way of influencing health services, or more responsive services which attract consumers	Rely on legally or administratively defined rights, and access to judicial and semijudicial institutions	Rely on ways for consumers to participate individually and collectively in health decisions
Consumers are subjects of research	Consumers are informed choosers	Consumers are citizens with rights	Consumer are equal partners and citizens
Strategies: – standards – outcomes – guidelines – variations – classification – patient surveys	Strategies: – information on providers – marketing – statement of expectations – consumer surveys	Strategies: – health charters – right to complain – legal redress – legislation – transparent decision making – advocacy	Strategies: – consultation – involvement in decisions – participation in planning – hand-held records – representation on committees – accountability to consumers

Source: Draper and Hill (1995).

Note: These authors note that the table was derived from one developed by the Health Issues Centre. *Casemix, Quality, and Consumers.* Melbourne, Australia 1992.

SOME CURRENT AND EMERGING OPPORTUNITIES
FOR CONSUMER INVOLVEMENT

Regionalization

There is some question about whether the recent regionalization of Canada's health care system in every province except Ontario allows more opportunity for consumer involvement in health care decision making. In fact, it is questionable whether increased decision-making authority is truly desired by the public (Charles and DeMaio 1993). A recent study in Ontario found that fewer than 30 percent of the District Health Council members sampled were willing to assume more authority, preferring to remain in an advisory role to the Minister of Health (Abelson et al. 1995).

In those provinces with regionalized systems, the process was at least partly envisioned to facilitate greater local community participation, including more consumer input. However, it is not clear whether this has actually occurred.

In Alberta, for example, many individual hospitals used to be governed by boards which had partly elected membership. These boards have now been replaced by regional boards whose members are political appointees. Although Alberta intends to elect two-thirds of its health board members, beginning with the municipal elections in 1998, opportunities for demo-cratic participation appear to have decreased with regionalization in the short term at least. There is also some question regarding whom the current health board members represent—consumers or the government.

Regionalization can also mean a decline in the absolute number of citizen boards governing health care. In Saskatchewan, for example, the number fell from some 400 separate boards to 30—which could mean less, rather than more, opportunity for consumer participation. Now eight of 12 members of Saskatchewan's health boards are elected, implying more direct accountability to the local population for their performance. After the first round of elections in October 1995, a large number of health care providers took seats on the boards, perhaps illustrating that those with the greatest stake in the system are more likely to seek control over its destiny than those with more diffuse, public interest concerns.

On the other hand, regionalization in Saskatchewan has been accompanied by some very deliberate attempts to increase consumer input. The Prince Albert Health District, for example, is creating new vehicles for consumer involvement including a rural health advisory committee, a community development committee, and an Aboriginal health working group.[4]

---

4. Personal communication with Stan Rice, CEO, Prince Albert Regional Health District.

In Quebec, regionalization did not replace institutional boards but rather introduced an additional layer in the decision-making hierarchy. The transfer of authority from the province to regional bodies has steadily increased as the regions have developed technical and managerial skills. In the latest set of reforms, the boards were given authority over resource allocation for most of the health care budget, although the Minister of Health and Social Services retains a veto over these decisions. In addition, extensive changes were introduced regarding the conduct of elections to the councils governing these regional boards and the other health care establishments in the province.

Regionalization (with its potential for increased local input) is also supposed to result in better decision making. There is little research evidence, however, to support this assumption (Charles and DeMaio 1993).

Nor is it clear that governance should be the focus for increasing consumer participation, given the extent to which providers manage to keep the upper hand. Two articles by consumer advocate Barry Checkoway (1980 and 1982) describe how consumers managed to take control of an Illinois Health Service Agency board in the late 1970s and how quickly this was reversed when the local hospitals and physicians organized to rout them at the next election and reasserted provider control over health planning.

The Cochrane Collaboration and Consumer Network

The Cochrane Collaboration is an international attempt to review the research literature on the effectiveness of health care interventions to facilitate evidence-based medicine and the development of clinical guidelines. One guiding principle is that decisions to abandon health care therapies determined to be ineffective according to the evidence should not be made by professionals and service providers alone, but require input from, and collaboration with, consumers as well. This openness by researchers to public input suggests a new and welcoming environment for those willing to become involved.

And yet, a recent paper by consumer advocate Hilda Bastien (1994) was critical of the Collaboration. "In the consumer approach, removing barriers to participation therefore becomes a goal. This is in stark contrast with the Collaboration's statement in its *Handbook* that 'the disincentives that confront those who are wondering whether they should become involved are a useful screening test in themselves.'"

Ms. Bastien continued by pointing out how acutely consumers feel their lack of status when forced to ask for information, phones, and reimbursement for out-of-pocket expenses. She also noted that, "For individuals where health care is irrelevant to their livelihood and days of participation may mean losing pay, the situation is different."

On the other hand, Bastien also applauded the openness of the research community in inviting consumer input and outlined the development of a consumer network "to bring together in a broad coalition the individuals and groups concerned with public participation in the Cochrane Collaboration." The proposal for the Consumer Network identified two main aims: to help foster an environment within the Collaboration which encourages and facilitates consumer input and to promote consumer groups' participation in, and use of, systematic reviews of the effects of health care.

Future plans for the Network include mechanisms to develop accountability for consumer representatives on the various review groups associated with the Collaboration. Bastien also suggested that consumers could be involved in more participatory research and noted the growing trend toward consumers conducting their own research.

Consumer Representation on Health Professions' Regulatory Bodies in Ontario

Another opportunity which theoretically opens the door for increased public participation was created when Ontario passed its Regulated Health Professions Act (RHPA). This legislation requires that public members (lay representatives) comprise up to 49 percent of the governing councils. Since each of these bodies is legally responsible for setting standards of practice for the profession in question, there appears to be new opportunity for consumer input into the process.

Certainly, in the case of midwifery, consumers have had a major influence over setting the standards of practice for this newly recognized profession in Ontario. Indeed, without consumers' strong support and backing, it is doubtful whether midwifery could have become a regulated profession (Tyson 1989).

Even before this increase in consumer representatives on regulatory boards, public members have occasionally been able to win concessions over professional objections. For example, one of the public members at the Royal College of Dental Surgeons of Ontario (RCDS) fought for a regulatory change that would permit dentists to work for nondentists—a change which would allow full dental care to be provided in community health centres, for example. Despite sharp attacks from some professional members, this regulation did pass the RCDS Council.[5]

INTRODUCTION TO THE CASE STUDIES

The following case studies of consumer involvement in health care decision making include one subnational example (long-term care reform in Ontario),

---

5. Personal communication with Michele Harding, the former public member of the RCDS of Ontario who fought for this regulatory change.

one national example (Breast Cancer Survivors in Canada), and one international example (the Consumers' Health Forum of Australia, Inc.).

They were selected because all three demonstrate the promise of consumer input, in that health care policies have changed as a result of their involvement. However, each also provides its own cautionary tale regarding some of the limitations and barriers which can interfere with consumer participation.

Each of the case studies begins with a brief background history, followed by a section detailing the evidence of consumer influence over policy, a section dealing with issues regarding consumer representation, and one dealing with resource issues. Each study concludes with a section highlighting its fit with the analytical frameworks described earlier.

CASE STUDY NO. 1: CONSUMERS AND LONG-TERM CARE IN ONTARIO[6]

Background

The Senior Citizens' Consumer Alliance for Long-term Care Reform was formed in 1990 in response to government proposals to change long-term care in Ontario. The Alliance was a coalition of three very large consumer organizations, representing the majority of seniors in the province:
- the Ontario Coalition of Senior Citizens' Organizations (OCSCO) with 39 member organizations representing more than 300,000 seniors;
- the United Senior Citizens of Ontario, with more than 1,000 seniors clubs from all areas of the province; and
- the Consumers' Association of Canada (Ontario).

The government's initial approach to reform included a very broad public consultation process, aimed specifically at garnering consumer input. The Alliance members believed that senior citizens should have influence over the ultimate policy direction. As the group most affected by long-term care changes (numerically, at least), its members believed that their voting strength could convince politicians to side with their wishes. However, the Alliance did not like the government's initial policy proposals and worried that the consultation process being designed by the government would not lead to the kind of policies preferred by its members.

---

6. Much of the information for this section comes from one of the authors of this paper, Carol Kushner, who was involved as a consultant to the Senior Citizens' Consumer Alliance for Long-term Care Reform between 1990 and the end of 1992.

With its own project funding—mainly from government,[7] the Alliance conducted a variety of initiatives related to long-term care reform, including:

- hiring consultants to conduct research, prepare briefs, raise funds and assist with communications strategy;
- sponsoring policy conferences where consumer groups, government decision makers, providers, and researchers could exchange views and debate the issues in the search for direction and consensus;
- running public hearings into long-term care during which consumers, providers and voluntary organizations, and government officials were invited to make oral presentations or written submissions to a panel of Alliance representatives;
- publishing and broadly disseminating several papers concerning long-term care reform, including a detailed alternative comprehensive policy proposal; and
- effecting a range of advocacy activities including direct lobbying of government officials, policy advisors, and ministers responsible for the decisions affecting the sector.

One of the Alliance's key policy proposals was to create a network of nonprofit, neighbourhood-level, multiservice agencies (MSAs). The MSAs would determine an individual's eligibility for service, provide initial and ongoing assessments, and deliver a wide range of community-based services. These new MSAs were to be governed by community boards, including consumer representation. This MSA model proved to be most controversial with providers because it represented a major shift away from the brokerage model, where intermediaries arrange for, and purchase, necessary long-term care from organizations such as the Victorian Order of Nurses and the Red Cross.

To bolster support for this key element, the Alliance commissioned an analysis of the economic advantages of the MSA model. The hypothesis was that integrating services under the MSAs would involve less spending on administration and overhead and permit more long-term care resources to go into direct service. The analysis (Price Waterhouse 1995) showed that MSAs would put approximately $44 million more into direct service delivery than the system as currently organized.

---

7. Ontario government funding to support the Alliance came from the Ministry of Health, the Ministry of Community and Social Services, and the Ministry of Culture (which was also responsible for the Office of Seniors' Issues at the time). Additional resources came from a number of private foundations and industry.

Evidence of Policy Influence

The Alliance did directly influence government policy, though for only a short time (Kushner 1996). Following the release of the Alliance's policy recommendations (Senior Citizens' Consumer Alliance 1992), the government put out a series of discussion documents and subsequently introduced new legislation which very closely mirrored the Alliance's advice (Ontario Legislature 1993; Ontario Ministry of Health 1993a,b,c,d).

Even before this occurred, however, Ontario's Health Minister, Frances Lankin, acknowledged in a private meeting with the Alliance that their proposals offered "a practical alternative" to the directions her government had largely inherited from the previous administration, and she hinted strongly that she intended to follow the seniors' advice.[8]

Political support for these proposals continued under the next Minister of Health, Ruth Grier, although by now, some of the difficulties with the new law had become evident. For example, consumer influence alone was proving insufficient to overcome resistance from providers. The consumers' perception that support from government officials was also relatively weak is understandable, given that the original proposals (which had been rejected by consumers) had originated with many of the same public servants. That being said, the new policies were outlined in government discussion documents and, ultimately, drafted and passed into law. However, this legislative victory did not translate into the creation of any MSAs as implementation never occurred.

Following the most recent provincial election, the long-term care act was repealed, as the new government had promised to do if elected. This was not politically difficult, as there were no MSAs to dismantle. The Alliance has continued its work with one less member (OCSCO dropped out to work on other priorities). However, on the issue of their preferred model for integrated service delivery, consumers have largely lost their leverage with political and bureaucratic decision makers. The new government is not particularly interested in consumer input. The opportunity to challenge the interests of providers seems to have passed.

Other Issues: Who Is a Legitimate Consumer? How Are They Accountable? Whom Do They Represent?

One common criticism of the Consumer Alliance was that it did not truly represent "consumer" interests, because its leaders were not care recipients themselves. (We will return to this issue again in both the other case studies.) A related complaint was that the Alliance members were really "professional"

---

8. Personal communication with Sylvia Cheuy, a consultant to the Alliance.

consumers, and somehow not "grassroots" enough. A third criticism was that the consumers were overly reliant on their consultants, who were "using" them to further their own policy ends.

To address these questions, we must look at the Alliance's structure and its mode of operation. It was essentially a group of groups—a coalition. (In fact, one of its members was itself a coalition of groups—OCSCO.) Each participating organization "donated" four of its senior representatives to join the Alliance as it addressed long-term care reform. Each organization had democratic mechanisms for selecting its own leadership, which in turn selected the participants in the Alliance. In some cases, the leaders of the organization took on this responsibility themselves. It is important to note that the Alliance was established to deal exclusively with long-term care. It was expected to "self-destruct" when this work was over. The Alliance members worked hard to address the complexity of policy issues and to think through a responsible "consumer perspective." They hired consultants to advise them, but remained very much in charge of the agenda. They communicated extensively with their own members and were responsible to them for the positions taken.

Other Issues: Resources

Resources for the Consumer Alliance came largely from the Ontario government, although negotiating for these monies required significant time and energy on the part of the seniors and their consultants. Additional support for activities also came from the charitable and private sectors. The consumers identified a number of issues associated with the continuous need to raise funds. One was that it tended to divide their attention between "bouts of fund-raising to support their activities" and "the policy work we had all joined forces to accomplish."

A related issue was the concern about potential co-option by the funder. For some consumer organizations, this is sufficiently worrying to reject business or government sponsorship as a matter of policy. For others, recognition that co-option can be a problem may prompt steps to reduce the likelihood of undue influence. For example, some groups insist on clarifying up front their right to independent action and their need to represent consumer interests rather than industrial or governmental ones. Satisfied that these measures can work, some consumer organizations now feel they can accept such offers of help without fearing compromise. There is no question, however, that consumer groups are very vulnerable to changes in funding sources. Co-option is only one aspect of this vulnerability.

One consumer advocate put it like this:

The lack of sustained core funding from governments for consumer organizations seems to be based on the assumption that consumer groups enjoy a degree of stability and capacity which parallel that of industrial groups and professional organizations. This is incorrect. The fact that governments appear to want our involvement has not always translated into their willingness to cover even our travel expenses and other out of pocket costs associated with our voluntary participation. As for resources to conduct our own research, publish position papers, or network among ourselves, we're often left scrambling to find a funder. The truth is in my organization today, what we're spending on fundraising is about equal to what we're raising through the effort. This is not a sustainable arrangement.

The increased use of the designation "special interest group" as a pejorative term has also been highlighted as a serious problem. The term has been used in Canada to delegitimize a wide variety of public interest groups. The Consumers' Association of Canada, for example, used to receive substantial core funding support from the federal government. It is no coincidence that the CAC no longer publishes its own magazine and has, as a result, lost its main mechanism for communicating with its members.

Interest groups of all types risk being disqualified for public funding on this basis. However, cutting them off fails to distinguish between those who have a vested interest and those who have a public interest perspective. The former groups, who stand to profit from policy directions, can—and usually should—pay for their own advocacy efforts. By contrast, consumer groups who have a public interest perspective in addressing the disposition of public goods, and representing the broad interests of the people usually cannot manage to fund themselves. This supports Yale University political scientist and professor Ted Marmor's analysis of concentrated versus diffuse interests (Marmor and Christianson 1982). Most consumers are really potential consumers of care rather than actual patients or clients of the system in an ongoing way. Occasional use of the health care system is not enough to produce a concentrated interest in the system. Even though, theoretically, everyone is a potential user of, for example, long-term care, most Canadians have only a diffuse interest in the system. On the other hand, those who work in the system, and in particular, those who have the most power within it, have a concentrated interest in its direction. Diffuse interests need substantial resources to compete effectively with concentrated interests.

Relevance to the Analytic Frameworks

In this case study, the Consumer Alliance was able to influence the direction of public policy very dramatically. The strategies conformed to the "democratic participation" approach in the Draper and Hill framework (table 1).

With reference to Charlotte Williamson's categories, the Alliance began as a consumer group with a specific mandate. However, its members quickly developed the consumerist's perspective looking broadly at the issues of access, equity, choice, continuity of care, and coordination of service. In the words of Alliance president, Jane Leitch, "We felt we were acting, not only on our own behalf, but also for our children and our children's children. A better system, that would be our legacy."

This case study also appears consistent with Alford's framework for looking at interest group politics, confirming that dominant structural interests (i.e., those people that work in the system) are usually well served by current arrangements and have more influence over its direction than the repressed interests, which include consumers, their family members, and consumer organizations. Similarly, it supports his view that enormous political energy is needed to organize these more diffuse and disorganized sectors. For example, early in its history, two of the three groups were in conflict over issues unrelated to long-term care. Although they set aside these differences and managed to work together, the process required time, energy, and strong leadership.

For a time, the Consumer Alliance attempted to become what Alford called "a challenging structural interest." It seized the opportunity created by the new government's decision to involve consumers more directly in policy development. Access to financial support from government for Alliance activities allowed the consumers to mount a concerted campaign for "a new way of doing things around here."

Paul Sabatier's work is germane to this case study as well. Part of his theory of the policy process is that fundamental policy change occurs only when beliefs change. To bring about changes in beliefs, according to Sabatier, requires "policy-oriented learning"—most often involving a public debate between at least two coalitions with adequate resources to put forward their views. He also argued that debates are most fruitful when organized around differing beliefs rather than ideologies.

Through publications, public hearings, and especially at the well-attended policy conferences, the Alliance was able to challenge existing beliefs with new perspectives and new evidence.

The impact, however, was short-lived. When it comes to major change in public policy, information plays a relatively minor role. Far more important in this case was the change in government and the declining government funding support for the Alliance.

CASE STUDY NO. 2: THE INFLUENCE OF CONSUMERS ON BREAST CANCER POLICY[9]

Background

Perhaps no disease or condition, except AIDS, has stirred more consumer activism than breast cancer. Survivors of the disease have begun to influence health policy in a number of spheres, including research and the development of clinical guidelines. This disease, according to research evidence, is destined to afflict one woman in nine over the course of her lifetime. It is estimated that in 1996, 18,600 women will be diagnosed with breast cancer and 5,300 will die from the disease (National Cancer Institute of Canada 1996).

Breast cancer presents a number of unique challenges. In the first place, unlike many other cancers, the factors which cause breast cancer remain largely a mystery, making primary prevention virtually impossible.

Then too, there are controversies over the effectiveness of various screening approaches (mammography, clinical breast examinations, and breast self-examination) as well as of current treatment options which include surgery, chemotherapy, and radiotherapy. Overall, although screening programs are turning up cancers at an earlier stage, mortality rates from the disease have remained almost stable over the past 30 years. While this might suggest progress, given the rising incidence of the disease, this may well not be the case. Although mammography is discovering more tumours and at an earlier stage than could be detected by physical examination, many of these "new" breast cancers are very slow growing and might never pose a threat to life. This not only raises questions about mammographic screening[10] but also suggests that science has not really made much progress against those "older" types of breast cancer which still cost lives despite early detection and treatment efforts.

From a public policy perspective, dealing with breast cancer presents a minefield of complexity. Many consumer groups have formed to address what are seen as major inadequacies in responding to the disease. First and foremost are the hundred or so local support groups peppered across the country whose raison d'être is usually to provide newly diagnosed women with a source of information and the chance to connect with other women

---

9. This case study was constructed from a series of telephone interviews with consumers, policymakers, advocates, researchers, and health care providers involved in the breast cancer issue (see appendix for list of interviews).

10. Canadian guidelines for breast cancer screening call for women to receive mammography from age 50 on, based on research indicating that this can reduce breast cancer mortality by about 30 percent. Evidence suggests that younger women do not obtain additional benefit from mammography screening.

with the disease. Other consumer-driven breast cancer groups emphasize their advocacy role. For example, the brochure for Breast Cancer Action in Montreal identifies it as an activist group. BCAM's founder and president, Sharon Batt says the goal is to "increase the power of women with breast cancer and have an impact on the policies that affect us."

One of the high points in the efforts of breast cancer survivors to influence public policy occurred at the National Breast Cancer Forum held in Montreal in November 1993. There, for the first time, 150 breast cancer survivors and their families were able to challenge the research and treatment community with a series of issues they felt were receiving too little attention.

Communications problems with providers were a major concern. Survivors and advocates wanted to have family doctors more involved in the prevention, detection, and treatment of their disease (Babinski 1993). Asked to indicate how their input might change clinical practice, for example, one survivor responded, "Well, a few physicians at the conference seemed surprised to find out how much information some survivors wanted. Some actually said that what they'd heard from survivors would change how they dealt with breast cancer patients."

Survivors also argued for a stronger role in all aspects of the breast cancer continuum—from research through to treatment (Babinski 1993). For example, survivors asked researchers to pay more attention to investigating what causes breast cancer—particularly its connection with estrogens and environmental pollutants. And they argued for more money for research rather than a reallocation of resources from other research initiatives. Another issue concerned alternative therapies. A large proportion of breast cancer patients use both conventional and alternative therapies but little information is available about the effectiveness of the alternatives. "Women need this information to make good choices," was how one survivor put it.

The three-day event was hailed by many who attended as historic. The conference ended with a long list of recommendations, many of which originated with the breast cancer survivors who attended.

Evidence of Policy Influence

One concrete indication of survivor influence is the existence of the Canadian Breast Cancer Network (CBCN). This consumer-driven network encourages education, public awareness, and research to improve the quality and length of life of breast cancer survivors. The federal government has provided CBCN with extensive technical support and expertise as well as financial and in-kind support for the network's outreach activities.

Also demonstrating consumer influence are the priority areas developed by the Canadian Breast Cancer Research Initiative (CBCRI): improving provider/patient communications at the time of diagnosis and afterward, establishing evidence on alternative therapies and health services research.

This is the group that sets the research agenda for breast cancer and it includes survivors, patients, researchers, ethicists, and policymakers. The management committee for CBCRI had their monthly meeting in Montreal so they could all attend the Forum.

"Based on what they heard at the Forum," said Louise Liao, research program director for CBCRI, "they wanted to take action." At the March meeting following the Forum, the management committee invited the Forum's organizers to a full-day workshop—asking them to identify underserved areas for research. "They, too, asked for more work on communications and alternative therapies."

> There's no question that advocacy and survivor groups have had an influence on the research agenda for breast cancer. But it isn't just the agenda. The processes for conducting research have been challenged by survivors, as well. For example, in setting aside funds for communications research, our sub-committee released an RFA (request for applications) which explicitly asked for applications that included survivors as part of the research team in developing the project, implementing the research and analyzing the results. It was our understanding that consumers and advocates could be involved in helping to frame the research question, helping to design the study, and interpret the results. In addition, when it came to reviewing the applications for funding, the review panel included a breast cancer survivor in order to tap her experiential expertise.

Of the eight projects ultimately funded, one is participatory action research. Breast cancer survivors will be fully involved—not just advisory to the project but actually conducting it and getting paid as part of the research team. The researcher, Professor Abby Lippman from McGill, agrees that this is a significant departure from traditional approaches, "but the logic behind this concept—that women with breast cancer find it easier to talk to other women with breast cancer than with a professional researcher— is compelling."

When the information exchange projects were being set up, 50 percent of the positions on each advisory panel had to be survivors, signalling the government's intention to put consumers more in charge of the projects' management. However, calling the panels "advisory" seems to imply that some other group would actually manage the projects and make the important decisions. That, in fact, appears to be the case in Atlantic Canada where an executive committee has been set up in addition to the advisory panel. Also, even though survivors on advisory panels have a strong influence over project operations in other regions, actual management of these projects is in the hands of paid coordinators. It is difficult to see an alternative to these arrangements given that the advisory panels typically meet only twice a year, too rarely to permit hands-on, continuous leadership.

Consumers are involved as well in advising the Canadian Breast Cancer Initiative about clinical guidelines for care and treatment. Breast cancer survivor, Dr. Maria Hugi feels strongly that no one could replace the important role survivors play in this process. "No one who hasn't been a breast cancer patient has the same insights," she said. She is the sole consumer on the clinical guideline committee and, although she would love to have others involved, she definitely feels that she has made an impact. "Perhaps because I am also a medical doctor, I'm not that easy to intimidate, and it's been possible for me to convey to other committee members the importance of seeing the bigger picture." She has tried, for example, to bring to the table the wealth of concerns related to what happens after the disease has been diagnosed and treatment has been received.

> There's a legacy of issues related to our daily lives and coping with the complications of treatment—what happens to younger women dealing with early menopause, for example, and their concerns about heart disease and osteoporosis? What about diet? What about pregnancy? What about implants? What about emotional issues, and getting back to work? What about lymphoedema? The experts weren't planning to address most of these issues, but I bring a sense of street smarts to the table—I'm in the trenches, they're in the ivory towers and we're learning to value one another.

The process being followed by the clinical guidelines committee involved the selection of 10 topics. The committee must agree about the content to be included under each topic. When position papers for the topics have been developed, they will be shared with other survivors for their reactions and feedback. Hugi pointed out "I'm really just a conduit in this process of sharing information and checking back with the broader survivor network."

Dr. Cindy Bell, who has the breast cancer portfolio at the Medical Research Council, agreed that advocates, survivors, and researchers have also had an impact in moving the research agenda forward. The management committee of the Canadian Breast Cancer Research Initiative has taken these issues very seriously. "We've been reminded of the importance of survivor perspectives." She argued for the need to strengthen the role of advocacy noting that advocates will be an important voice when the breast cancer research initiative comes up for renewal next year. (The federal government's commitment of $25 million for breast cancer over five years was established in 1992.)

On the other hand, some survivors and policymakers are more cautious about the influence consumers have had. For example, Pat Kelly, one of the organizers of the National Forum in Montreal and a breast cancer survivor herself, said she is worried that the five or six site-specific programs for breast cancer research in Canada are not working together or sharing information.

In addition, Kelly, who helped set up Ontario's breast-screening program, now has some doubts about whether mammography may cause more harm than good, "given that nine out of 10 mammograms identified as 'suspicious' are actually false positives causing women enormous anxiety."

Sharon Batt, president of Breast Cancer Action Montreal and policy advisor to the Canadian Breast Cancer Network, also believes that consumers are not having as much impact as she would like. In some cases, she noted, projects that do not reflect consumer priorities have been rubber-stamped for funding. She also worries about tokenism—the tendency of government processes to add a single consumer to a group of professionals and then feel that consumer input has been ensured.

Other Issues: Who Is a legitimate Consumer? How Are They Accountable? Whom Do They Represent? What Issues Can They Tackle?

Pat Kelly said she is concerned about who really wields the power at the CBCRI, noting that consumers are on the management committee but not the steering committee where she believes the real decisions are made. Dependence on government funding is part of the problem, said Kelly, "because you want the money, but then government wants to pick and choose the individual participants which skews things their way....I'm not passive enough to suit government-controlled processes." Despite her long involvement with the issue and her role in planning the Forum, she maintained that she was not invited to help establish the Canadian Breast Cancer Network, a contention hotly denied by Sharon Batt and several others active in CBCN, who insisted that Kelly was invited to help set up the network.

While it may, perhaps, be natural for those new to the experience of sharing power to select people who will be less adversarial, Kelly is worried this can mean losing the advocacy role she values so highly. However, Kelly said, "Until consumers have an understanding of their own values and identity and manage to nurture that sense into a forceful body, I think we will keep losing the battle against co-option."

She also feels strongly that survivors involved in public policy must be accountable to a group or an organization. "They need to represent more than simply their personal issues; survivors must be advocates for change and tied into a broader group for input and reporting back."

Another interviewee mentioned that although survivors were for the most part eager to participate in policy setting, there was one area none wanted to address, for understandable reasons—palliative care. It is possible that this issue (and perhaps there are others) might be better addressed by consumers who are not survivors—perhaps by affected family members or other advocates who do not have breast cancer. On the other hand, both

Kelly and Batt warned against accepting any arguments that may exclude survivors a priori and rob them of their advocacy rights.

It was pointed out by several researchers and policymakers that consumer involvement took more time but that the time invested was worth it because of the extreme relevance of the input. Some, however, cautioned that it was often difficult for individual survivors to move beyond their personal issues to become effective advocates.

Other Issues: Resources

What consumer advocates want and need is money—a level of funding that can be used to support our activities—and an agenda that reflects our perspectives which are understandably diverse given the multicultural nature of our society. We want the advocacy community to continue influencing the research, diagnostic and treatment communities. We need to build these partnerships.

Ms. Kelly contrasted the situation for survivors and advocates in Canada with what is happening in the United States and finds the United States further ahead in terms of the respect and support consumers receive there. For example, one of the key American initiatives involves training survivors to sit on peer review committees, something almost unknown here in Canada.

However, a key limitation to more consumer advocacy in Canada is that nonprofit charitable organizations must, by law, limit their advocacy work to 20 percent or less of the budget to retain their charitable status. This financial disincentive discourages many organizations from becoming more involved in advocacy and, in general, weakens the consumers' opportunity to push for change. To address a similar difficulty in the United States, the National Breast Cancer Coalition there has set up two separate nonprofit organizations: one for advocacy education and the other one for advocacy. Donations to the former are tax deductible, while those to the latter are not.

Pat Kelly said she recommends creating stronger links to breast cancer advocacy organizations in the United States. She also thought the private sector should be paying more of the shot. "There is a huge amount of profit going to industries involved with this disease that's not benefitting us at all."

By contrast, Sharon Batt thinks that reliance on industry support would increase consumer groups' vulnerability to exploitation and make it even harder for them to advocate for policies opposed by business. However, without adequate support for advocacy, she said "consumer groups are also ripe for exploitation by governments who are more than willing to offload service responsibilities to them as long as they don't have to pay for it." She noted for example, that although the Canadian Breast Cancer Initiative has a five-year budget of $25 million, the federal government only provided

$75,000 this year to support the Canadian Breast Cancer Network, with no guarantees of continued funding for it. And she went on to note the enormous challenge of trying to build a network of support groups that barely exist, they are so starved for resources. "It would have been better to begin at the beginning and get these groups up and running on a more solid footing. You can't network nothing."

Besides resources to reimburse expenses, or to purchase supplies and pay for consulting services, some consumer advocates raise the prospect of payment for their participation. However, although both Pat Kelly and Sharon Batt were paid as consultants to help plan the National Breast Cancer Forum, Batt said that in general there is high resistance in Canada to the idea of paying advocates. And Kelly noted: "When I work in the United States, I get paid as an 'expert,' as do all of the other experts on the panel, because I've lived with breast cancer and because of my involvement with survivor issues and advocacy. Here, I don't even get invited when I ask to come for free!"

Relevance to the Analytic Frameworks

Survivor involvement in breast cancer covers each of the four approaches outlined by Draper and Hill: scientific, market, legal and democratic participation. However, their influence on the research agenda suggests an impact well beyond the usual, with the example of consumers participating on an equal footing with professional researchers in conducting research.

With respect to Williamson's categories, consumer involvement in health policy for breast cancer centres mainly on survivors and their carers, with an understandable focus on individual needs. The consumer support groups which formed to address their concerns are getting help to make linkages, and have been involved in some policy activities. However, concerns over the accountability of individual survivors on decision-making bodies perhaps suggest the need for stronger democratic processes for selecting consumer representatives.

Consumers had an impact during and following the Breast Cancer Forum in Montreal. This suggests that they succeeded in transforming themselves from a group of patients with a "repressed interest" in the system into a group with a "challenging interest" as Alford said can sometimes occur with the addition of additional resources from government and lots of organizational energy on the part of survivor support group leaders. Alford, however, also pointed out that there are often conflicts within an interest group, and these have been highlighted as well. It is possible, however, that the value consumers place on receiving better information concerning the disease and more effective treatment is perhaps the glue that holds breast cancer survivors together in spite of their differences about how to arrive at these ends.

Paul Sabatier's analysis regarding policy-oriented learning is perhaps most relevant here. The National Breast Cancer Forum in Montreal was a perfect opportunity for the treatment, research, and consumer communities to meet and share their perspectives. In effect, each represents a coalition, and the sharing certainly involved numerous challenges to commonly held beliefs in each group. As a direct result, two of consumers' key concerns were identified as priorities for research, and a survivor was appointed to participate on the guidelines to treatment committee. The role of consumers as researchers is yet another concession to what was heard at the Forum about the desire of survivors to be partners in the search for better answers to this disease.

CASE STUDY NO. 3: THE CONSUMERS' HEALTH FORUM OF AUSTRALIA

Background

The Consumers' Health Forum of Australia, Inc. (CHF) was established in 1987 (Palmer and Short 1994). It began with a petition to the common-wealth (federal) government from consumer and community groups who wanted more representation in health policy development to balance the views of professionals, governments, and industry. Its creation more or less corresponded to recommendations from a review of community parti-cipation in the Commonwealth Department of Health in 1985. The health minister of the day, Neal Blewitt, believed the Forum might be a useful foil in dealing with provider groups and, after some serious lobbying, he agreed to fund it.[11]

Representatives from 16 consumer organizations formed the original core of the general committee (the Australian term for board of directors) of the CHF.[12] The first board meeting emphasized that the group was not

---

11. Personal communication with Kate Moore, the fourth executive director of the Consumers' Health Forum. At the time of the Forum's creation, Ms. Moore headed Neal Blewitt's political staff.

12. The original list is telling—they were representative of the women's environ-mental, consumers', and health movements in Australia: Australian Community Health Association, Australian Conservation Foundation, Australian Con-sumers' Association, Australian Council of Social Services, Australian Council on Rehabilitation of the Disabled, Australian Council on the Ageing, Australian Federation of Consumer Organisations, Australian Pensioners' Federation, Australian Women's Health Network, Collective of Self-Help Groups, Disabled Peoples' International Australia, Federation of Ethnic Community Councils of Australia, Health Issues Centre, National Aboriginal and Islander Health Organisation, Victorian Mental Illness Awareness Council, Youth Affairs Council of Australia (Baldry 1992).

to become elitist, and that its role was primarily one of networking, bringing in new consumer groups, working on matters and questions the Forum members identified as having high priority and helping individual groups to work on matters they saw as essential.

The goals of the CHF (Consumers' Health Forum of Australia 1994) are:

- to be a national voice for health care consumers by promoting the role and importance of consumer perspectives on health policy and practice, and by nominating to national health committees, consumer representatives who can promote consumer views;
- to develop and respond to a network of Australia's consumer and community groups with interests in health, and to identify areas of common concern by enabling member organizations to meet, work together, and pool knowledge and resources on issues of common concern at a national, state, and local level; and
- to develop policies and actively pursue their adoption and implementation, so that inequalities are reduced, universal access is enhanced, and consumer rights are upheld by ascertaining the needs, views, and priorities of health care consumers and member organizations, and by facilitating, stimulating, and encouraging research and evaluation by consumers, and advocating for the vital role of consumers.

Voting members include representatives from peak consumer councils, national organizations, self-help groups, specialized interest groups, and advocacy organizations. It is also possible for individuals and other organizations not representing consumers to be members, although they do not have the right to vote. President Ros Wood comments that "the structure of the Forum is very important in permitting small consumer organizations like the one I helped found [the Endometriosis Association of Melbourne] to have a voice alongside the large peak groups like the Council on the Ageing. Together we can cover a lot of territory."

Any voting member can bring an issue forward for consideration by the general committee and every vote has equal weight. At the end of its first year, the Forum's voting membership numbered 81 and its associate membership 35. By September 1990, these had increased to 108 and 75 respectively, making CHF one of the largest consumer organizations in Australia (Baldry 1992). Today its activities are coordinated by a core group of 13 organizations which make up the general committee, elect an executive committee of not more than five, and employ a secretariat.

Kate Moore, CHF's executive director, heads a small staff including a policy/liaison officer, a departmental liaison officer, an office manager, and a secretary. The Forum also hires consultants as required to handle special projects and has established a good relationship with several academic researchers. She noted that the CHF only tackles "those projects which other consumer groups want us to take on. We're not in the business of duplicating what's already being handled and this has helped preserve our relationship with existing groups. We're meant to be a support and an adjunct, not a replacement."

The Forum does, however, speak for all its members on broad issues, such as doctors' fees and pharmaceuticals, while providing access to government decision makers for those matters specific to the member groups' interests.

The work and responsibilities of the Forum have expanded considerably since it was first established. "It democratically selects, organizes and supports consumer representatives on over 80 national committees, including most committees and working parties in the Department of Health, Housing, Local Government and Community Services and the National Health and Medical Research Council" (Palmer and Short 1994).

Evidence of Policy Influence

Shortly after the creation of CHF, Nancy Milio (1988) observed that there was perhaps no other country in the world where an organization representing consumer interests had such direct access to national policymakers.

In their book, *Health Care and Public Policy: An Australian Analysis*, authors George Palmer and Stephanie Short (1994, 317) suggested that the CHF:

> … and its consumer consultations have contributed to policy development on a number of issues including breast implants, and other therapeutic devices, pharmaceutical education programs, and the establishment of divisions of general practice. The CHF would appear to be achieving its aim of increasing access by consumer and community groups to decision making on policy, research priorities, budget allocations and regulatory and legislative change.

They also singled out the CHF's popular quarterly journal *Health Forum*, the major vehicle through which the organization stays in touch with the public.

John Loy, who is first assistant secretary to the Hospitals and Health Financing Division of the Commonwealth Department of Human Services and Health, is the government official who oversees the budget from which CHF is funded. Asked about CHF's influence, he said they were "well plugged in at the overall delivery level—although their influence is felt more at the national than at the state level." He felt the Forum's role was useful, positive, and generally well accepted—although "at first there was resistance and a general underestimation of what consumers could do; but they have been particularly helpful as a policy broker, helping to resolve some intractable disputes with providers."

One specific area where CHF has had a clear influence is in the development of standards of GP practices as part of a process for accreditation. The idea of accrediting general practices arose in 1991 in discussions between the profession and the Minister of Health and was initially seen as involving only physicians and government. As the project developed, however, consumers began to take an active role.

The Royal Australian College of General Practitioners (RACGP) established a working group to develop standards of practice for GPs in 1992 and has been engaged in an interactive process with the profession, government, and consumers who have been reviewing and commenting on successive drafts. The introduction to the *Response by the Consumers' Health Forum to the Discussion Paper: Draft Standards for General Practice*, dated April 1993 noted: "CHF congratulates the RACGP on the progress it is making… It is apparent that considerable thought has gone into assimilating comments made on the previous draft." The criteria and indicators supporting the standards have been extensively reworked since the 1993 draft as a result of the process of trial and consultation.

Assistant secretary general of the RACGP, Dr. Michael Crampton noted that the process "has revealed… a full range of views about what constitutes quality" and that different stakeholders have different perspectives (Consumers' Health Forum 1996).

Dr. Col Owen, president of the Royal Australian College of General Practitioners, thought the CHF influence had been positive: "The groups I have been involved with who have dealt with the Forum have found that a) their input has been very useful because they have experience in things such as standards and accreditation which we are still only coming to terms with and b) the consumer groups in general are supportive of general practice" (Richards 1995).

In November 1995, CHF hosted a conference on health care quality attended by consumers, researchers, providers, government officials, and other interested parties. It was an opportunity to explore policy proposals for reform in light of their impact on quality and offered numerous chances for debate and discussion. At the conference, Dr. Michael Crampton gave an update on the GP standards development process noting that the new 1996 version is undergoing its final development and "that includes specific consultation with representatives from the Consumers' Health Forum" (Consumers' Health Forum 1996).

Other Issues: Who Is a Legitimate Consumer? How Are They Accountable? Whom Do They Represent? What Issues Can They Tackle?

While many health professionals have welcomed the consumer movement's involvement, former chairperson, Janne Graham, said that some do seem uncomfortable with it and the pivotal role the Forum was playing. "What we are talking about is a cultural shift and we are always uncomfortable with that sort of change" (Richards 1995). Australian Medical Association president, Dr. David Weedon, for example, said the Forum is "too politicized" and that "one needs to be removed from government to be truly representative of consumers," suggesting that the funding relationship with government necessarily compromises the Forum's independence.

By contrast, the Doctors' Reform Group, a small group of physicians, who support universal public health insurance and want to pilot different types of non-fee-for-service reimbursement for doctors, supports the CHF and its growing influence. Its president, Dr. Con Costa, thinks being politicized is fine. "If the Forum is going to take its involvement on these committees seriously, then without it being tokenism, like any other group they need to be very politicised" (Richards 1995).

Within the consumer movement in Australia, these issues occasionally arise. However, the structures of CHF were very carefully and deliberately developed to ensure accountability and open lines of communication. These strategies have helped CHF avoid some of the difficulties mentioned earlier.

Other Issues: Resources

As noted earlier, CHF is funded by the commonwealth government for its core operations—approximately AUS$315,000.[13] CHF also receives support from member organizations and, this year, has grants for special projects totalling some AUS$700,000.

The biggest concern about resources for CHF was what would happen when the Labour government, which got it started, lost office. And indeed, Labour lost the most recent election in 1996. Before the election, the *Health Forum*, CHF's newsletter, arranged an interview with the opposition spokesperson on health, Dr. Michael Wooldridge. He said he believed consumers had a role to play in determining health care policies and practices and he indicated that existing support arrangements for the organization would be maintained in the event of a Coalition victory (Consumers' Health Forum 1995). Dr. Wooldridge is now the Minister of Health. Although CHF had to wait until the first budget was announced to know for sure, Kate Moore said she was hopeful that government support for the organization would be maintained and that, if cuts are coming, they will most likely apply to all sectors without singling out CHF.

---

13. The Australian and Canadian dollars were almost at par when this was written.

Relevance to the Analytical Frameworks

CHF's work to clarify consumer perspectives in research and promote participatory research (scientific), to improve the quality of information available to consumers concerning how to get good care (market), to establish complaints bodies and other mechanisms for redress (legal), and to promote consumer participation in all aspects of health care decision making (democratic participation) covers the full range of approaches outlined by Draper and Hill in table 1.

The Forum has had very insightful leadership (Palmer and Short 1994; Baldry 1992) at both the elected and executive levels, an effective process for developing consumers' capacity for participation (e.g., orientation, policy training, etc.) which has allowed it to move well beyond the interests of individual patients and carers (although this is a key starting point). CHF has been able to provide effective linkages among a wide assortment of consumer groups, large and small, and encouraged their active participation. In addition to issues brought to the table by the members, CHF has also tackled a set of broader issues on behalf of the whole consumer community— issues related to access, quality, and continuity of care. The CHF therefore meets Williamson's definition of "consumerist."

As noted by Palmer and Short (1994), "The principle behind the CHF is that the best way to ensure better representation of the repressed community interest is through resourcing and networking consumer and community organizations that have an interest in health issues." As they further pointed out, CHF's presence has allowed interest groups with concentrated interests, such as the Endometriosis Association or the Maternity Alliance access to policy tables where they can articulate and strengthen the interests of their members.

"It acknowledges that the community interest is repressed because the existing structure guarantees that its interests will not be furthered unless an extraordinary amount of political and organizational energy is expended to counteract its structural disadvantage" (Palmer and Short 1994).

As for Paul Sabatier's framework, CHF really is a coalition of interests within the consumer health sector. The policy conference on quality of care which it hosted last November is only one example of the opportunities for public debate encouraged by the organization, considering the large number of policy tables at which CHF consumers play a role. Leading health professionals and government officials have acknowledged that this involvement has resulted in "policy-oriented learning" for all.

LESSONS FROM THE CASE STUDIES

The most significant lesson from the case studies is that meaningful changes to the structure of health care delivery are extremely unlikely unless consumers' potential and repressed interests can be transformed into challenging interests. This, in turn, is unlikely to occur unless extraordinary efforts are made to organize and resource the consumer sector. In short, if it has been established that more consumer participation is desirable, where is the money? The Canadian case studies signal that consumer input can be hampered by sporadic or insufficient funding. The Australian example shows what can be done when funding for consumers' core operations is stable and sufficient.

The Canadian case studies suggest a particular difficulty with respect to Canada's taxation rules for charitable groups. As government support for consumer groups has diminished, these policies, which limit advocacy work to 20 percent of the budget to retain charitable status, impede the ability of consumer groups to raise funds in the private sector. Consumerism is unlikely to be much of a force in policy development if funding opportunities are thus limited in both the public and private sectors.

On the other hand, the case studies also demonstrate that given adequate financial support and opportunities for consumers to "get in the game," consumer perspectives can help to change beliefs and policy, too. (This is not to deny that consumer perspectives can be changed by challenges to their beliefs, as well.)

The case studies warn, however, that consumer groups may feel co-opted by their funders, whether the money comes from government or business, and fear being accused of being "bought and paid for." This can only be countered by clarifying that advocacy has a legitimate role in the policy-making process and by demonstrating that criticism (or praise) of policy directions by consumers does not affect funding support. This may seem too much to ask in a political arena where so much is at stake. However, it does appear more likely that governments can comply with this condition better than private sector firms.

And so, while more consumer participation can be helpful to governments who want to introduce structural reforms to health care, it cannot be assumed that the actual policy directions envisioned by government at the start of a policy development process will automatically be accepted by consumers. Similarly, if pharmaceutical companies become the alternative source of finance for consumer groups (several interviewees suggested that they were the only ones with deep pockets these days), consumers would likely find it difficult to speak out about drugs and the behaviour of the industry.

In addition, the case studies also clarify a number of issues related to representation. First is the need for processes to ensure that consumer representatives on policy-making bodies are not acting on an individual basis but are accountable to those whom they represent. Groups need to have democratic processes for selecting representatives and strong mechanisms for seeking input and feedback as policies develop.

The case studies also suggest that, although one need not have an illness or health condition to advocate for better services, those who do have direct experience of the system may be in a better position to judge its quality of service and, in some cases, its quality of care. On the other hand, they may also be less able to participate because of their illness. There may also be issues that "survivors" themselves do not wish to address directly (such as palliative care) which could be tackled by other consumer advocates, such as family members. Such arrangements, however, should not be used to preclude survivor involvement.

The case studies also demonstrate the challenge facing consumer groups in addressing their information needs, both in terms of managing incoming information and publishing their own newsletters, position papers, policy critiques, and alternative proposals. Although adequate resources are part of this challenge, there are also technical challenges related to the complexity of many health care issues and numerous administrative challenges. And while computer use and Internet connections are permitting wider access to some consumers, the increasing reliance on these newer forms of communication may be excluding many potential participants.

With respect to creating linkages and forming alliances, all three case studies point to strength in numbers and the greater potential in sharing resources and working together. Shared values appear to be important in maintaining such alliances over the long term and their absence may doom an alliance's longevity. Also, the potential for information sharing should not be overlooked. Policy analysis in one jurisdiction may well have relevance to another group or geographical location.

The analysis of regionalization (and Canada's experience with hospital boards, more generally) suggests that governance mechanisms provide relatively weak levels of accountability and have not necessarily enhanced opportunities for consumer participation. The lesson is that creating more boards, or more consumer positions on boards, or introducing elected boards, will not likely have much impact on increasing consumer influence—although these initiatives may be worthy for other reasons including the desire of the organization to reflect its own community more accurately.

The case studies also identified some approaches related to government consultation processes which have been rejected by consumers as inappropriate:

- "rigged" processes in which the outcome is predetermined are unhelpful—consumers are not there to rubber-stamp;
- "tokenism"—the tendency to appoint a solo consumer representative and assume the participation base is covered—it is not; and
- "undue haste"—the failure to recognize that consumer involvement adds to the time required for policy development (the time may well be worthwhile if it results in better policies).

The case studies also allow us to derive some specific measures that would increase and strengthen consumer participation in policy development here in Canada:

- creating more opportunities for public debate;
- helping consumer groups network with one another, sharing information, analysis, and resources; and
- helping consumers to become more knowledgable about the policy process.

As a final lesson, it seems clear that although consumers tend to organize around a single issue or condition, (breast cancer, long-term care, disability, AIDS, etc.), some proposals for reform, if implemented, would provide better service to all these groups. Bringing small and large groups together in a broad-based coalition and encouraging them to develop a united position regarding specific health reform proposals, could dramatically change the political balance of debates.

WHAT GOVERNMENT CAN DO

1. *Clarify the goals of consumer participation:* The consumer organizations in our case studies were very clear about their goals and objectives, but government processes involving consumer input have not always been quite so explicit. A starting point would be for governments to clarify their goals for consumer participation. This would allow consumer groups to evaluate both their desire to participate and what might be expected of them if they choose to do so.

   Governments cannot really reform the delivery system without consumer involvement. Many provinces have made a start through regionalization and hospital rationalization processes to attempt to improve their system's cost-effectiveness. However, many of the recommended policies for resource reallocation have been frustrated by opposition from provider groups. For example, experts have been recommending for years the need for a stronger, more coordinated and integrated primary care system. It has been the subject of national debate. However, reform in this area has, so far, proved elusive.

   The theoretical literature suggests that reform will not happen without expending enormous energy to organize the repressed and potential interests in the system. So the ball is very much in government's court.

2. *Ensure government funding for consumer interest groups:* The involvement of government as a funder of special interest groups is generally unnecessary. Most industrial and professional interest groups can pay their own way. Many disease-specific groups established primarily to raise funds for research are also in a position to finance themselves. However, consumer interest groups with a major focus on advocacy (in addition

to member services) are different. To function effectively, they need reliable core funding from government. This support must not involve co-option to a particular agenda or partisan position, but it need not be entirely without strings. One acceptable "string" might be to tie funding to the consumer organization's willingness to meet the government's goals of consumer participation as well as its own. The requirement to participate in the policy process, to contribute to the debate, to build and foster a consumer coalition of interests through networking, and policy orientation for consumers—all of these could be part of the "contract."

To help advocacy groups raise private sector resources, government should also seriously consider changing the current rules for charitable giving to permit these groups to retain their charitable status although more than 20 percent of their resources are spent on advocacy activities. Without this change consumerism will lose even more ground in Canada, from its already quite weak position.

3. *Support and mandate more consumer participation in decision making:* While increased government funding for consumer advocacy appears essential if health reform is to move forward, the support required is not only financial but also structural. Governments are in charge of designing processes which can either include or exclude consumer participation. They can further the opportunities for consumer impact by explicitly mandating consumer participation. It should be noted however, that the capacity of consumer representatives to participate meaningfully also needs to be ensured. This could involve, as just one example, sponsoring policy orientation sessions for consumers to become more informed about the policy process.

4. *Develop and fund a national consumers' health forum:* The Consumers' Health Forum of Australia provides an excellent organizational template for strengthening consumer participation in health policy development. Many officials in the Australian government, as well as politicians, acknowledge the useful role of consumers in moving forward the health policy agenda.

However, even if an organization modelled on the CHF were seen as desirable in Canada, there remain questions about whether such an organization would work here. What are the similarities between our two countries, our respective health care systems, institutional arrangements, and policy processes? In short, can the impact in Australia be applied generally to the Canadian scene?

Both countries are modern industrial states with parliamentary democracies. Both involve large territories. As to the details of our respective health care systems, there are both similarities and differences. Perhaps one of the key differences is that in Australia many health policy decisions affecting service delivery occur at the federal level. This is not the case in Canada, where provinces have almost exclusive jurisdiction over health care delivery, both constitutionally and in practice. However, in the case of breast cancer, the federal government has found ways to support the development of a national network of breast cancer survivors. Perhaps this can be the precedent that leads to federal support for consumer coalition building at the national level.

5. *Sponsor a consumers' health conference:* A developmental step to explore the potential of these recommendations would be for the federal government to host a national consumers' health conference in 1997. The focus would be on engaging consumer advocacy organizations across the country to review their current perspectives on health reform and their willingness to work together on a joint agenda.

CONCLUSIONS

It is important that these initiatives be viewed as national, but not necessarily federal, given the dominant role of provinces in health policy development.

While support for consumer participation can be politically useful, it also appears to be in the broader public interest to engage the perspectives of these important, but often neglected, stakeholders. Public support, in the form of funding for advocacy and other consumer group activities is not merely a contribution to another interest group but an investment toward a more civilized and civic society.

While the decision to move forward on these issues is obviously a political one, the consequence of failing to act also has political implications. Canada's health care system is a treasured national resource which badly requires structural reform. The reforms are currently stalled, largely because dominant interest groups object to them. Consumers—particularly those with chronic illness—stand to benefit from a better-organized system, but they are poorly organized and poorly funded. They could be a much more potent voice in advocating for change, if given the chance.

Carol Kushner *is a writer, researcher and health policy analyst, probably best known for having coauthored* Strong Medicine: How to Save Canada's Health Care System *(1994), and* Second Opinion: What's Wrong with Canada's Health Care System and How to Fix It *(1989). Her recent policy experience includes work on international health care reform, consumer health issues, quality of care, primary care, and labour adjustment. She works as a health policy consultant in Toronto.*

Acknowledgements

The authors would like to acknowledge the invaluable assistance of those who agreed to be interviewed for this paper. Thanks are owed particularly to Andrew Aitkens, Sharon Batt, Pat Kelly, and Dawne Rennie for their helpful comments on an earlier draft of this paper.

BIBLIOGRAPHY

ABELSON, J., J. LOMAS, J. EYLES, S. BIRCH, and G. VENESTRA. 1995. *Does the Community Want Devolved Authority? Results from Deliberative Polling in Ontario.* McMaster University, Centre for Health Economics and Policy Analysis. Working Paper 94–19.

ALFORD, R. R. 1975. *Health Care Politics: Ideological and Interest Group Barriers to Reform.* Chicago (IL): University of Chicago Press.

BABINSKI, B. 1993. Breast cancer patients want more input from FPs. *Family Practice* December 6.

BALDRY, E. 1992. *Health Consumer Movement in Australia.* Canberra.

BASTIEN, H. 1994. The power of sharing knowledge: Consumer participation in the Cochrane Collaboration. The Cochrane Collaboration. December.

BRENNAN, T. A, L. L. LEAPE, N. M. LAIRD, et al. 1991. Incidence of adverse events and negligence in hospitalized patients: Results of the Harvard Medical Malpractice Study I. *New England Journal of Medicine* 324: 377–384.

BRITISH COLUMBIA ROYAL COMMISSION ON HEALTH CARE AND COSTS. 1991. *Closer to Home* (Chair, Mr. Justice Seaton). Victoria.

CHARLES, C., and S. DEMAIO. 1993. Lay participation in health care decision making: A conceptual framework. *Journal of Health Politics, Policy and Law* 18(4): 881–904.

CHECKOWAY, B. 1982. The empire strikes back: More lessons for health care consumers. *Journal of Health Politics, Policy and Law* 7(1): 111–124.

CHECKOWAY, B., and M. DOYLE. 1980. Community-organizing lessons for health care consumers. *Journal of Health Politics, Policy and Law* 5: 213–226.

CHURCH, W. J. B., L. D. SAUNDERS, M. I. WANKE, and R. PONG. 1995. Component 2: Organizational models in community-based health care: A Review of the literature. In *Building a Stronger Foundation: A Framework for Planning and Evaluating Community-based Health Care in Canada.* Conference of Federal, Provincial and Territorial Deputy Ministers of Health, Health Human Resources Committee, Ottawa.

CONSUMERS' HEALTH FORUM OF AUSTRALIA. 1993. *Response by the Consumers' Health Forum to the Discussion Paper: Draft Standards for General Practice.* Lyons, ACT.

———. 1994. *Health Forum.* October.

———. 1995. Profile: Michael Wooldridge. *Health Forum.* October, p. 14.

———. 1996. *Making Quality Count.* Proceedings of Consumers' Health Forum's National Conference 1995. Canberra.

CUPPLES, M. E., and A. MCKNIGHT. 1994. Randomized controlled trial of health promotion in general practice for patients at high cardiovascular risk. *British Medical Journal* 309: 993–996.

DEBER, R. 1995. From paternalism to consumerism. Eighth Annual Centre for Health Economics and Policy Analysis (CHEPA) Conference, May 18–19.

DRAPER, M., and S. HILL. 1995. *The Role of Patient Satisfaction Surveys in a National Approach to Hospital Quality Management.* Melbourne (Australia): Department of Human Services and Health. October.

HALL, N., P. DE BECK, D. JOHNSON, K. MACKINNON, G. GUTMAN, and N. GLICK. 1992. Randomized trial of a health promotion program for frail elders. *Canadian Journal on Aging* 11: 72–91.

HEALTH ISSUES CENTRE. 1992. *Case Mix, Quality and Consumers.* Melbourne, Australia.

HENDRIKSEN, C., E. LUND, and E. STROMGARD. 1984. Consequences of assessment and intervention among elderly people: A three-year randomized controlled trial. *British Medical Journal* 289: 1522–1524.

KUSHNER, C. 1996. Consumers and health policy development: Confessions of a guarded optimist. *Inernational Journal for Quality in Health Care* 8(5): 1–6.

LINTON, A. 1988. Would Hippocrates accept cost containment? *Annals of the Royal College of Physicians and Surgeons* 21: 21–24.

LOMAS, J. 1990. Finding audiences, changing beliefs: The structure of research use in Canadian health care policy. *Journal of Health Politics, Policy and Law* 15(3): 525–542.

MARMOR, T. R., and J. B. CHRISTIANSON. 1982. *Health Care Policy: A Political Economy Approach.* Beverly Hills: Sage Publishers.

MARMOR, T. R., and J. A. MORONE. 1980. Representing consumer interests: Imbalanced markets, health planning and HSAs. *Milbank Quarterly* 58: 125–162.

MILIO, N. 1988. *Making Policy: A Mosaic of Australian Community Health Policy Development.* Canberra (Australia): Commonwealth Department of Community Services and Health.

NATIONAL CANCER INSTITUTE OF CANADA. 1996. *Cancer Statistics 1996.* Ottawa (ON).

ONTARIO HEALTH REVIEW PANEL. 1987. *Towards a Shared Direction for Health in Ontario,* Toronto. p. 31.

ONTARIO LEGISLATURE. 1993. Bill 173. *An Act respecting Long-Term Care in Ontario.*

ONTARIO MINISTRY OF HEALTH. 1993a. *Partnerships in Long-Term Care: A New Way To Plan, Manage and Deliver Services and Community Support: A Policy Framework.* Toronto (ON): Queen's Park, April.

_____. 1993b. *Partnerships in Long-Term Care: A New Way To Plan, Manage and Deliver Services and Community Support: A Local Planning Framework.* Toronto (ON): Queen's Park, May.

_____. 1993c. *Partnerships in Long-Term Care: A New Way To Plan, Manage and Deliver Services and Community Support: An Implementation Framework.* Toronto (ON): Queen's Park, June.

_____. 1993d *Partnerships in Long-Term Care: A New Way To Plan, Manage and Deliver Services and Community Support: Guidelines for the Establishment of Multi-Service Agencies.* Toronto (ON): Queen's Park, September.

PALMER, G. R., and S. D. SHORT. 1994. *Health Care and Public Policy: An Australian Analysis.* 2nd ed. Melbourne (Australia): McMillan Education Australia. pp. 316–317.

PATHY, M.S.J., A. BAYER, K. HARDING, et al. 1992. Randomized trial of case finding and surveillance of elderly people at home. *Lancet* 340: 890–893.

PICA, L. A., M. M. BOUCHER, R. GRIGNON, R. GUIBERT, and V. DERY. 1993. Hypertension follow-up survey. Laval, Quebec, 1988. *Canadian Journal of Public Health* 84: 174–176.

PRICE WATERHOUSE. 1995. *The Revised Price Waterhouse Report on the MSA Model of Long-Term Care Reform, December 1994; With a Preamble by the Senior Citizens' Consumer Alliance.* Toronto (ON). February.

RICH, M. W., V. BECKHAM, C. WITTENBERG, C. L. LEVEN, K. E. FREEDLAND, and R. M. CARNEY. 1995. A multidisciplinary intervention to prevent the readmission of elderly patients with congestive heart failure. *New England Journal of Medicine* 333: 1190–1195.

RICHARDS, J. 1995. Conflicting diagnosis on health forum. *Australian Doctor* July 14.

SABATIER, P. 1987. Knowledge, policy-oriented learning, and policy change: An advocacy coalition framework. *Knowledge: Creation, Diffusion, Utilization* 8(4): 649–692.

SENIOR CITIZENS' CONSUMER ALLIANCE FOR LONG-TERM CARE REFORM. 1992. *Consumer Report on Long-Term Care Reform* (advance copy). Toronto (ON).

STUCK, A. E., H. U. ARONOW, A. STEINER, et al. 1995. A trial of annual in-home comprehensive geriatric assessments for elderly people living in the community. *New England Journal of Medicine* 333: 1184–1189.

TAMBLYN, R. M., P. J. MCLEOD, M. ABRAHAMOWICZ, et al. 1994. Questionable prescribing for elderly patients in Quebec. *Canadian Medical Association Journal* 150: 1801–1809.

THE ROCHON COMMISSION. 1988. *The Commission of Enquiry into Health and Social Services.* Quebec.

Toronto Star. 1996. Asthma suffers must take more care MDs warn. March 20.

TYSON, H. 1989. Presentation to 2nd Annual Centre for Health Economics and Policy Analysis (CHEPA) Conference. Hamilton. June 2.

VETTER, N. J., D. A. JONES, and C. R. VICTOR. 1984. Effect of health visitors working with elderly patients in general practice: A randomized controlled trial. *British Medical Journal* 288: 369–372

WILLIAMSON, C. 1995. A manager's guide to consumers. *Health Services Journal* November 30: 28–29.

APPENDIX

APPENDIX

Interview List

The following people were interviewed for this project by phone in June 1996.

Andrew Aitkens
Research and Policy Coordinator
One Voice Seniors Network
Ottawa, ON

Sharon Batt, Founder
Breast Cancer Action Montreal and
Policy Advisor to the Canadian Breast Cancer Network
Montreal, PQ

Dr. Cindy Bell
Medical Research Council of Canada
Ottawa, ON

Barbara Mains, Executive Director
Willow
Toronto, ON

Lin Grist
The Lyra Group
Toronto, ON
(former political advisor to Ontario health ministers,
Frances Lankin and Ruth Grier)

Michele Harding
Health Strategies Group
Ministry of Health
Toronto, ON

Dr. Maria Hugi
Consumer representative
Clinical Guidelines Committee
Canadian Breast Cancer Initiative
Whistler, BC.

Pat Kelly, Cofounder
Burlington Breast Cancer Support Services, Inc.
Burlington, ON

Louise Liao, Director
Research Program
Canadian Breast Cancer Research Initiative
Ottawa, ON

Professor Abby Lippman, Researcher
McGill University
Montreal, PQ

Lise Mathieu
Program Manager
Disease Prevention Division
Health Canada

Margaret Ann McHugh
Manager, Women's Health Bureau
Ontario Ministry of Health

Dr. Phillip Mickelson
Medical Consultant
Health Standards, Disease Prevention Division
Health Promotion and Programs Branch
Health Canada, and Facilitator of the
Clinical Guideline Committee
Canadian Breast Cancer Initiative
Ottawa, ON

Dawne Rennie
Coordinator
Canadian Breast Cancer Initiative

The following people were interviewed in November 1995 in Australia:

Dr. Michael Crampton
Assistant Secretary General
Royal Australian College of General Practitioners

Dr. Con Costa
Doctors Reform Group
Sydney, Australia

Janne Graham
Former Chairperson
Consumers' Health Forum of Australia, Inc.
Lyons, ACT

John Loy
First Assistant Secretary
Hospital and Health Financing Division
Commonwealth Department of Health and Human Services
Canberra, ACT

Kate Moore, Executive Director
Consumers' Health Forum of Australia, Inc.
Lyons, ACT
(also interviewed in July 1996)

Ros Wood, Chairperson
Consumers' Health Forum of Australia, Inc.
Melbourne, Australia

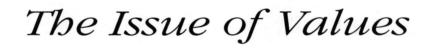

The Issue of Values

Research on Canadian Values in Relation to Health and the Health Care System

FRANK L. GRAVES, M.A.

President, EKOS Research Associates Inc.

PATRICK BEAUCHAMP, M.A.

Director, Qualitative Research, EKOS Research Associates Inc.

DAVID HERLE, B.A., L.L.B.

Partner, Earnscliffe Research and Communications

SUMMARY

Health Care and Values: Current Consensus and Emerging Divisions

It has become something of a truism to note that public debate about the health care system must ultimately confront the issue of values. But beyond the broad consensus that the health care system is profoundly linked to core societal values, what are the nature of these connections? More importantly, what are the real-world implications for the future of the health care system?

These are difficult questions which are made even more challenging by the somewhat amorphous nature of the notion of "values." A rational economic framework may provide more precision in estimating the cost/benefit ratios of various options, but it also runs the risk of missing the essential foundations of the debate in the public's mind. The current research vividly underlines the difficulty of applying a purely rational calculus to these complex problems.

The National Health Forum has squarely acknowledged the centrality of values in the debate about health care. This research project examines the role of values in the debate about health care. It attempts to refine our understanding of the way that values shape public preferences for the future of health care in Canada. This research builds on existing quantitative research on values and health care conducted under the aegis of the Rethinking Government project. Quantitative survey research provides a useful but limited vehicle for understanding this problem. The current project uses a combination of linked qualitative and quantitative research tools in order to secure a deeper insight into this problem.

If we understand values to broadly refer to relatively stable cultural propositions about what is deemed to be good or bad by a society, then we are close to the definition used in this study. This normative domain can only be roughly approximated in survey research. The current research uses qualitative focus groups to approach this problem. It also uses concrete scenarios specifically designed to provide real-world examples of the nature of the trade-offs involved in deciding about the future of health care. Both the discussion and the actual decisions made by the groups are designed to illustrate the underlying values (or interests) which are most instrumental in shaping public judgements. It is important to note that values do not operate in isolation. It is the potent interaction of strong values and high vested interests which produces such high levels of concern about health care. Once we combine various images and knowledge about health care, with a general sense that the system is under pressure, we have an incendiary combination.

The current research also includes a hybrid quantitative design. The broader communities where groups were conducted were surveyed in order to provide statistically reliable data. We also measured focus group participants before and after the discussion sessions to assess the impact of talking about these questions. Finally, we rotated the application of a basic package of "objective" information in order to test the impact of this knowledge on attitude formation. Together these design refinements provide a strong basis for assessing the role of values in this debate. Following are some of the key themes emerging from this exercise:

Basic Images and Concerns: The Emerging Defining Issue?

The groups revealed an unusual mixture of concern and eloquence. Few topics we have researched generate such a blend of articulate and passionate responses. It is the powerful interaction of strong vested interests (everyone can get sick, all will die) and powerful values (pride, equality, compassion, national identity) which produces the capacity for more heat than light in future debates.

Images of the health care system are incomplete and dominated by the more visible, traditional institutional structure (viz. hospitals, doctors). There is a broad consensus that the Canadian health care system is a collective accomplishment, a source of pride, and a symbol of core Canadian values. The values of *equality, access, and compassion are salient to perceptions of the system and often held in contradistinction to perceptions of the American system. Moreover, the system is seen as relatively effective and sound. It may be the only area of current public endeavour which is seen as a clear success story.*

It may then be ironic that this singular public success story is also seen as under clear threat. There is a consensus that the system is under acute pressure. The public are increasingly wary of the signals and actions they see in this area and feel frustrated with changes which are clearly producing declining confidence. Unlike other areas of public endeavour, where there is a sense that the system does not work, or costs far too much, the public are actually satisfied, comfortable and even proud of the health care system. It is therefore not surprising that they feel frustrated and frightened by ominous signals about its fragility.

This sense of declining confidence is fuelled by a barrage of messages and real-world examples of declining service. The public perceptions of problems in the health care system reflect many of the themes evident in broader concerns about government. One of these themes is a growing wariness of "expert" prescriptions for the health care system. Participants spoke of conflicting interests of different expert stakeholders (e.g., doctors advising on the use of alternative medical practitioners with whom they compete). Although trust in individual doctors remains high, there is deteriorating trust in the broader profession. The expert-public gap on the debate about health care is a recurring theme of broader research. With the stakes so high, and strong perceptions of mixed motives amongst various experts, the public are insisting on inclusion and real influence on these issues.

The participants seemed to believe that the affordability problems currently plaguing the system are the legacy of abuse and mismanagement. Much like broader views on government overspending, it is much easier for participants to attribute this to waste or inefficiency than a fundamental shortfall in public resources against services delivered. This conviction of abuse and inefficiency was pervasive and often alloyed with numerous real-world examples (e.g., doctors overprescribing, patients burdening the system with frivolous ailments).

Does Dialogue Matter? Does Information Matter?

The research design supports the conclusion that talking about these problems has a significant impact on attitudes and judgements. It also shows a modest but somewhat puzzling impact from providing basic information. Further testing of "deliberative" impacts, however, is necessary before drawing conclusions about the impact of information.

By far the more important influence was the simple process of sitting down and talking about these issues in a small group. Three major impacts were detected as a consequence of discussing the issues:

1. People became more confident in the system. The sense of imminent decline (and perhaps collapse) of the current system was significantly lower after these discussions occurred. This suggests that there are exaggerated fears about the system which can be somewhat calmed through a process of dialogue.

2. *The role of values increases and the role of economics declines. Participants are more likely to see the debate as essentially about values rather than economics following the discussion. This reflects a broader tendency for the groups to reject a rational calculus in approaching health care. This may partly reflect the social psychology of small group discussions where moral imperatives are more "socially desirable" than pecuniary criteria.*

3. *Issues around two tier produce polarization. Of those going to groups, the clear majority changed their views about two-tier issues. Unlike the change in values or confidence (which produced greater consensus), the groups generated stronger polarization on the two-tier issues. This may well serve as a harbinger of the eventual divisiveness of the two-tier issue in the real world. Interestingly, most of the other values and attitudes tested were fairly stable.*

Soft Resolve around Hard Choices

The groups had great difficulty with many of the choices. In summary, we can conclude that most groups eschewed a rational calculus of decision making where real human welfare (i.e., illness) was seen as threatened. Despite the apparent plausibility, or even inevitability, of many of the trade-offs and choices presented, the groups were ingenious at avoiding the hard choices. Often the basic premises of the exercise (e.g., we simply cannot afford to do this anymore) were rejected. We get the sense that public and experts do not share a common universe of discourse about the public policy issues.

Whatever the reasoning or judgement involved, this finding has important implications for the Forum. If the public reject hard choices even in the controlled environment of a small group, with specific scenarios designed to illustrate the points, then the prospects for a rational debate in the broader public arena are even lower. This finding reconfirms a consistent conclusion of other research in this area — the gap between expert rationality and public values. It would be prudent to acknowledge the public's entrenched resistance to a purely economic mode on health care.

The Priority of Values over Economics

Another way of seeing this question is by noting the preeminence of moral considerations over economic considerations. The core values which seem to be impervious to economic questions are accessibility and the quality of the system itself. These link to other values such as security, well-being, and compassion. It is also important to note that these issues are being connected (spontaneously) to issues of national identity and national unity. In the aggravated unity environment following October 30, and in a world where federal withdrawal is registering uncertainties and anxieties about our societal character, the issue of health care assumes even greater symbolic significance. Particularly in English Canada the connections of preservation of health care to the maintenance of a distinct Canadian identity is an important issue.

Innovation: Pragmatism, Scepticism, and Guarded Receptivity

The groups tested attitudes to a number of forms of innovation (e.g., shift to a more prevention-based approach, more family responsibilities for caregiving, private clinics, "alternative" medical approaches). A number of key conclusions are evident. First, people were generally loath to trade-off elements of the current system against the promise of better or fairer future performance. This reflected a general scepticism that reform and innovation may well be code for withdrawal. It also reflects fairly high attachment to the current system, which is seen as successful. Why trade the uncertainties of potential improvement in results, fairness, or costs against the proven security of a working system? It was not that people could not appreciate the value or logic of innovations, but rather that they were reluctant to exchange innovations for the core system. Receptivity varied by area tested.

Alternative medical approaches received relatively strong support — although not as a replacement for the traditional system but as a complement, the key criteria here were pragmatic (what works). Preventive approaches and social programming to reduce health costs were understood in principle, but rejected in practice. The logic was too speculative, the payoff too delayed, the potential for abuse too high, to justify a major shift from current approaches to prevention. These approaches were fine, up to the point where they threatened treating sick people (the way we currently do). This reflects our earlier quantitative research showing that enthusiasm for innovation declines as one worries about one's personal health.

The issue of increased family responsibility for the care of sick family members was rejected outright. It was seen as a particularly offensive and intrusive form of off-loading broader societal responsibilities.

The issue of private clinics and "two-tier" systems deserves special attention. Although championed by many (including a growing number of doctors) as a solution to the fiscal problems confronting the health care system, private clinics are clearly rejected by most participants. They are seen as a part of a slippery slope which will lead to an American-style system and sacrifice the core values and merit of our system.

Although this conclusion is largely consistent with our earlier research, we offer the following caveat. There is evidence of growing support for private clinics and other two-tier features, particularly in the quantitative component of this research. The potential support for two tier may well be understated in the focus groups. In fact, those supporting these approaches are rather meek in the face of strenuous group support for more socially desirable values such as compassion and equal access. Yet the quantitative data show growing (albeit still minority) support for two tier. Moreover, there is heightened polarization which is clearly connected to one's sense of economic and health security. Health and wealth are also strongly interdependent.

In general, we find that enthusiasm for terms such as innovation, efficiency, freedom of choice, and prevention is systematically higher amongst the more secure members of society. Stripped of the moderating influence of the group, the quiet power of the checkbook may well provide a more rapid tilt to two-tier approaches, once these options take root in the medical marketplace.

Final Synthesis

The public is highly concerned about the health care system and it may well be emerging as the defining issue for governments in the near future. People are proud of the existing system and see it as a source of collective values and national identity. They are worried about the future viability of the system and are resistant to many of the options/alternatives currently on the table. Cynicism about change is high and the public reject many of the premises for "reform." They believe cost problems are rooted in mismanagement and abuse and would prefer to see these dealt with first. Failing this solution, people prefer fuelling the system with new public resources in order to preserve its integrity and core values.

The public will be resistant to a rational discourse on the costs issues because they are more likely to see these issues in terms of higher-order values. The evidence suggests that further dialogue will tilt the debate more to values than economics. The public will insist on inclusion and influence in this crucial debate and they will reject elite and expert authority. Finally, we predict growing division around two-tier questions with heightened support for those who see this option serving their personal economic or health interests.

TABLE OF CONTENTS

APPENDICES

LIST OF FIGURES

LIST OF FIGURES (APPENDIX 3)

TABLE

INTRODUCTION

Study Objectives

In establishing the broader public policy context within which health care issues are currently situated, the drive to reduce public indebtedness looms large over the horizon. At both the federal and provincial level, the 1990s have confirmed deficit reduction as the dominant factor over program and resource decisions. The dominance of the deficit reduction agenda has been premised, however, on the promise of something more tangible than a clean balance sheet. At the federal level, for example, great emphasis has been placed on the linkage between deficit reduction, economic prosperity, and sustainability of cherished programs such as health care.

In pursuing these principles, governments have attempted to prioritize their existing spending habits requiring extremely difficult choices over what to preserve, what to reduce, and what to eliminate. Inevitably, health care, as the single largest consumer of public expenditures, has been central to this debate and both provincial and federal governments have begun to struggle with these tough choices.

At the same time, there can be little doubt that the issues surrounding the country's health care system have gained significant currency in recent years because they touch cherished and core values of Canadians. Indeed, at a time when other traditional elements of the Canadian value system have been placed under demonstrable stress, health care has increased in both importance and prominence as a shared and common value. In fact, health care has always engendered strongly positive characteristics among Canadians: shared risk, compassion, fairness, and common responsibility. In recent years, however, its significance has broadened into symbolic terms as a defining characteristic of being Canadian, one of the national tenets of our citizenship.

The purpose of this research was to help decision makers and stakeholders understand the values and priorities that Canadians want to see reflected as health care in Canada evolves to meet the public policy challenges of the coming years. Specifically, the two prime research objectives of this study were:

1. to conduct a focused dialogue about health with a cross section of Canadians; and
2. to identify underlying values and trade-offs.

Organization of This Report

The qualitative and quantitative results are presented separately. The following section presents the findings of the focus group research. The section "Quantitative Findings" is devoted to an analysis of the quantitative data produced by this study. The final section of this report contains a synthesis and integration of the key focus group and quantitative findings and presents the conclusions of the study. This report also contains five appendices. Appendix 1 includes the text of the eight scenarios which were discussed in the focus groups. Appendix 2 contains the moderator's guide. The handout used in the deliberative exercise is presented in appendix 3. The survey questionnaire used to collect all of the quantitative data is found in appendix 4. Finally, verbatim comments on the health care system are found in appendix 5.

QUALITATIVE FINDINGS

This section presents the findings of the focus groups. A brief discussion of the methodology is followed by summary findings for each of the eight scenarios tested in the groups. A separate summary of the focus group with Aboriginal Canadians is provided. Where appropriate, notable differences according to group composition (e.g., location, age, activist vs. general public) are highlighted.

Focus Group Methodology

Location and Composition of Groups

A total of 18 focus groups (including two pretest focus groups) were conducted in five different regions of Canada between April 9 and May 7, 1996. Table 1 presents the details regarding focus group location and composition.

As indicated in the exhibit, the design of the research aimed to include the participation of a cross section of Canadians. Additional details on the selection criteria are presented below.

Centre size – Both large cities (e.g., Vancouver, Toronto, Montreal), as well as smaller centres (e.g., Regina, Quebec City, Sudbury) were selected as it was anticipated that residents from smaller centres may have different views/concerns about the health care system.

Age – People under 25 years of age were excluded because they were expected to be somewhat detached from the issue of the health care system and, thus, would be less involved participants in the groups. Four groups with individuals aged 60 years and up were formed to ensure that the particular views of this important segment of the population, especially in the context of health and the health care system, were collected in the research.

Language – Four groups (in Quebec) were conducted in French with the remaining groups being conducted in English.

Activism – We conducted four groups with a subset of the Canadian population who are more involved in current issues as past research has

Table 1

Language and composition of focus groups

Location	Group type	Deliberative exercise
Ottawa (2) (pilot)	General population (25–60 years)	
	General population (25–60 years)	√
Halifax (2)	Activists (25–60 years)	√
	General population (25–60 years)	
Montreal (2)	General population (60+ years)	
	General population (25–60 years)	
Quebec City (2)	Activists (25–60 years)	√
	General population (25–60 years)	
Windsor (2)	Activists (25–60 years)	√
	General population (25–60 years)	√
Sudbury (2)	General population (60+ years)	√
	General population (25–60 years)	√
Regina (2)	General population (Aboriginal)	
	General population (25–60 years)	√
Edmonton (2)	Activists (25–60 years)	√
	General population (25–60 years)	
Vancouver (2)	Activists (60+ years)	
	General population (25–60 years)	√
TOTAL	18 focus groups	10 deliberative exercises

demonstrated that this third of Canadians tends to have a significant influence on public policy debates.[1]

Aboriginal Canadians – A focus group with Aboriginal people from the Regina area was conducted.

Focus group participants were drawn randomly from the general public. Potential participants were contacted by telephone at their homes during the evening. Using a script, recruiters introduced the study to the people contacted, applied the screening criteria and invited those who met the criteria to participate in the study. Participants were offered a $50 honorarium for participating in the study.

---

1. Involved Canadians were determined on the basis of whether they had ever made a speech to a public audience, written an article for a publication, served as an officer of a club or organization, written a letter to the editor, or called a television or radio talk show.

A total of 145 people participated in the focus groups; there was an average of approximately eight participants per focus group.

Focus Group Implementation

All the group discussions were conducted in the evening (two sessions per evening) with each group lasting two hours. The focus groups were held in dedicated focus group facilities (where available) or hotel meeting rooms.

The two focus group moderators relied on discussion guides based mainly on questions provided by the National Forum on Health (appendix 2). The guide was designed to measure the depth of core attitudes and beliefs held by the study population with respect to the values involved in the debate around health and health care.

A core group of questions were used to initiate the discussion in all of the focus groups. These initial questions allowed participants a chance to begin thinking about the broader issues of values and health and the health care system and to provide spontaneous reflections on the study issues before the scenarios were presented.

Participants' views about underlying values were obtained by using eight "scenarios" (i.e., short stories; appendix 1) designed to highlight one or two key issues. The eight scenarios were selected by the research team, in consultation with the National Forum on Health, from 12 scenarios designed by the Forum. The eight chosen were those which the research team felt would be the most appropriate for use in the group discussions. While the scenarios were tested across all the focus groups, only two were discussed in any one particular group. This ensured that each scenario and its accompanying questions received adequate time for processing and reflection by focus group participants. Each scenario was tested in four different groups.

Participants were provided with a text version of the scenario and an audiotape version. Participants were able to follow the scenario using their written version as the tape was played. The inclusion of the audiotape version made it easier for participants to digest the content of the scenarios.

In 10 of the 18 focus groups, a "deliberative" exercise was conducted. This involved providing participants with some basic factual information about the Canadian health care system (appendix 3). The moderator walked participants through six graphs and solicited their reaction to the material. The purpose of the deliberative segment of the groups, which lasted 10 to 15 minutes, was to assess whether or not providing participants with information had an impact on their views. Impact was measured in terms of participants' subsequent comments in the groups, as well as by comparing their responses to the pre- and postsurveys. (A description of this survey component is presented in the next section.)

Caveat: Some Limitations of This Study

Focus group research has a number of inherent strengths and weaknesses. In comparison to survey research, one of the main limitations of focus groups pertains to the external validity of the findings. That is, the extent to which a finding is generalizable to the study population as a whole. Of course, focus groups are not meant to provide representative results; surveys are used for this purpose. Focus groups, rather, provide in-depth information about the core beliefs and felt experiences of people, particularly on complex topics.

The overall research design of this project was strengthened by the addition of a quantitative component (this component and its results are described in the section "Quantitative Findings"). It is important to note, however, that even with the addition of the quantitative component, the results are still not, strictly speaking, generalizable to the Canadian population. This is particularly the case when one begins to narrow the unit of analysis to specific types of participants. This study included dedicated groups with seniors and one focus group with Aboriginal Canadians. This was done in an effort to ensure that a wide range of people had an opportunity to participate in the study, not as a way of ascribing the results generated from these groups to the broader population. Similarly, the data were not analyzed based on other participant characteristics (e.g., gender, race, etc.). Particular caution should be exercised with respect to the findings generated from a single group of Aboriginal Canadians.

Findings

This section begins with a brief analysis of participants' general perceptions of the health care system followed by a synthesis of participants' reactions to each of the eight scenarios examined in the groups. Complete texts of the scenarios are contained in appendix 1. The moderator's guide, which includes the questions posed to participants, is included in appendix 2. We suggest that the reader familiarize himself with the scenarios and related questions before proceeding.

Perceptions of the Health Care System

The initial series of questions posed to participants were aimed at obtaining information to help understand participants' "going-in" position on the broad topic of health care and values. Participants were ask to discuss, in a general way, their views of the health care system based on their personal experience. More specifically, they were asked to identify the key positive and negative aspects of the current system.

There was a tremendous amount of consistency in the views of participants (appendix 5) about what the strengths and weaknesses of the health care system were. In a number of cases, participants took the opportunity to voice their concerns about the future of Canada's health care system.

Perceived strengths of the health care system – Many participants prefaced their comments by stating that Canadians were very fortunate to have benefitted from such a good system. Participants tended to describe accessibility/universality and quality as the twin pillars of the health care system, with accessibility being somewhat more important for the majority. Participants expressed approval and took pride in the fact that "both rich and poor" received the same quality of health services in Canada. Doctors were often praised for their expertise and ability, if not, as we shall see later, for their altruism and objectivity.

Perceived weaknesses of the health care system – Participants' discussion of weaknesses was deeper, more varied and expressed mainly in terms of concern about the future. Participants agreed that the health care system was showing numerous and obvious signs of stress and, in some instances, deterioration. Increases in the time patients must wait for treatment, hospital closings, reductions in service, the imposition or contemplation of user fees by governments, visibly overworked staff (mainly nurses), lack of specialists, and the loss of doctors to the United States were most often mentioned as symptoms of stress.

When participants spoke about the future of the system, almost all did so in bleak terms. Taken together, participants' vision of the Canadian health care system in the twenty-first century was one which had become overburdened with aging baby boomers and "Americanized," complete with user fees and a growing gap between the level of care available to rich and poor. Few were optimistic about the possibility that breakthroughs in health research, medical technology, public awareness about health issues, or improved health care management systems might coalesce to counter some of the more ominous trends identified by participants.

There was general agreement that the stress on the system was the result of fiscal pressures. Yet, most participants felt that these fiscal pressures were the result of mismanagement of the system (e.g., political expediency, poor administration, duplication, lack of planning, etc.) and patient and doctor "abuse" and misuse of the system. Other sources of fiscal pressure identified by participants included the rapid development of expensive medical technology and an aging population.

Abuse of the system was raised as a main concern in all of the group discussions, particularly in the focus groups with seniors. With respect to abuse of the system by patients, participants identified fraudulent use of the system (e.g., nonresidents receiving treatment with health insurance cards) as a problem, but not the main concern. For most participants, the core problem was that too many Canadians were taking the health care system for granted: "People are running to the emergency room for things that could be handled in a clinic." A number of seniors remarked that too many of their friends and relatives paid unnecessary visits to their family doctor: "You know, sometimes these people are lonely and want someone to pay attention to them. They know their doctor will listen."

Most participants felt that patient "abuse," or misuse, was not usually the result of wilful misconduct, but, rather, the product of ignorance about the workings and costs of the system and, more importantly, the resulting poor judgement about appropriate courses of action to take when one is ill. Participants agreed that all Canadians needed to be educated about these issues.

Participants' views of doctors tended to be far less charitable. In all of the discussion groups, at least one or two, and often a majority of participants, felt that too many doctors were manipulating the system and their patients in order to further their own economic interests.

Participants identified two main types of "abuse" of the system by doctors. First, a number of participants complained that some doctors seemed to schedule "unnecessary" return visits. Seniors were said to be especially vulnerable to this practice: "They make you come back for return visits. You have to be vigilant and watch this. They prey on older people." The second prevalent example of abuse was the overprescribing of drugs by doctors: "I had a bad sun burn. The doctor prescribed this cream, but it came in a huge bottle. I only needed a bit, so almost all of it was wasted." and, "There is a reason why doctors prescribe so much medication, they own the drug companies."

The general perception of most participants that fiscal pressures on the health care system were mainly the result of mismanagement and abuse is very significant. As indicated in the following sections, many participants were doggedly unwilling to restrict themselves to the narrow options and tough choices put forward in the scenarios and related questions. This reaction was apparently conditioned by their rejection of the premise which underlies the rationale for having to make the difficult choices. In short, many participants felt that the alternative remedies of improving the management of the system and eliminating abuse and misuse had to be exhausted *before* some of the options described in the scenarios could be contemplated.

Scenario 1: Alternative Treatments and Medicines

There was consensus among participants that the cost of alternative medicines and approaches, such as acupuncture and chiropractic, should be covered by the health care system *if* they were proven to be effective. This pragmatic approach to the issue was largely based on participants' generally positive personal experience with alternative approaches. Many participants put forward anecdotes telling how they or someone they knew had benefitted from chiropractic, acupuncture, homeopathy, or other approaches: "My back bothered me for years. My doctor had me sleeping on a wooden board. I went to see a chiropractor and I've been okay ever since."

Despite participants' personal experiences and awareness of the existence of considerable anecdotal evidence to support the assertion that certain alternative approaches are effective, most agreed that consumer demand did not constitute sufficient grounds on which to base a decision to publicly fund an alternative health service, treatment, or medication. The notion that consumers/patients should have an important say in the process held a great deal of appeal to participants, particularly in light of their perception that the "medical establishment" has fought against the inclusion of alternatives into the mainstream of the health care system. After some deliberation on the issue, however, there was general agreement that "scientific proof" or "medical evidence" was required before funding a procedure: "You have to know whether it works or not. You have to study it." In the end, there was agreement that if there was enough consumer demand for an approach to be covered by the health care system, its effectiveness should be objectively studied. If it were proven to be effective, the procedure should then be covered, at least partially. This requirement for scientific verification of results was supported even in the focus group with Aboriginal Canadians.

The question of what should be considered "effective" was discussed in some groups. Here too, participants were able to reach general agreement. For most, a procedure that "helped" a patient, or was proven to have a significant "positive impact" should be deemed effective for the purposes of making a decision about coverage. In support of this view, a few participants noted that a higher standard of effectiveness (e.g., a cure) was not warranted given that traditional approaches sometimes had no positive effect on patients.

The issue of who or what should judge the effectiveness of a procedure was also debated. Participants quickly found themselves in a quandary. On the one hand, they agreed that *medical evidence* was necessary. On the other hand, most felt that the majority of "establishment" doctors were biased against alternative procedures: "It would be like putting the fox in charge of the chicken coop." Discussion led participants to suggest that an "independent" body or panel should be charged with the task of judging effectiveness. Many suggested that this body be composed of various stakeholders with different interests and perspectives, including some from outside of the medical profession. Specific suggestions for panel members included doctors, nurses, representatives of the Canadian Medical Association, alternative health practitioners, academics, government scientists and officials, lawyers, and patients/consumers.

Participants' openness to examining the possibility of funding alternative medical procedures, such as acupuncture, chiropractic and homeopathy, was not carried over into the discussion of multicultural health care.

Participants were given a number of examples and questions to react to, including examples of Native Canadian medicine and the idea of allowing ethnic groups an approximately equal share of money spent on health care. Regardless of the example or question, most participants reacted negatively.

The fact that acupuncture and other alternative medicines discussed previously in the groups were not Western medicines was seemingly lost on participants. Seniors in particular reacted negatively, as discussion of ethnic medical approaches and multicultural health care conjured up images of third world conditions and folk remedies. The issue was clearly disassociated from the other questions raised by the scenario about covering alternative approaches and negatively linked to immigration and Native issues: "If they choose to immigrate here, they should content themselves with the system that we have," was a typical response.

Scenario 2: Emphasizing Prevention or Acute Care?

Participants found the questions raised by this scenario very challenging. While people were drawn to the inherent appeal of the prevention argument, they also found it unconscionable that someone who was seriously ill should have to be put through the situation described in the scenario.

Understandably, many participants' first reaction to the question of which regional board had made the right decision (i.e., emphasize prevention or acute care), was that "both were important": "You need a large budget for prevention and a large budget for [acute] care." Quite a few participants tended to go outside the parameters of the scenario and related questions for solutions. These often revolved around "eliminating abuse and inefficiency" in the health care system. Other participants suggested that money for prevention not be taken from acute care budgets, but from other areas of government spending, such as foreign aid.

Most participants appreciated the prevention point of view. They believed that the system ought to focus more on the broader determinants of health. Many felt that more emphasis on prevention could both provide a healthier population and result in long-term cost savings. When forced to choose between one of the two approaches outlined in the scenario, however, the vast majority reluctantly said that emphasis should be placed on acute care. Almost all older participants and those who had indicated to the group that they had suffered a serious illness supported this choice. It seemed that when forced to choose, participants tended to see prevention programs as somewhat intangible in contrast to the awesome and concrete nature of acute care medicine. In addition, some participants expressed doubt about the effectiveness of prevention programs: "People will make [poor] lifestyle choices no matter what you tell them."

It was apparent from the discussions that most participants were uncomfortable with the idea of making choices in which a person's health would be negatively affected, perhaps to the point of dying. Similarly, there seemed to be an unawareness or denial among participants that these sort of choices are made every day: "You're talking about a human life!"

On the issue of regional variations in waiting lists, participants' initial reaction was one of puzzlement and some dismay. The situation described in the scenario struck them as "unfair." A broader discussion of decision making in the health care system, however, led most participants to conclude that regional/local health authorities were probably in the best position to assign priorities because of their more immediate knowledge and appreciation of "local needs."

Should private clinics be allowed to open? – The issue of whether or not to allow private clinics to open in order to give people more choice was discussed in depth. The issue was framed in terms of giving Canadians who face a medical dilemma similar to the one described in the scenario the option of paying for more timely health services. The issue generated a great deal of discussion among participants; it was clear they realized that the question of whether or not to allow aspects of private health care to take root in Canada was key to the future of the health care system.

On the whole, the views of participants were surprisingly mixed, at least initially. The discussion of pros and cons was most often characterized by pragmatism rather than principle and ideology. In the end, most participants opposed allowing private clinics to open. The question of whether these clinics should be partially subsidized was not discussed in detail since most were opposed to allowing people to pay for the *full cost* of private health services, let alone the partial cost.

Opposition to private clinics was rooted mainly in the fear that they would attract "all of the best doctors," particularly specialists, as well as the best equipment and support staff. Participants who opposed the suggestion mainly on principle feared that no matter how private clinics were run and regulated and despite assurances which might be given about the preservation and preeminence of the public system, the core value of equality of access would be compromised. Dilution of equality of access, these participants warned, would eventually cause the Canadian system to resemble its American counterpart, where "the rich get the best quality care and everyone else gets inferior care." Participants who mainly opposed private clinics on principle were more adamant in their opposition, while those who in the end opposed the idea on mainly pragmatic grounds tended to vacillate during the discussion.

Participants who supported the idea of allowing private clinics to open did not defend their view with vigour. Essentially, supporters indicated that private clinics were acceptable as long as the public system was maintained: "Private clinics are fine, as long as no one is denied medical treatment." Some participants talked about the importance of giving people a choice, others suggested that private clinics would relieve some of the pressure on the public system.

In response to a question on how health care was different from other commodities and services sold in the marketplace, participants agreed that its main difference lies in the fact that it was directly related to "life and death." Some also indicated that it was different because it was an important source of national pride and identity.

Scenario 3: Shifting Resources from Health Care to Long-Term Prevention

The majority of participants who were asked to react to this scenario tended to side with the character (Mariella) who opposed shifting resources away from direct health care in order to pay for programs aimed at promoting the general health of the population (e.g., job creation, cleaning up the environment). It is important to note, however, that a number of participants had difficulty following the counterargument in favour of channelling resources away from treatment towards improving the health of the general population. This difficulty was at least partially due to the fact that the positive correlation which exists between better health and higher levels of employment and education was not mentioned in the scenario. To some participants, therefore, the ideas of creating jobs and cleaning up the environment had merit, but they had some trouble seeing how they were related to cuts in health care.

Once participants understood the connection between improvements in the environment, education and other indicators of socioeconomic status, some supported a slight shift in funding aimed at promoting the general health of the population: "It makes sense. It's a long-term strategy about treating the cause rather than the symptom." Most participants were much less sanguine and remained reluctant to take funding away from health care to pay for "prevention programs writ large," as one participant called it. Some participants said their opposition was mainly based on their inability to countenance a policy which would reduce health services, no matter how promising the long-term impacts of a prevention strategy were. For others, opposition stemmed mainly from a lack of confidence in governments' ability to achieve the intended impact of prevention programs (i.e., a healthier population): "The government has wasted a lot of money on job creation." and "There is no certainty about the [desired] long-term effects."

Overall, participants were divided concerning how much weight should be given to what patients and consumers want, as opposed to what the "experts" think, in deciding the level of public funding for health care. Their comments here, as well as in other segments of the focus groups, suggested that their confidence in doctors' and other "experts'" ability to make choices in the interest of the public had been seriously eroded: "Doctors look after their own interests just like everybody else." At the same time, participants evinced a great deal of respect for the doctors and the other health care professionals they dealt with on a *personal* level, along with considerable confidence in the ability and judgement of doctors in treating the individual patient. They also appreciated the fact that knowledge and expertise were needed in making decisions in such a large and complex field as health care.

There was consensus among participants that Canadians had a right to health care. In terms of qualifying this right, participants tended to indicate that Canadians had a right to the level of services they currently enjoyed. When asked how they characterized the level of services currently available to Canadians, the vast majority described it as "quality" services.

When asked if it was reasonable for Canadians to continue to expect to receive the same level of quality services in the future as they do now, most agreed that it was. In fact, a few participants suggested that "we should aim higher." This positive attitude in relation to setting health policy objectives stands in contrast to the generally pessimistic prognosis given by participants when they described their vision of the future of health care in this country. This suggests that Canadians' personal pessimism of the future does not translate into softer expectations of those who design and administer the health care system.

Participants generally agreed that the health care system had a great deal of special importance to them as Canadians: "It's a basic, fundamental tenet of being Canadian." Many agreed that the universality of the system helped to distinguish Canada from the United States in a way that showed us to be a more generous and compassionate society. Others said they derived pride from the quality of the system.

The few Francophone participants who commented on the issue were less enthusiastic in their comments. They indicated that the accessibility and quality of the system generated a certain amount of pride, but did little for their sense of identity.

Scenario 4: Prevention vs. Treatment

This scenario directly tested the participants' understanding of the broader determinants of health and their link to the health care system and other social programs.

In virtually every group, the preliminary general discussion about the health care system and the state of health usually generated considerable talk about the value of prevention. Many participants bemoaned the lack of attention paid to prevention in the approach taken to health care. This scenario tested the limits of that belief.

There were some participants in every group who were strongly convinced of the merits of focusing on prevention and the very root causes of health problems, including those caused by social and economic factors. They were a minority, but a distinct presence. Most participants had a more limited view of what prevention constituted; they confined it to the context of the health care system. They tended to see prevention more along the lines of education about lifestyle or encouraging proper nutrition or fitness.

Most participants balked at the notion that the health care system would intervene in a direct way in the community to provide a material change in people's living conditions. With respect to the scenario, for example, almost all thought providing Jimmy with a furnace would be a smart thing to do. They could also see how it would result in cost saving to the state overall. However, they did not see it as the responsibility of the health care system. Rather, it was seen as the responsibility of social services departments or some other agency of government.

Part of the problem was that most participants did not see a solid connection between buying the furnace and health care. There might be a relationship, but not direct enough to justify the involvement of the health care system. This dichotomy really speaks to the scepticism many people feel about prevention issues, particulary as one broadens out those issues and tries to get at them in a more holistic way. Many people are uncertain about the actual results that accrue from prevention measures.

When they were asked whether they would prefer to save the lives of 10 heart attack victims or reduce the number of heart attacks, and thereby save 100 lives, participants' views tended to be roughly split. However, in our view, even that overstates the level of support that would actually exist for such a choice. The question is designed—by guaranteeing the saving of 100 lives—to overcome the basic problem that undercuts support for reallocation to prevention and the related uncertainty inherent in this shift.

The discussion surrounding this scenario brought into sharp focus the way in which participants think of health care and the health care system. Most drew a clear distinction between prevention issues that "made great sense" and would help to create a healthier population on one hand, and treatment: what the health care system ought to concern itself with. Most participants tended to see the health care system as an insurance policy, for themselves and their family. They pay into it expecting that one day they might need it and they will have a right to draw on it and to expect that it will devote the required resources at that point. The fundamental responsibility of the health care system is to treat the sick. Anything else is peripheral to this mission.

Support for prevention measures, within the health care framework, is strongest the more tightly connected the measures are to traditional understandings of health care and the more limited and focused they are in their scope. There were also clear undertones in the groups which indicated a belief among some participants that prevention in terms of making healthy lifestyle choices was largely a matter of *personal* responsibility. This view helped to contribute to the resistance to reallocating resources from prevention to treatment. Some of the problems that this scenario encountered were also related to concerns about the funding crisis in the health care system. People are inclined to think that the system is already stretched to the maximum and they were concerned that activities like the one contemplated could result in health care dollars being spent too broadly in society at the expense of its ability to be prepared for acute care.

Scenario 5: Meeting the Needs of the Dying Compared to Delivering Acute Care

Participants had a great deal of difficulty making the hard choices they confronted in this scenario. Initial discussion of the importance of ensuring that the needs of the dying were met as fully as possible compared to trying to save lives when chances of success are very poor, resulted in most participants saying that both were very important. Similarly, participants were reluctant to say whether they thought too much emphasis was placed on saving lives at any cost to the detriment of other needs. Generally speaking, participants exhibited a tendency to want to go outside of the parameters of the scenario and related questions for suggestions and solutions.

In some cases, participants simply reiterated the need to reduce waste and inefficiency and curb abuse as a way of finding the resources needed to properly fund both palliative care and acute care. The most interesting and often made suggestion, however, was that the chronically ill should be given the right to die, or at least made more aware of their right to refuse treatment. There was a surprising amount of consensus and an equally surprising absence of rumination surrounding this issue. Often basing their opinion on the personal experience of having known someone who had died of terminal illness, participants estimated that there were substantial numbers of people who would choose death over the continuation of treatment if this option were more openly discussed and available. The resources saved by not having to expensively prolong the lives of patients who choose to die, they reasoned, could then be spent on improved palliative care and acute care for those who choose to live.

When participants were asked to restrict their discussion to the relative merits of palliative versus acute care funding, the vast majority indicated that it was more important to focus on saving lives, even when the chances of success were small: "The needs of the dying are important, but the primary objective of the health care system has to be saving lives and curing people."

Participants' difficulty in making "hard choices" was unabated as discussion turned to identifying the grounds on which society should decide which needs should receive greatest priority. Together with finding the issue distasteful, a large part of the problem for many participants stemmed from their reluctance to accept the premise on which such a discussion was based.

Quite a few participants were simply not prepared to accept that Canada had reached the point where "rationing" of medical services was required. Their often passionate arguments pointed to numerous areas, both inside and out of the health care system, where they felt resources could be found: "Look at all of the money that is wasted in this country, whether it's perks for politicians or the cost of peacekeeping in Bosnia. Our health care system is the most important thing [that we have]."

In the context of the focus groups, the participants who accepted the premise for rationing health services sometimes became apologetic in explaining their support for using the amount of benefit produced per cost as the most appropriate criteria for deciding which, whether, and at what level health services should be funded: "I don't mean to sound callous, but..." In the eyes of these participants, using a "formula" or analytical technique to determine the cost-effectiveness of services seemed like the only thing to do under the circumstances.

In the end, participants remained about equally divided on the issue. The real point of debate, it is important to note, did not centre on what criteria should be used for determining funding levels for health services, as much as whether or not circumstances really warranted the adoption of any such measures.

Scenario 6: Guidelines to Encourage the Use of Less-Expensive Drugs

Participants had a moderate amount of difficulty in reaching a decision on the key question raised by this scenario. After initial discussion in which a few participants expressed moral indignation at what they considered to be "putting a price on a human life," participants generally agreed that it was acceptable to use cheaper, but slightly less-effective drugs, in order to save resources and channel the savings towards meeting other needs. Most participants qualified their response by stating that they had been swayed by the information in the scenario which indicated that the drug *would still be available* to doctors if the latter felt its use was necessary to save someone's life. Participants sought to make it clear that they were not compromising survival, but rather trading off comfort and speed of recovery for a substantial saving of resources.

Participants' response to this and other scenarios indicate that Canadians are willing to support cost-saving measures which reduce qualities such as choice, comfort and timeliness, as long as these measures do not jeopardize lives. This is how the majority of participants reconciled the conflict between providing the "best possible care" on the one hand, and making sure that there were sufficient resources to ensure that all Canadians can receive treatment. This view is strongly linked to the difficulty that many participants have in accepting the premise that the country has reached a point where it must consider rationalizing health services in a manner that might cost lives. In this scenario, for example, the hypothetical suggestion that the more expensive drug could increase patient comfort, but have no long-term impact on the patient's health, rendered the issue almost insignificant. Participants did not hesitate to say that if such a drug was significantly more expensive, then it should not be available to doctors.

Participants acknowledged the ethical dilemma faced by the doctors in the scenario, but there was a consensus that these doctors had not compromised their professional ethic. In considering the situation, participants once again adopted a pragmatic approach. Their response to the issue came easily: Physicians can only be expected to operate within the parameters set by the state: "They simply have to do their best with what is given to them." From this perspective, the choice is not made by the doctor, but by the state. Some participants also emphasized the importance of having the state set clear guidelines in order to relieve doctors of the burden of having to make choices which might make them feel like they are compromising their principles.

Participants were less certain about whether or not a doctor should have to disclose to patients the fact that the treatment they are receiving may not be the most beneficial. Some participants said that they would like to know this in order to have the choice of going to the United States to obtain treatment. Others said that they would maintain peace of mind by not knowing this information. A few took a less personal and more philosophical stance: "There is always going to be a treatment out there that is probably better that what we receive here, especially in the U.S. So what if what we receive here is not the absolute best available? It's still pretty good." Most ultimately felt that the patient had a right to know if there were alternatives available to the treatment they were receiving.

Finally, in some focus groups, the issue of whether or not people should be given the option of purchasing more expensive (and presumably more effective) drugs was discussed. Opinion was mixed, and varied according to region. In Quebec City, for example, participants rejected the notion out of hand. They saw this as akin to allowing private clinics to open and argued that giving people this choice would undermine the bedrock principle of universality. In Windsor, Ontario, on the other hand, participants were more pragmatic. For one thing, they were quite familiar with the practice of purchasing medicine across the boarder in Michigan. They were also apparently more familiar with the U.S. health care system. Even in this group, however, opinion was at best divided. Participants who were opposed voiced similar objections to those articulated by their Quebec City counterparts. Conversely, those who supported giving people this option said that it was far different than allowing private clinics to open. They pointed out that there was no potential for a shift in resources away from the public system because choice would be limited to medication and no portion of additional costs would be borne by the provincial health care system.

Overall, this was an issue that generated the most even split on the two-tier question because many people could not see how allowing people to purchase the more expensive drug could weaken the system for others. As a consequence, opposition was restricted to those (still a majority) who were philosophically opposed to allowing different levels of care, rather than those who worried about the practical impacts of introducing two-tier medicine.

Scenario 7: Increasing the Level of Responsibility That Families Have for Taking Care of Their Own

Discussion of this scenario was often emotional, but produced a clear consensus among both young and old. Participants strongly agreed that it was not fair to expect families to assume increased responsibility for caring for their own and that the state should in no way rely on such an assumption in making allocation decisions. In fact, the idea seemed outrageous to quite a few participants, despite the fact that a few had talked of having assumed these types of responsibilities in the past (e.g., feeding a hospitalized relative).

Participants listed a number of mutually reinforcing arguments against even a slight shift in responsibility away from institutions and health care professionals towards families. The main objection was that such an approach ran counter to dominant societal trends such as the growth of single-parent families, the increased number of families where both parents have to work, longer working hours, individualism, consumerism, and atomization of society: "Women have gone back to school, gone to work and seen their marriages break up." Participants emphasized the significance of these trends as a way of showing that most people were not equipped, either financially or emotionally, to take on the sort of responsibilities described in the scenario. Other arguments against assuming responsibility included the following:

- Parents have already been expected by the state to take on more responsibilities in other areas, such as the schooling of their children.
- Older participants agreed that they did not want to burden their children and spouses. They also emphasized that it was naive to assume that they would even want to be taken care of by their children.
- Younger participants echoed the above views, with many frankly admitting that they could not "handle" taking care of a parent;
- Some expressed concern about the ability of a family member of taking proper care of a recovering patient, especially when the family member was older: "What if something goes wrong? Would we get training?"

The idea of compensating people who assume significant responsibility for looking after someone, through a tax credit for example, produced mixed responses.

Some participants felt that this was fair and reasonable. They supported a policy which would provide such compensation, but would not require anyone to assume more responsibility for a relative unless they freely chose to do so.

Others rejected the idea. In some cases, participants were apparently still worked up by the earlier discussion. A few said they found the idea of the state "paying people" to take care of a relative distasteful: "You are bribing people to do the right thing." Others said that such a policy would open the door to abuse, particularly parent abuse. In the end, these participants preferred that the state stay away from the issue completely and leave matters to family members: "It has to come from the heart. People have to want to do it or else it won't work."

On balance, however, there was considerable scepticism that government would put the required resources into the hands of people or communities. Many saw it as a thin veil for service reductions.

Predictably, participants also unanimously rejected the idea of fostering more widely in society the expectation that families will look after their own. Participants, including seniors, said that this would prove to be a fruitless attempt at "turning back the clock." Many did not have fond memories of the days of more individual responsibility in this area. In this vein, several pointed out that it was in response to the inadequacies of that approach that the current system had evolved. Finally, some added that they doubted governments' ability to have any success in changing public attitudes: "What are they going to do? Put ads on TV? It was TV that helped to make us the way we are" (i.e., individualistic and materialistic).

Participants also strongly agreed on a final point. They encouraged government to facilitate and fund home care and other forms of community-based care in which health care professionals looked after people: "Everybody knows that people recover faster and are happier in their own home. It's also cheaper. But professionals should look after people, not family members."

Scenario 8: Principles of the Health Care System

The scenario about competing values generated remarkable consensus among participants in all groups in which it was discussed. With one exception, all values were considered to be valid principles around which to organize the health care system.

The one exception was equal shares for groups. This was dismissed as an operating principle by virtually all, and expressed with a fair degree of vehemence. Part of this opposition is likely driven by the connection that was made between this kind of approach and different ethnic or religious groups. Other research shows that the rapidly changing face of Canada is fuelling some backlash or intolerance on the part of some people and this would have coloured some responses on this point.

For many other people, however, it was simply an invalid criteria on which to base resource allocation. Other discussions indicated that many people were quite open to alternative forms of medicine provided that effectiveness could be established. They were not open to funding alternative medicines as a way of achieving a sense of balance between groups.

None of these concepts can be understood outside of the context of real angst about the financial viability of health care and diminishing levels of access and quality. People have a well-defined hierarchy of values as demonstrated in discussions of this scenario.

Overwhelmingly, equal access and quality of care were the most important criteria for virtually all participants. There were divisions about which one was more important of the two, but no real belief by most that anything else was of equivalent importance. Participants also tended to think that they reflected a consensus in Canadian society about values and health care. It was a badge of some nationalistic pride that there was a "Canadian" way of looking at these issues.

Some of those most concerned about fiscal issues would rank efficiency very highly. They were concerned that the absence of a cap on health care spending would have a negative impact on government deficits and tax rates. Most participants, however, tended to disagree with these participants' "sense of priorities." It was not that others were unconcerned about efficiency in health care, they were, and often this would lead to discussions about causes of inefficiency, such as the practices of physicians or overuse by patients or poor administration. Most simply did not want efficiency to be the driving force in health policy. Similarly, the concern of virtually all participants about government deficits did not lead them to think that the health care system was the main problem. Most felt it was the highest priority and savings should be found elsewhere.

Most people did think that maximum benefit for dollar had to be a consideration for society. As discussed elsewhere, they did not like the trade-offs inherent in that approach and did not confront them easily. However, there was a sense that health care dollars were not being spent in the wisest fashion. Combined with the belief that dollars were now very limited, this created an acceptance among many that tough allocation decisions would have to be made to preserve the elements of real value in the system.

The prime areas of conflict that people saw emerging from the different principles were between equal access, on the one hand, and quality of service and maximum return on the other hand. They expressed combative resistance to giving up on either quality or access. When pushed, most tended to look for solutions that compromised equal access but did not eliminate it. Examples would be the willingness by some people to accept user fees for doctor or hospital visits, or the willingness by some to think that private clinics might be a way to get more money into the system. Most did not advocate these approaches as desirable. Rather, if convinced (and this constitutes a large "if") that governments could not afford to maintain the status quo— maintaining the status quo was the first choice overwhelmingly—ultimately they felt more comfortable looking at solutions that introduced more resources into the system to forestall a diminution in quality.

Summary of Focus Group with Aboriginal Canadians

A special focus group consisting of Aboriginal Canadians was held in Regina. The issue of Aboriginal health and the relationship of Aboriginals to the health care system is obviously a subject that cannot be done justice in one focus group in one region. However, we felt that our research in this area would not be complete without some insight on this subject. The composition of the group included some Métis and some First Nations, both Status and Nonstatus.

This particular group was conducted along different, more traditional lines than were the other groups. Rather than use the scenarios to stimulate discussion, more direct and focused probing was used to elicit the views of participants on core principles and values as they relate to health care.

Even more so than participants elsewhere, these participants were focused on decline in the health care system. There was a very strong feeling that the service delivered to them had diminished in both quality and access, as had the infrastructure through which they receive services.

As were the other participants in this project, those in the Aboriginal group were very attached to the health care system and the underlying principles of that system. In keeping with Saskatchewan attitudes on this subject, there was some pride of ownership over medicare. They tended to talk of the system, its values and what it represents about Canadians as a people, in very similar ways to other participants.

Most tended to be pessimistic about the future of health care. Perhaps as a consequence of the health care restructuring that had gone on in Saskatchewan—or perhaps that restructuring has taken a more serious toll on them—there was a real sense on the part of participants that the decline they felt was already occurring would continue into the future.

Participants in this group were anxious that the federal government continue to have a strong role in health care. This might be thought to be anomalous in a province which has traditionally had a lot of faith in its provincial government to protect and advance health care. However, like many Canadians, these participants' fears about lack of sufficient health care funding led them to want all of their governments to focus on that area. More particularly, however, these participants felt that they had a special relationship with the federal government and that the federal government had a special fiduciary responsibility to them.

All that being said, there was very little understanding of the federal role in the area of health care. While the principles of the Canada Health Act were understood by them to be the principles underlying the health care system, there was little understanding of the Canada Health Act itself.

Few had heard of it or what it represented. When the principles embodied in the act were presented to them, they felt that they were appropriate and that it was important for the federal government to be playing that role.

They had an interesting take on alternative medicines. Many in the group felt there ought to be a role for a more spiritual aspect to medicine. There was a sense that modern, science-based medicine did not place enough emphasis on "healing" in a true sense. They tended to view traditional or alternative forms as complementary to science-based medicine—not as a replacement. For instance, allowing an Aboriginal Canadian to have a spiritual advisor in the hospital room with them to help with prayer. They also felt, similarly to participants in other groups, that ultimately the alternative forms ought to pass some test of effectiveness.

Participants in this group seemed somewhat more aware of the broader issues of health than did other participants. As a consequence they had a different understanding of what prevention meant in a health context. They did not conceive of it only as education, which is what others tended to do. Rather, they tended to focus on the role of poverty and lifestyle problems and the relationship between those issues and health.

Despite their enthusiasm for prevention, they shared other participants' reluctance to reduce the priority placed on acute care. There was even less acceptance of the paradigm that said that there were only so many dollars to be spent on health care and choices and allocations had to be made within that envelope. They were more willing to challenge that assumption and to suggest that what was really required was more money in the system.

In wanting to see more money in the system, though, they were more resistant than other participants to any form of private involvement. The commitment to public administration and to universal access was very strong and willingness to look at any compromise of access was limited to one participant.

QUANTITATIVE FINDINGS

Background

One of the principal advantages of focus group work is the capacity to iteratively refine and test research issues in a much more open-ended, naturalistic, and flexible fashion. However, the capacity to generalize (external validity) is severely limited by both the nature of recruitment, very small sample sizes, and the somewhat reactive and artificial social psychology of the focus group.

A quantitative enhancement was added to help redress this problem (appendix 4). A mini quantitative survey was conducted during the recruitment period and after completion of the groups focus. Several of the questions included in this miniquantitative study were already asked of a representative sample of Canadians under the auspices of the *Rethinking Government* study.

The five key objectives of this quantitative component are outlined below:

1. enhancing the generalizability/external validity of the findings from this study;
2. mapping differences between members of the Canadian population as a whole (respondents of the *Rethinking Government* study) and respondents of this survey;
3. providing a method of measuring attitudinal and demographic differences between those who were willing to participate in a focus group and those who were not;
4. providing a method of determining the causal influence of focus group sessions on public judgements; and
5. measuring the impact of deliberative focus group sessions on public judgements.

Methodology

The methodology used in conducting this quantitative component of the study is outlined below.

Screening questionnaire – During the recruitment of focus group participants, potential participants were screened using a four-minute (14-item) questionnaire examining attitudes concerning the study issues (e.g., values surrounding health care, perceptions of health care in Canada), as well as general demographic characteristics. After the potential participants had completed this battery of questions, they were asked if they would be willing to participate in a focus group session. A total of 800 individuals were asked this battery of questions.

Postparticipation questionnaire – At the conclusion of each focus group session, participants were asked to respond to another short attitudinal questionnaire, which basically encompassed the same set of questions as the screening questionnaire.

The quantitative component yielded the following two data outputs:
- 14-item survey of 803 people living in and around the nine centres in which the focus groups were conducted; and
- 93 matched pre- and postsurveys of focus group participants.

Findings

Findings from the quantitative research are organized around the following four major themes:

- differences between the survey findings and the findings of the *Rethinking Government* survey;
- differences between focus group participants and nonparticipants;
- influence of participating in the focus group sessions based on the pre- and the postsurvey results; and
- influence of the deliberative exercise on participants' attitudes based on the pre- and postsurvey results.

Survey Findings

The findings detailed below encompass both the Health Forum survey and selected replicated questions from the *Rethinking Government* study. A number of differences between the findings from the two surveys are discussed below. Prior to moving to this discussion, we would like to provide some possible explanations for the presence of differences in responses to these identical questions:

- *Sampling effect*: The *Rethinking Government* sample was randomly selected to represent the Canadian population. The Health Forum sample was limited to the nine centres in which the focus groups were conducted. A comparison of the two samples reveals that the latter sample is overrepresented by urban dwellers, people under 60 years of age, and females. Income and education indicators, however, are representative of the population as a whole.
- *Time effect*: The two surveys were conducted approximately seven months apart. People's attitudes may have been influenced by events related to health care which occurred between the two time periods.
- *Questionnaire design effect*: The *Rethinking Government* questionnaire was approximately 35 minutes long and addressed a number of topics. In contrast, the questionnaire used in this study was short (four-minute telephone interview) and focused uniquely on health care issues.

Approximately 800 respondents were first asked a battery of attitudinal questions about the health care system (figure1).

Respondents are split in their views about whether economics or values should be paramount in the health care system. The same percent agree (40 percent) as disagree (38 percent) with the notion that the health care system is more about values than economics. Activists, those over 60 years of age, men, and lower-income Canadians are more likely than others to feel that health care is about values.

Respondents express concern about the sustainability of the health care system. Over two in three (68 percent) disagree with the statement, "I have more confidence that the health care system will take care of me than I did five years ago." Activists, women, those with high school education, and those with higher income are particularly pessimistic about the future of health care. A similarly high level of concern about the sustainability of the

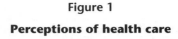

Figure 1

Perceptions of health care

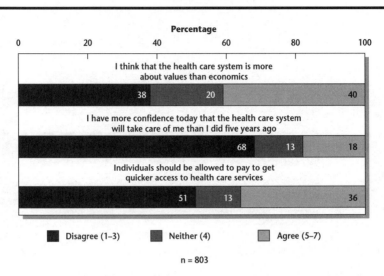

n = 803

system was expressed in the focus groups. This concern is fuelled by what participants viewed as *tangible* signs of stress and strains on the system.

This question was also asked of *Rethinking Government* respondents (the general public). The Canadian population as a whole is slightly more optimistic about the future of the health care system than respondents to this study: 60 percent of *Rethinking Government* respondents disagree that they have more confidence in the system.

Most survey participants do not endorse the concept of a two-tiered health care system. A majority (51 percent) disagree that individuals should be allowed to pay to get quicker access to health care services. Those under the age of 60 are particularly negative in their views of two-tier health care.

This question was also asked as part of the *Rethinking Government* study. The general public are more opposed to a two-tier system than respondents to this study. Sixty-one percent of *Rethinking Government* respondents disagree that people should be allowed to pay extra to get quicker access to health care services.

Respondents were also asked to rate the importance of a range of values in shaping the health care system (figure 2). All values are believed to be of importance in shaping the health care system; however, efficiency, performance, and equality of access are assigned highest priority by the Canadian public.

Figure 2

Importance of various values in health care

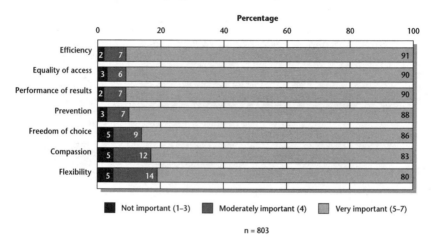

*How important should each of the following values be
in shaping the health care system?*

Percentage

Value	Not important (1–3)	Moderately important (4)	Very important (5–7)
Efficiency	2	7	91
Equality of access	3	6	90
Performance of results	2	7	90
Prevention	3	7	88
Freedom of choice	5	9	86
Compassion	5	12	83
Flexibility	5	14	80

Not important (1–3)   Moderately important (4)   Very important (5–7)

n = 803

The importance assigned to each of these values differs across the demographic and attitudinal characteristics examined in the study. These differences are outlined below.

- Those under the age of 60, women, and those who rate their health as good are the strongest supporters of freedom of choice as a value.
- Those under the age of 60, those with higher education, and those living in households earning $60,000 or more are the strongest proponents of an efficient health care system.
- Those under the age of 60 and women are the most likely to feel that flexibility is an important value.
- Those with university education, those living in households who earn more than $60,000 per year and who rate their health as good are more likely than their counterparts to assign importance to the performance of the health care system.
- Those under the age of 60, women, and those living in households earning less than $20,000 are particularly likely to endorse compassion as a value for health care.
- University educated, those living in households earning $60,000 or more, and those who rate their health as good are the strongest supporters of prevention.
- Few subgroup differences are exhibited with respect to the importance of equality of access.

Respondents were then forced to choose which one aspect of health care was of greatest importance to them (figure 3).

Figure 3

Most important feature of health care

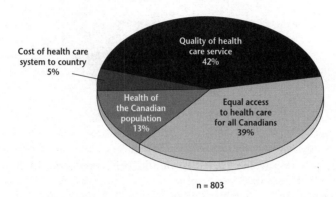

Which one of the following aspects of health care is of greatest importance to you?

Cost of health care system to country 5%

Quality of health care service 42%

Health of the Canadian population 13%

Equal access to health care for all Canadians 39%

n = 803

Quality of health care (42 percent) and equality of access (39 percent) are seen as the ultimate goals of the health care system. It is interesting to note how few respondents selected the cost of the health care system to the country (5 percent). This finding is very consistent with the qualitative results. In the focus groups, participants reiterated the view that these two values were the twin pillars of the Canadian systems.

The quality of health care is assigned greatest importance by women and higher-income earners. Equal access is given highest priority by those with high school education and those with lower income.

The same forced choice was asked of *Rethinking Government* respondents. The pattern of responses is quite similar for the general public (equal access and quality of service are considered to be of paramount importance). However, respondents to the *Rethinking Government* survey as a whole assign higher priority to equal access (53 percent) and survey respondents accord higher importance to the quality of health care.

Finally, respondents were asked who should be responsible for health care (figure 4).

The findings indicate that survey respondents feel that both the federal and provincial governments should be actively involved in health care (although they indicate a slight preference for a federal lead role). This reflects a general desire for partnership (and a corresponding fatigue with

Figure 4

Responsibility for health care

Who should have responsibility for health care?

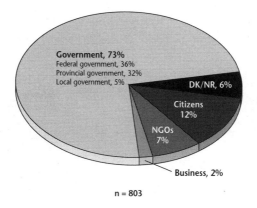

n = 803

territorialism) among the Canadian public. It also reflects a preference for checks and balances in this area of profound importance for Canadians.

This thirst for partnership is also revealed in the *Rethinking Government* findings, although among the general public as a whole the lean is to a slight provincial preference.

Differences between Participants and Nonparticipants of Focus Group

In order to gain a clearer understanding of the similarities and differences between the people who participated in the focus group sessions and those who did not, a comparison of focus group participants and those who refused to participate was conducted. This comparison encompassed both the attitudinal and demographic questions addressed in this survey.

On an overall basis, few differences were found across the attitudinal and demographic questions, indicating that focus group participants were similar to the general public. However, some differences were exhibited as outlined below.

Few differences were found with respect to whether health care is about economics values (figure 5). However, those who participated in focus group sessions were less likely than the general population to express confidence in the future of the health care system and to feel that individuals should be allowed to pay to get quicker access to health care.

A similar comparison was done across the preferred values for shaping the health care system (figure 6). Across virtually all options, nonparticipants assigned slightly higher importance to the values.

Figure 5

Comparison of general public and focus group respondents—
Attitudes

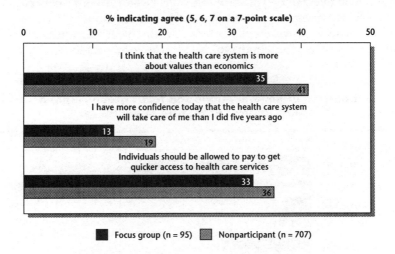

% indicating agree (5, 6, 7 on a 7-point scale)

Focus group (n = 95)   Nonparticipant (n = 707)

Figure 6

Comparison of general public and focus group respondents—
Values for health care

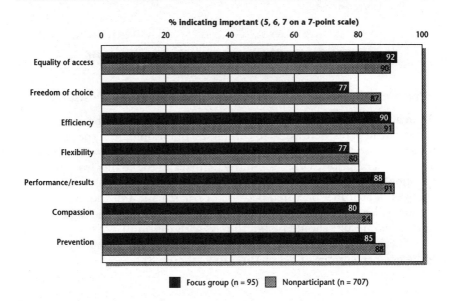

% indicating important (5, 6, 7 on a 7-point scale)

Focus group (n = 95)   Nonparticipant (n = 707)

The two groups exhibit similar preferences with respect to the most important aspect of health care (figure 7) although nonparticipants more strongly endorse the quality of health care as being the paramount feature of the system. It is also interesting to note that the focus group participants were more likely to be unsure about which aspect is most important.

The two groups were also compared across demographic characteristics. Men, participants with higher education, and older Canadians were more likely than their counterparts to attend focus group sessions.

Figure 7

Comparison of general public and focus group respondents— Most important feature of health care

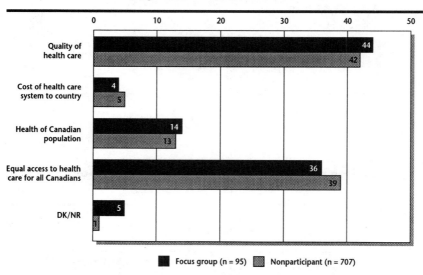

Focus group (n = 95) ▨ Nonparticipant (n = 707)

Influence of Participating Focus Group Session (Pre- and Postsurvey)

As an additional feature of this quantitative component of the study, focus group participants were asked to complete a questionnaire at the end of the focus group session. This questionnaire was composed of the same questions as those asked prior to the session. By comparing the results from the pre-questionnaire and the postquestionnaire, it is possible to establish if any changes in attitudes occurred because of participation in the focus group session. (Please note that because the sample sizes used in these analyses are quite small, results should be interpreted with caution.)

The findings indicate that taking part in the focus group sessions did influence perceptions of health care issues (figure 8).

Figure 8

Changes in attitudes about health care

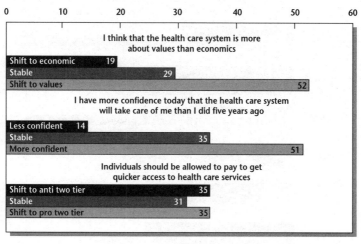

n = 95

The focus group discussions augmented the belief that health care is more about values than economics. Participation in the focus group sessions also increased confidence in the health care system.

Participation in the focus group session resulted in a polarization of attitudes surrounding a two-tiered health care system. Respondents were as likely to increase as decrease their support for a two-tiered system. It is interesting to note that all of those over the age of 60 changed their views about two-tier health care (33 percent strongly endorsed the two-tier system and 67 percent more strongly opposed this system).

The responses of participants concerning the values which should define our health care system were also examined both before and after the focus group sessions (figure 9).

Equality of access, efficiency, and prevention are largely stable between the two time periods. Flexibility and compassion have a tendency to become more important to participants. Freedom of choice exhibits a slight diminishment in importance. The importance of flexibility is as likely to decrease as increase between the pre- and the postsurvey.

Participants' top value preference for health care changed markedly between the two time periods, as summarized below.

- The majority of respondents who selected quality of health care in the presurvey either continued to select quality or changed their selection to equal access.

Figure 9

Changes in importance of values for health care system

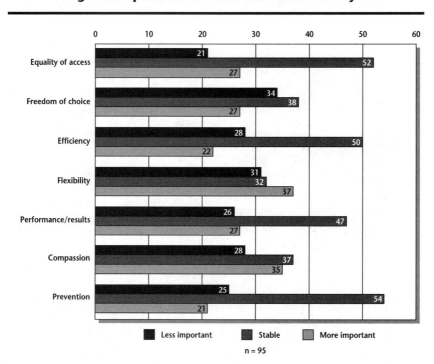

- All (four) of those who initially selected the costs of the system changed their preference to either quality or equal access.
- The majority of respondents who initially selected health of the Canadian population changed their selection to the quality of the health care system.
- The majority of those who initially chose equal access to health care for all Canadians either maintained this preference or changed it to the quality of health care.

Influence of Deliberative Exercise (Pre- and Postsurvey)

Further analyses were conducted with respect to the impact of participation in deliberative focus group sessions on attitudes. Participants in these deliberative groups were given basic factual information about Canadian health care (see appendix 3) and asked to briefly discuss their reaction to this information. Changes in attitudes which occurred between the pre- and postsurvey for both the deliberative and nondeliberative sessions are outlined below.

Figure 10 illustrates the impact of participation in the deliberative focus group sessions across the questions addressing values versus economics, confidence in the system, and two-tier health care. In general, the "deliberative" test was a much weaker test than the test of the effects of group discussion. The "deliberative" stimuli were relatively modest and focused on economic indicators. The results of the tests are inconclusive and require further testing.

Figure 10

**Changes in attitudes to health care
(deliberative vs. nondeliberative sessions)**

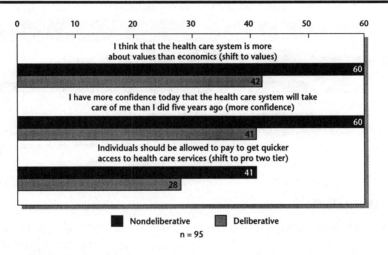

Nondeliberative　　Deliberative

n = 95

Individuals who did *not* participate in a deliberative focus group session became more values oriented than those who attended a deliberative session. Confidence in the health care system increased by a larger margin among those who did not participate in a deliberative session. Those who did not participate in a deliberative session were also somewhat more likely to support a two-tier health care system. This somewhat anomalous finding is of marginal statistical significance and probably should be treated with suspicion until replicated in a more robust test.

Attitudes about which values should define the health care system were also examined across the deliberative and nondeliberative groups (figure 11).

Across the majority of these values, participation in a deliberative session increased the importance that respondents attached to values, particularly the performance of the system.

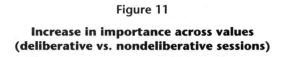

Figure 11

Increase in importance across values
(deliberative vs. nondeliberative sessions)

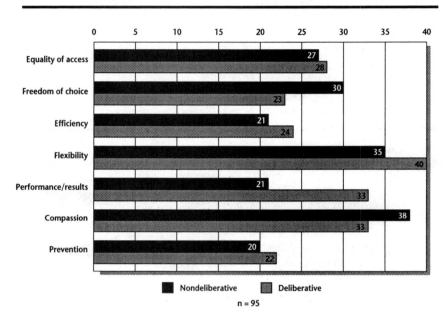

Nondeliberative ■   Deliberative ▨

n = 95

CONCLUSIONS

The combination of the focus group discussions and the two waves of survey research have helped to provide real insight into the underlying values and principles with which Canadians approach issues of health and health care.

It is important to note that these issues are very much at the forefront of what Canadians are thinking about, in terms of public policy, at this time. There is overwhelming evidence (see *Rethinking Government*) that health care concerns are at the top of the priority list for most people in the country. What was revealing about the focus group work was how much prior thought participants had put into the issues being discussed. Relative to other research of this type, participants in this project had remarkably fully thought-through ideas and opinions. At the same time, the fact that participants had given the issues considerable thought prior to attending did not mean that their views were cast in stone. On the contrary, the difficulty of the trade-offs and choices that the scenarios forced on them often shook their core beliefs and forced them to reassess long-held attitudes. Arguments put forward by some participants were often persuasive to others. It made the case very strongly that the debate over health care policy in this country exists in a very dynamic environment, one in which conflicting powerful forces are at play. The debate itself has the potential to shape opinion.

Health care has become top of mind for Canadians because it is something about which they care deeply, something about which they are very concerned, something in which they understand significant reforms are occurring, and something in which they believe dramatic changes will occur. They want health care reform to reflect the values they believe in and to be undertaken with an eye not of dismantling what exists, but toward improving and preserving what they consider to be important about it.

Some broad findings emerged from the research.

Pride in the Canadian Approach to Health Care

The vast majority of those who participated in the focus groups were immensely proud of the type of health care system that has been built in Canada. It was considered by almost all participants to be strongly reflective of *Canadian* values and was often contrasted with the American system of health care.

Although other competing priorities emerged over the period of the discussions, it is *equality of access* that serves as the primary source of this pride. The "Canadian" values are wrapped up in equality of access—everybody gets relatively equal care when they are sick and nobody has to lose their house to pay their hospital or doctor bill. It is this feature of the system which is seen to most distinguish it from the American model (which is the point of comparison).

Many people readily acknowledge that their belief in egalitarianism is restricted to health care and that they are not troubled by wide discrepancies based on ability to pay or status in other areas of society. They have no trouble isolating health care in this way because they see health care as something of a completely different character than housing or automobiles or vacations. It is also clear that many, perhaps most, feel that they *personally* might be worse off if the system evolved into two tiers.

One of the ways in which it is different is the fact that being as healthy as possible is seen to be fundamental to having the kind of quality of life that is believed to accompany being Canadian. It is simply seen as being more important and more fundamental. It is one thing that one person lives in a larger house or takes better vacations than other people as a result of higher income levels. Few people are willing to intervene to stop that result. It is another thing entirely that one person not receive the same treatment for a physical ailment that another person does on the basis of income. Few respondents were willing to tolerate that.

Second, equality of access is seen to be an essential component of opportunity. Variances of income or other accoutrements might be end results of the market economy, but being physically healthy is seen to be a precondition to having a fair chance at success. If there is to be equality of opportunity, to the extent possible, everyone should start from a position of good health.

Third, many people see it as a smart investment on the part of our country; one that gives us some economic comparative advantages and makes society more stable. In an era when the rapidity of change is proving deeply unsettling for many people and when economic change is having an adverse effect on many families, the fact that Canadians need not worry about either not being able to afford necessary medical treatment or being bankrupted by medical bills is seen as a sensible approach.

Concerns about Future Viability

Many participants were concerned that health care would not remain as it is in future. Those concerns were driven by the following factors:

- A sense that the health care system was in decline and that its viability was threatened. A significant portion of participants in the research felt that health care in Canada was not as good as it had been. Anecdotal evidence presented to support this contention centred around government cuts in health care spending, waiting lists for doctors or procedures, and the number of Canadian doctors going to the United States.

- Regardless of whether one believed that there had already been a diminution in service, almost all believed that the future of the system was threatened. Levels of government indebtedness have convinced most that greater cuts are possible in the future. That expectation is positioned against an understanding that health care costs will continue to rise, especially things like drugs and technology-aided diagnosis and/or treatments.

- Worry by some that the will to maintain the system was not strong enough; perhaps there were other ideological agendas that were at play in undercutting the system. These were people who did not quarrel with the principle of governments getting their fiscal houses in order, but felt that some governments had agendas to diminish medicare by subterfuge—that the need for spending cuts provided cover to those who did not believe in the principles of the health care system.

- Some believed that the system design contained the seeds of its own lack of viability. This *minority* saw medicare as a generous impulse but ultimately unrealistic and unsustainable.

A Reluctant Willingness to Consider Change

Notwithstanding the priority placed on equality of access, a large minority of participants were either prepared to contemplate some form of "two-tier" health system or were resigned to its eventuality. Two forces seemed to be driving people in that direction.

- First, as discussed earlier, many people felt that the money to sustain the system was increasingly not available and that injecting private money into the system was one of the few options for preserving some semblance of what we have in terms of health care. Not all were of the view that "two tier" would be the end of quality care for those unable to afford private care. The arguments presented in favour of "two tier" seemed to make intuitive sense to many people. This was especially true of two arguments. The contention that those who paid privately would free up space in the public system and resources for that system was an argument that had some persuasive effects in the focus groups. The idea that some form of user charge would discourage abuse and overuse was also noted. Virtually everybody was of the view that this type of abuse existed and constituted a real problem for the system. Even some of those who felt that the problems associated with user charges outweighed the advantages felt that the system could benefit from some measure that put some responsibility back on to users to help control costs. Many felt this could be done simply by informing people what the actual costs of the services are.

- Second, for the first time, quality of care is starting to conflict with the higher-minded principles of medicare. In health care, as in Ford cars, "quality is job one." The quantitative portion of this research found that equal numbers of people felt that equality of access and quality of care were the most important things to them personally. There is an overwhelming consensus among Canadians about the importance of equality of access as the defining characteristic of our system. That consensus is premised upon the assumption that quality is a given, as they have perceived it to be in the past. The research revealed that the consensus over equality is much less firm when it conflicts with quality of service. Participants felt that historically, our health care had been better than or at least equal to anything in the world—with the possible exception of the care available to the very wealthiest Americans. Most felt that was still the case. Most also felt that condition was threatened. As stated earlier, either through personal anecdotal experience or through their understanding of larger trends, there was a profound sense of a system in decline. Many people were prepared to entertain significant changes in the way the system is designed and administered in order to preserve quality of care. There did not appear to be a similar willingness to accept significant reductions in the quality of care in order to preserve access. It would appear that attempts to preserve the values that are important about the Canadian health care system must be premised upon continued high quality.

The standard of quality that was demanded by most participants appeared to be "among the highest in the world." As part of the constant comparisons to the American system, people tend to accept that the very highest level of care available is of a higher standard than what is available in Canada. The trade-off that makes this acceptable is that the median level of care is seen to be higher in Canada. Almost all seemed to accept that in the world of endless technological advances and spiralling health care costs, not everything would be doable in our system. As an example, most had no problem with the use of the cheaper heart drug in exchange for a minor increase in risk. On the other hand, participants volunteered concerns about the "brain drain" of doctors as evidence of people's worries about the ability to maintain quality in our system with decreasing or insufficiently increasing dollars.

Values and Change

The philosophy of "two tier" did not seem terribly persuasive to people. Arguments about freedom of choice, or the right of people to access the exact care they want at the time they want it—if they can afford it—did not have many adherents around the table.

To the extent that people were prepared to contemplate a "two-tier" system, it was because they felt practical considerations were overwhelming compared to what they considered to be the right set of principles—not that we had the wrong set of principles. The overwhelming preference would be for change that preserved both the quality of service and the principles of medicare as Canadians have come to know them.

There are some important assumptions built in to the value choices that people make about health care. The debate about two-tier health care is a clash between individual priorities and communal priorities. One has to be careful in interpreting the priority people place on the communal values of health care, such as equality of access, over individual ones, such as freedom of choice or quality. The truth is that most people feel free to place a higher priority on the communal values because quality and choice are taken as a given.

As a consequence, they are not choosing between competing values so much as they are layering communal values on top of a baseline expectation of service. This does not diminish the communal values—they are strong and, given that they are not found in every country or society, the priority placed on them does speak to a Canadian value system. It is also true that, since Canadians recognize that a truly private system like the U.S. version might provide even greater levels of quality or freedom of choice to at least some citizens, they are choosing to sacrifice some of that from the system in order to provide equality of access to a universal system.

All this is to say that there is self-interest involved in decision making on this issue. If people's assumptions about quality or freedom began to prove incorrect because of attempts to maintain equality of access or universality, it is not clear that the value consensus would hold. If put to a real choice, rather than the somewhat false choice people make now when discussing this issue, those to whom equality of access is less important personally might well prefer a system that delivered the product—quality service and freedom to choose one's doctor—that they expect from a health care system.

Health Care Is Fundamentally about Acute Care

Many people support putting greater emphasis on prevention conceptually. In the initial general discussion of health care, many people volunteered that greater emphasis on prevention would be beneficial and likely generate cost savings over the long run. However, the number of respondents who can follow it through all of the ramifications is considerably smaller. As either discussion or the scenarios force people to confront trade-offs, particularly reductions in acute care, they tended to back off of prevention and to articulate that ultimately the system had to be there for sick people, whatever else it was doing.

There is a fairly narrow definition of prevention within a health context. It tended to be limited to traditional things like education, vaccination, and fitness. Some of the broader examples raised by the scenarios (e.g., job creation and environmental programs) seemed to most people to be good ideas but not directly related to health care and more properly the responsibility of social services departments.

Once one scratches the surface, there is significant scepticism about the efficacy of prevention measures. Many people felt the results were hard to quantify and not certain to happen. Moving resources from acute care to prevention seemed to be giving up the bird in the hand.

For most people, it was fundamentally unacceptable to deny critical care because resources had been expended on prevention. While a minority felt the other way, most people felt the priority of the health care system had to be to provide care to the sick. As a consequence, prevention, for most people, was an add-on, not a replacement option.

Health Care Is Whatever Works

Opinions about alternative forms of health care were negative when linked to ethnicity or religion. Some, who were strong adherents to "scientific" medicine, felt these alternatives had no place in the system. Others thought that perhaps there were useful approaches not utilized in our type of health care. These respondents tended to feel that "scientific" medicine had some flaws, or that other approaches seemed to work for some people.

Demand and proportionate allocation of resources were rejected as appropriate considerations by participants in the research. It needs to be noted that while visible minorities were present in every group, these issues were not tested in such a way that would allow one to gauge accurately the extent to which they might or might not share this consensus. However, the perspective on this issue among the participants in the Aboriginal group was essentially the same. Health care is not a multicultural program and there is no place for remedies that will not be effective just because somebody wants them. The vast majority felt that any alternative form would have to pass a test of some scientific rigour.

There was a point of consensus that covered most people on this issue. The bottom line for all participants was that any approved procedures had to be demonstrably effective. People felt that unless new treatments could pass a rigorous scientific test for effectiveness, they should not be funded. Many people could draw a distinction between what ought to work and what actually works. The important consideration is whether it helps patients heal.

The Line-Up Starts with the Most Ill

People had difficulty priorizing patients by ranking principles or criteria. People pay lip service to the idea that some decisions or trade-offs are necessary but find it virtually impossible to make them themselves. However, there are some considerations that are clearly not valid considerations and others that most could agree ought to be primary factors.

- Two considerations that were clearly off the table that people felt were essentially without merit were *financial ability to pay* and *first come, first served.* In rejecting *first come, first served,* respondents are implicitly acknowledging the need for choices. That is, the person first in line is not necessarily the person whom the system ought to service first. Rather, the person more in need should receive the service first.
- To the extent that there was a consensus about the most important criteria, it revolved around need or medical urgency. Most people felt that this criteria trumped all others. This fits with the earlier finding about critical care—participants' bedrock point is that the health care system cannot turn people away. The only other consideration which had potential with some people to qualify as the absolute priority of medical need was age or the linked criteria of benefit to society.
- Age was the most controversial criteria. Participants were quite literate about the high cost of critical care for the elderly and the drain on health resources that exercises in extending life for the elderly ill can be. On the other hand people were quite troubled by the idea of making a decision that a person no longer merited every attempt—it seemed to contradict their belief about the value of life. Ultimately, most felt it had to be a consideration. Many felt that if patients or families were informed, a lot would make the decision themselves. The most prevalent view, however, was that at some point, the value per dollar to society had to be considered. This is certainly an issue people are more com-

fortable not having to confront. They want health care administrators and doctors making commonsense decisions and judgements and, on issues like this, not confronting them with the decision. Many felt it had to be a consideration, few wanted to personally have to face the consequences of that logic.

- Another area of controversy was whether lifestyle ought to be a consideration in treatment or priority. The common examples that leapt to mind for people were smoking, drinking, and not wearing seatbelts. A minority felt very strongly that people who wilfully create their own health risks should be penalized. Most ended up in the opposite camp. They tended to feel that this criteria was too intrusive and led to a slippery slope of conformity and state intervention with which they were not comfortable. They felt that probably everybody is harming themselves in some way and that can not invalidate a person's claim to what is considered a right of Canadian citizenship—access to quality health care.

What Does It Mean to Be Canadian and Can We Afford It?

At the conclusion, one has the feeling that health care is a primary battleground for many of the larger issues, all value laden, confronting Canada.

People said that medicare was an essential part of the definition of Canadian identity. The different approach to health care was one of the main things that distinguished Canada from the United States. In a period when the unity of the country is perhaps more fragile than at any previous period and when people from coast to coast are struggling to find the common values and shared enterprise to keep the country together, it is both symbolic and disquieting that people perceive medicare to be as threatened as this study suggests.

It may be that the anxiety that many Canadians feel about the future of Canada and the anxiety felt about the future of the quintessential Canadian enterprise of medicare are linked, and so may the solutions. Certainly, the Canadian approach to health care is so central to Canadian identity that if the core principles of medicare were to disappear, one of the most effectively unifying concepts and rights of citizenship would have disappeared.

In some important ways, the debate over the future of health care in Canada and what is required to fix it is a surrogate debate for a broader one. The underpinnings of the Canadian system—that it ought to be run by the government and not run on a profit basis; that money is not the primary consideration and that all are entitled as a matter of citizenship to equal access to quality care—are examples of the typically Canadian approach to problem solving. It is an approach that for many people is emblematic of a Canadian commitment to compassion, equality of opportunity, a sense of community and common purpose. Those types of approaches are under attack every day from the forces driving change in society: high levels of government debt, the globalization of the economy, and the influence of international money markets as a result of the first two factors.

These factors argue against government solutions and against the kind of tax rates required to fund universal health care. Since health care is the most valued of all the examples where this approach has been implemented in Canada, it stands to reason that if they cannot be maintained in this policy area, it is doomed elsewhere.

Ultimately, the Canadian health care system, as it has operated for the past three decades, continues to enjoy broad and strong public support. In an era when belief in government efficacy is at a low ebb, medicare is a government program that is popular and thought to be sensible. As popular as it is, people understand it to be threatened. They are not confused about what is threatening it either. They do not think it is threatened because it is not a good idea or because a new approach is required. They understand it to be threatened by steadily rising costs and by the inability of government finances to absorb those costs. For the most part, however, abuse, misuse and poor administration are foremost in Canadian minds as the main engine of spiralling costs. They will want to see these core problems addressed before contemplating other approaches to medicare.

Canadians understand that change is coming—not out of desire, but out of necessity. Much will have to change if health care is to remain the same. What Canadians desire out of the process of program reform is a program that is consistent with the one that exists now: a high-quality health care system founded on the principle that health care should be accessible on an equal and affordable basis to all who need it. They like how it works. They like the security and peace of mind that it provides. They like what it says about Canadians as a people.

The Evolving Context and Implications for Communications

The period of time since the establishment of the National Health Forum has witnessed a number of important shifts in the environment, shifts which have the potential to impact upon how the recommendations of the Forum are received. Among the more important shifts are the following:

- The aging of the population continues apace, and with it the rising levels of personal preoccupation with health issues, personal and familial in nature.
- Heightened speculation about the future of the CPP and government pension support, combined with an aging population, has aggravated feelings of insecurity, which in turn makes the debate about future availability of quality health services more tense.
- Several years of continued government cutbacks and stories of the impact of cutbacks have made people somewhat less convinced than they were

to assume that there is rampant waste and abuse in the system. This is more likely to be felt in those provinces where major cutbacks have been the focus of acrimonious debate, but it is generally true in most parts of the country. Election outcomes, and political debates in Ontario, Alberta, Saskatchewan, and Quebec have probably been most noteworthy in this regard.

- The strains on the health care system are more apparent to more people over time. A greater number have witnessed firsthand the stresses evident in emergency wards, doctors' offices, etc., which makes the debate about the future of the health care system less theoretical and much more practical for those people.
- There is a modest minority of the population who are starting to feel that governments are gaining the upper hand in the fight against deficits, and beginning to wonder about the kinds of choices which balanced budgets or budget surpluses might afford in the future. At the top of most people's wish list is an effort to strengthen the health care system, a "luxurious" thought which seemed previously unaffordable.

The implications of these shifts could include the following:

- The notion that there is a gap between public "irrationality" about the choices facing the health care system pitted against elite "rationality" may not apply. Instead, it may be the case that the public is increasingly aware and accepting of the difficult decisions which lie ahead. Rather than assuming that the public needs to be educated about the fact that there are difficult choices which need to be made, the Forum may want to consider assuming that the public has already moved beyond that point, and indeed may have started to come to their own conclusions already (see below).
- Similarly, the notion that the public's values and their economic self-interests are clashing or incompatible when it comes to the health care system may not apply. Rather, it may be the case that the public has concluded that it values the health system over all other public services, and is willing to support increased investments (and public borrowing) if necessary to avoid a situation where further rationing/erosion/tiering options are contemplated. The Forum should be cognizant of the fact that the public may no longer be conflicted about their desire for deficit management and a good health care system.
- For many people, the health system is increasingly a personal benefit or entitlement question, rather than an abstract symbol of Canada, or an interesting public policy debate. Consequently, ideas or institutions which purport to "reform" the health care system are put under more scrutiny by the public, and on balance people are worried that they too often begin with the goal of reducing expenditures, rather than the betterment of health care. To some degree, the language of reform has

become associated with problems, strains, and bad news stories in health care, rather than solutions and good news stories.

In summary, we would recommend that the Forum approach its communications requirements:

- Taking care not to adopt the stance of educators of an ill-informed public, at least about the need to make hard choices.
- Seeking to prove its bona fides as a reform-minded institution by avoiding the deficits versus health care paradigm.
- Ensuring that its message is developed to fit not only worthy minorities, but also the broad, self-defined Canadian middle class. Stress how ideas will work not only to protect the entitlements of those who are least able to fend for themselves, but also those who are presumed to be reasonably comfortable, but who in reality are feeling quite insecure about their futures.

Frank L. Graves *studied sociology and anthropology at Carleton University, Ottawa. In 1980, he founded Ekos Research Associates, an applied social and economic research firm. Mr. Graves is one of Canada's leading public opinion and social policy experts. He has examined public attitudes in key policy areas such as employment and labour markets, national identity and unity, health care and governance. His groundbreaking research on the evolving relationship between Canadians and government,* Rethinking Government, *has for the last three years yielded a number of fresh insights into the way Canadians view their governments and each other.*

APPENDICES

APPENDIX 1

SCENARIOS

Scenario 1: Alternative Treatments and Medicines

Although she tried to hide it, Charlie could see that his mother was in pain. The physiotherapy wasn't doing her any good. It had been almost a year since her back began troubling her, and nothing they had tried so far had helped. It was getting worse.

Mrs. Wong had come to live with her son Charlie and his family two years ago, after her husband died. It had been difficult for her to adjust to the way of life in their small, northern city. She missed Chinatown and her friends there, and all the comforts it provided her, especially since she had become sick.

When the first symptoms of her back problem appeared, Charlie's mother knew what it was at once. "I had this problem 10 years ago," she had told him. "I went to the Chinese healer and right away he could tell what was wrong. After four weeks of acupuncture, the pain was gone. But he told me it would probably come back again, and now it has."

There was no Chinese healer in the city in which Charlie lived, but there was a naturopath who practiced acupuncture. He had a good reputation, but his treatments were not covered under the province's health insurance plan. Treatments didn't cost much—four weeks of treatment might cost about $500—but Charlie and his family didn't have that kind of money. They were having difficulty making ends meet as it was.

It was because of lack of money that Charlie had persuaded his mother to see his doctor almost a year ago, and after that another doctor, and then a physiotherapist.

It had gone on too long. Looking at his mother, he decided that in the morning, he would take his mother to the naturopath. And if the naturopath thought acupuncture would help, he would go to the bank and borrow the money.

It doesn't make any sense, he thought to himself. If my mother was in Chinatown, 600 miles away in the same province, the acupuncture treatments would be paid for because the Chinese healer belongs to a publicly funded clinic. Here in my city, the public system will pay much money for treatments that do not help her, but it will not pay for the treatment that probably will.

Scenario 2: Emphasizing Prevention or Acute Care?

After waiting three weeks for an appointment, Mr. S., a 55-year-old independent truck driver, met with a heart specialist, who advised him he needed coronary bypass surgery. Unfortunately, it would take up to 10 weeks before he could have the surgery. Mr. S. was told that his angina was stable and not immediately life threatening, but serious all the same. For his safety, and the safety of others, the specialist said he should not return to work, and that she would review his fitness to work following the surgery.

Mr. S. complained that being laid up would bring him financial ruin, and that it would be maddening to live under the shadow of the operation for that long. The doctor listened carefully and sympathetically, but responded that there was nothing she could do.

Dejected by this news, Mr. S. pulled some strings with an old friend and got a meeting with a specialist in another major city. That specialist said he could get him in for surgery in about two weeks.

Mr. S. was pleased about this, but curious about the reason for the difference in waiting lists between the two cities. He investigated, and discovered that five years earlier the regional board for the city in which he lives decided to spend more money on prevention, and consequently to spend less on acute care. The regional board in the other city, however, considered and rejected this option, and decided instead to ensure that programs like the coronary bypass program were well funded.

According to a recent newspaper article, the prevention program has been very successful. The incidence of heart disease in Mr. S.'s region has decreased by 5 percent, and is a full 10 percent lower than in the region to which he travelled for the bypass. "Maybe the board in my region made the right decision," he remarked to his wife, "but I'm sure glad I won't have to suffer its negative consequences."

Scenario 3: Shifting Resources from Health Care to Long-Term Prevention

Walking home from the community meeting, Mariella and Pablo continued the discussion about health care funding that had begun there.

Mariella: I can't believe you supported the cuts to health care.

Pablo: It's not that I don't think health care is important. But I think we could get better value for our money—more health for our money—by spending this money on other things. That money would do a lot more good if we spent it on job creation and cleaning up the environment.

Mariella: I think it's much more important to look after the people who are sick right now than to improve the health of the general population. And besides, I doubt that the money saved would be spent on making a difference in health. Our health care system is one of the things that makes this country so special, Pablo, and I'm very worried about the impact of these cuts.

Pablo: You heard what the experts at the meeting said. There's lots of waste and inefficiency. If we get rid of that, there's plenty of money to fund the system.

Mariella: I'm not so trusting. Maybe there is lots of inefficiency, but do you really believe that quality won't suffer? These cuts will make it very difficult for the provinces to ensure that all Canadians have equal access to high-quality, medically necessary care.

Pablo: That term "medically necessary" is so broad it can mean anything. The health care system has expanded beyond its original intent, and beyond what we can afford. Sure, we have to see that no Canadians will lose their houses or burden themselves with debt in order to meet their medical needs, but maybe the government just can't afford to meet all the lesser needs and wants.

Mariella: Well, who's going to decide what we can and cannot afford, and which and whose needs are greatest? People like the ones at the meeting who supported the cuts? Most of those people were very well dressed and pretty healthy looking. Not very typical of the people I work with every day in the chronic care unit. And not very typical of the people in the neighbourhood where you and I grew up Pablo. Those are the people I care most about.

Pablo: We agree then Mariella, because it's these people I care most about too. I want them to have jobs, and I want their children to have good schools and safe streets. Those things don't come from doctors and hospitals.

Scenario 4: Prevention vs. Treatment

Jimmy was terribly sick, but Nurse J. could tell from the faint smile he formed as she entered the room that he was very happy to see her familiar face. Young Jimmy Brown, nine years old, was no stranger to her care. This was his third visit to the emergency department since the fall. She clutched his hand and said, "Everything will be all right now, Jimmy. We'll look after you."

Jimmy Brown has chronic asthma, and his condition had deteriorated since his last visit. This time Nurse J. was very worried from the signs she saw. They would look after him and give him the best care possible, and probably he would get better. But everything wouldn't be all right. In a week or so, if everything went well, he would go home, but that wouldn't make everything all right. Far from it. That was where the cycle would begin again.

Since his father had abandoned him and his mother two years ago, Jimmy had lived in a dilapidated old house on the outskirts of town. And in that house—a shack others might call it—was a wood stove that served as the only source of heat. Jimmy's mother knew that the fumes from the smoke aggravated his asthma, but there was nothing she could do. She didn't have the money to buy a furnace or to move into a better place. And the welfare system wouldn't cover it. Nurse J. and the social worker had tried their best to intervene on the Browns' behalf, but to no avail.

Nurse J. felt frustrated and angry. The system could not or would not do anything to remedy the problem that was causing Jimmy's sickness, but whenever he got really sick the system would go into high gear and spend many times more money than the cost of a furnace to fix him up. And the cycle would begin again.

It didn't make sense: not for Jimmy, not for his mother, and not for society. They wouldn't look after him, not really. It wouldn't be all right. It was only February, and there were cold months ahead.

Scenario 5: Meeting the Needs of the Dying Compared to Delivering Acute Care

The newly formed Springdale Regional Board is responsible for health services, including hospitals and chronic care facilities, for a community of 300,000 people.

Each year, the Board receives a fixed sum of money from the province, which it must divide among health institutions, agencies, and services in its region. Money is tight, and the Board has learned that it must make do with 10 percent less money than it got last year. It has ordered an extensive review of all services to assist in setting priorities.

The study disclosed that many health needs were not being adequately met by existing services. The needs of people who were dying were identified as an area of special concern especially in light of the region's mission to ensure that people who choose to do so will be able to have a good death in the personal environment of their homes rather than in institutions. The study found that, overall, very little money was spent on palliative care compared to other health services and to acute care in particular. The report concluded, "We spend a tremendous amount of money trying to save lives even in cases where the chances of success are very slight. Money is no object here, it seems. But once it is decided that further aggressive treatment is futile or undesirable, we turn our backs on the dying and spend very little money to ensure that they have as good a death as possible."

Board members agreed that the needs of the dying were not being adequately met, and also agreed about ways to improve the situation. However, these strategies would require additional money, and, given the cuts to their budget, there wasn't even sufficient money to fund existing programs. "The bottom line is that we cannot go on leaving these needs unmet," one member said. "We have to find the money to do this, and regrettably this will mean shifting it from other services. A good part of our budget goes to acute care, and I see little choice but to reallocate some money from acute care to palliative care. Given the other demands on our resources, maybe we can't afford that heart-lung transplant program at the main hospital. Very few people benefit from it, and the money could accomplish a lot more good if we spent it on the dying."

Scenario 6: Guidelines to Encourage the Use of Less-Expensive Drugs

"It's hard to say at this time how serious the heart attack was," the younger doctor said. "I think she'll be fine with the streptokinase."

"Let's hope so," the older doctor replied. "I'm not happy with the new guideline. If this happened a week ago, we would have used TPA, and I would have felt better about that."

The doctors must not have realized that the woman in the elevator with them was Mary S., the daughter of the 62-year-old woman they were talking about. Mary had eavesdropped intently on their conversation, but hesitated to identify herself and ask the questions that were burning in her mind. She had decided instead to return to the floor and ask the nurse. The answers she received troubled her.

The nurse explained that there are currently two drugs available for treating heart attacks: streptokinase and r-TPA (tissue plasminogen activating factor). R-TPA is slightly more effective in severe heart attacks. Some research shows that it saves about one additional life for every 100 uses. However, the cost difference between the two drugs is great. Whereas streptokinase costs $460 per dose, r-TPA costs $2,500 per dose, more than five times as much.

The costs of a policy of using r-TPA in every case would be enormous, the nurse explained. Given budget constraints, the hospital pharmacy had recently examined its policy in this area, and debated whether the benefit, in terms of the number of lives saved, was worth the cost. This money, it was claimed, could be used to better effect in the hospital. Some people thought the hospital pharmacy shouldn't carry the more expensive drug at all. A compromise was reached that the hospital would carry it, but that doctors would only use it when they thought the heart attack was very severe. That was probably the guideline Mary heard the doctors talking about, the nurse figured.

Mary went back into her mother's room. She was sleeping now, and her vital signs were looking good. She was a strong woman, Mary thought. She'll be home and back out in her beloved garden in no time at all. Still, it troubled her to think that her mother might not have received the best treatment possible.

Scenario 7: Increasing the Level of Responsibility That Families Have for Taking Care of Their Own

There was a profound sadness in the cafeteria. After months of rumours, it was final now. The hospital would be closing.

"They say this community doesn't need two hospitals," Nurse L. remarked. "We're bursting at the seams with more people than we can look after, but the hospital isn't needed? Obviously we're meeting somebody's needs. How will those needs be met when we close? I don't get it."

"Oh, I get it all right," Nurse S. said. "That's where community-based care comes in. These needs will be met in the community, closer to home. You know, self-help and all that—families taking more responsibility to look after their own. That's the story the public is expected to buy, hook, line, and sinker."

"I think you're being a little too cynical," Nurse J. broke in. "Community-based care makes a lot of sense. You know as well as I do that many of the people we care for could just as well be cared for in the community or in their homes."

"Oh, I agree that a lot of them *could* be." Nurse S. replied, "if there were a community support system, or a family able to look after them. But the reality is that in too many cases there just isn't. And until there is, it's not right to dump sick people into the community."

"I agree," Nurse L. joined in. "And it's not just the patients I'm concerned about, it's their families—the mothers, sisters, and daughters who will bear the burden of caring for their needs. Undoubtedly this hospital isn't the best place for elderly people like Mr. J. in room 312. Nothing we can do will cure old age. But there's nowhere else for him to go except home, and then the burden of care will fall on Mrs. J. At her age it would be too much for her. Next thing you know, she'd be the one in the hospital. Community-based care—I'm all for it… if the community supports are in place. They say they're going to transfer some of the money saved from closing the hospital to the community and build up the support system. Why don't they do that first?"

"I'll tell you why," Nurse S. volunteered. "Because they have no intention of building up the support system, that's why. We've seen all of this before. Saving money is the name of the game here, and community-based care is just a smoke-screen."

Scenario 8: Principles of the Health Care System

Joe was a feeling a little nervous. As a respected leader in his community, he had been asked by the Regional Health Board to hold a meeting with his people to gauge their values about priorities for health spending in the region. He examined the list of values they had prepared for him to go over at the meeting:

i)   *Efficiency* – The health system should be as efficient as possible. Services and programs should be effective, used appropriately, and delivered at the least cost possible.

ii)   *Comprehensiveness* – The range of services should include all treatments and services that meet health needs.

iii)   *Quality of care* – The quality of care available to all Canadians should be as good as, or better than, what is available in other countries.

iv)   *Patient autonomy* – Patients should have maximum choice in deciding what services and treatments are available to them, and under what terms they will receive them.

v)   *Equal access for individuals* – Every Canadian should have equal access to health care. Ability to pay should not be a barrier.

vi)   *Equal shares for groups* – Resources should be distributed such that different communities and population groups get equal shares.

vii)   *Neediest first* – Resources should be distributed on the basis of need: the needs of the neediest should be met before or ahead of the needs of the less needy; resources should be distributed to individuals and populations in proportion to their need for them.

viii)   *Maximum benefit for dollar* – We should strive to get the most "bang for buck," or benefit for health care dollar.

ix)   *A healthy population* – We should strive to make as great a positive impact on the health and well-being of the Canadian population as possible.

Important issues were at stake. The budget for the Health Board has been cut back, and there were some difficult choices to be made. His community would be affected. He thought it was important that these choices be based on values instead of politics, and that the Board was wise to try to gauge the values of the communities it represented. Even so, values are hard to capture, and Joe wondered how well the values on the list captured the values of people in his community and whether the meeting would succeed in bringing their values to the surface.

APPENDIX 2

MODERATOR'S GUIDE

I   Introduction and Warm-Up   5 minutes

II   Preliminary Questions and Discussion   15 minutes

1. As you know, we will be talking about health and our health care system tonight. First off, I would like to know what you include in your understanding of "health care system."

   What are some of the main things that are part of "health" or the "health care system"?

2. We can all relate to the health care system based on our personal experience. Think about your own experiences and perhaps those of the people who are closest to you. I would like you to characterize/describe the health care system in one sentence or two.

   [participants should be encouraged to jot down their response on a piece of paper to avoid yea-saying]

3. Describe the three best and the three worst things about the health care system.

   [participants should be encouraged to jot down their response on a piece of paper to avoid yea-saying]

III   Scenario Discussion   1 hour, 40 minutes

Scenario (as designed by the Forum) will be presented for discussion by participants. The moderator will provide a written copy of the scenario and play an audiotape version as well. The moderator will ensure that at least two scenarios are discussed in each group. More will be added if time permits.

Discussion pieces for each of the eight selected scenarios will be as follows:

Scenario 1: Alternative Treatments and Medicines

1. Do you think the health care system should pay for acupuncture for Charlie's mother?

2. On what grounds do you think the system should decide which health services will be publicly funded? Evidence of effectiveness? Consumer demand for them? Medical opinion?

3. Western medicine is but one of many different healing methods developed over the years by different cultures. In a multicultural society, should we be more willing to embrace multicultural health care?

4. State whether, and why, you agree or disagree with the following statement: "The decision whether to fund a given health service should be based on evidence

of effectiveness. If traditional cures and therapies from other cultures meet these standards, they should be funded. If not, they should not be."

5. Does fairness mean that different population groups, and in particular ethnic groups, have a right to an approximately equal share of money spent on them for health care?

Scenario 2: Emphasizing Prevention or Acute Care?

1. Given the information above, which board do you think made the right decision, and why?

2. Is it consistent with equal access that there should be such great variation in waiting lists between different regions in the same province?

3. How would you rank the various criteria listed below for priorizing people in a waiting list for a medical service? Are there any that you feel should definitely not be used and why?

    a. medical urgency

    b. benefit to the individual

    c. benefit to society

    d. age

    e. lifestyle factors

    f. first come, first served

4. Supposing there were a private clinic where Mr. S. could get quicker treatment,

    a. Is private clinics delivering more timely health services to those able to pay for them inconsistent with the principle of equal access?

    b. In deciding whether private clinics are a good or a bad thing, how much difference does it make whether they are in part subsidized by the government?

    c. Is it unfair if people with money can get more timely or higher-quality health care than people who have to rely on the public system?

5. How would you feel about the inequality that would exist in a two-tiered system in which the public system funded only the most basic and essential services and a second, private system, delivered more "Cadillac" services to those with the ability to pay?

6. How important do you think it is for people to have the freedom to purchase health care privately if they can afford to and believe that the additional benefit is worth the cost?

7. If everyone's basic needs were met in the public system, but some people could get more timely treatment by paying for it privately, would this be a serious inequality? Would you be prepared to accept this inequality in order to allow those with means the freedom to spend their money as they wished?

8. How is health care different from other services in our society that are bought and sold in the marketplace? What, if anything, is so special about health care?

9. We tolerate many inequalities in Canadian society. Some people have big houses, other live in the street. Some people drive fancy cars, while others cannot afford to buy a car at all. Is inequality in health care different than in other areas of life? If so, why?

Scenario 3: Shifting Resources from Health Care to Long-Term Prevention

1. Which of the two speakers do you most sympathize with, and why?

2. Mariella is concerned about the consequences of funding cuts for poor and needy people. How important is the government's obligation to help these people? Is there anything else more important?

3. State whether, and why, you agree or disagree with the following statement: "We can't afford to pay for everything the public wants; we have to concentrate on what the public really needs."

4. In deciding the level of public funding for health care, how much weight should be given to what patients or consumers would like as opposed to what experts think they need?

5. Do you believe that all Canadians have a right to health care, and if so, how would you qualify this right? A right to basic services? A right to quality services? A right to the best health services possible?

6. Mariella thinks our health care system has special importance for us as Canadians. Do you agree? What significance or value does our health care system have for you as a Canadian citizen? Is there anything else about this country that you think is more important?

7. Some people claim our health care system is vitally important to our national identity. Do you agree? What is it about our health care system that makes you most proud as a Canadian?
   a. its high level of quality
   b. its efficiency
   c. its success in meeting the needs of the sick and vulnerable
   d. its equality

Scenario 4: Prevention vs. Treatment

1. Would it be appropriate to redirect money from sickness care to prevention if the money spent on prevention would produce more benefit, and perhaps even save money in the long run?

2. Do you think it is more important to ensure that people who are sick and disabled are able to achieve the best level of health possible or to ensure that people who are healthy do not become sick and disabled?

3. If the same amount of money could be used either to save the lives of 10 heart attack victims over a five-year period, or through preventive measures to reduce the number of people who would suffer heart attacks over the same time period and thereby save 100 lives, which would you choose? Why?

4. In some cases, the costs of treating someone who is sick and in need are enormous, and the anticipated benefit is uncertain and slight at best. In other cases, however, tremendous benefits can be had for very little cost. If you had to choose between producing very slight benefit for one very sick person, and a greater benefit for 10 people who were less sick, which would you choose, and why?

Scenario 5: Meeting the Needs of the Dying Compared to Delivering Acute Care

1. How important do you think it is to ensure that the needs of the dying are met as fully as possible compared to trying to save lives when chances of success are very poor?

2. Interventions to save lives are often very expensive. Do you think we put too much emphasis on saving lives at any cost at the expense of not meeting other important needs?

3. If we cannot afford to meet all health care needs, on what grounds should we decide which needs will receive greater priority?

4. Is the amount of benefit produced per cost an appropriate criterion for deciding which, whether, and at what level health services should be funded? What alternative criteria would you suggest, and how would you compare their importance?

5. If two services are compared in terms of how much benefit each produces in terms of cost, and both cannot be funded, should we fund the one with greater benefits per cost?

6. In deciding where to allocate health care resources, how important is it to you that the benefits are distributed fairly among various populations? How important is this consideration compared to ensuring that the greatest amount of benefit possible is produced, regardless of who gets what and how much of it?

7. How does information about how much money per person is spent on people in different groups bear, if at all, on fairness?

8. If you had to choose between funding a service that delivered three healthy meals a week to shut-ins and needy seniors, and a school lunch program that provided lunches for needy children, which would you choose? Why?

9. What does fairness mean to you, and how important do you think it is for health care resources to be distributed fairly? How do you see the relationship between fairness and equality?

Scenario 6: Guidelines to Encourage the Use of Less-Expensive Drugs

1. Suppose the money saved from this guideline could be used to achieve greater benefit (save more lives) in the hospital by being allocated in other ways. Do you think it is acceptable to use the cheaper but slightly less effective drug? Why?

2. Suppose that the money saved by using the cheaper drug was enough to fund a nurse to offer low-income families prenatal care in their homes, and that more lives could be saved by such a program than by always using the more expensive drug. If you had to choose between these options, which would you choose, and why?

3. If the more expensive treatment slightly increased patient comfort, but would have no long-term impact on the patient's health, do you think it should be offered, even though the benefit for this additional cost would be relatively small compared to other uses to which the money could be put?

4. All of us want the best care possible for ourselves and our loved ones. We also want to ensure that there is enough to go around, and that everybody gets a fair share. Do you think these two wants are ever in conflict? If so, how would you resolve the conflict?

5. Should we always do what is best for the individual patient, regardless of costs, or should we try to ensure that scarce health care dollars are used to produce as much benefit as possible?

6. Do you feel that the doctors have compromised their professional ethic by using the arguably second-best treatment?

7. If a physician is aware of a treatment that would be more beneficial for you than any he is able to offer, is he obliged to disclose this information to you?

8. Should physicians ever be put in a position where they are required to do anything less than what they believe is in the best interests of their patients?

Scenario 7: Increasing the Level of Responsibility That Families Have for Taking Care of Their Own

1. Do you think it is fair to expect families to assume increased responsibility for caring for their own? Is it fair to rely on such an expectation in making allocation decisions?

2. In some cultures there is a greater expectation that families will look after their own than in others. Is such an expectation something that we should try to foster more widely in our society?

3. When the burden of caring for someone is transferred from an institution to a family, should some part of the money thus saved be transferred to the family to assist them?

4. If costs can be saved by relying less on professional caregivers and more on family members and informal care groups, is it justifiable to pass this burden onto them? On what grounds?

5. Should charities and volunteers be expected to assume more of the burden of care currently being delivered in institutions or by the publicly funded health care system?

Scenario 8: Principles of the Health Care System

1. How would you rank the principles listed above, and why? Are there any values you think should be added to the list?

2. What conflicts do you see as potentially developing among or between these values, and how would you resolve them?

3. Do you think most Canadians share the same values about health care and health care funding, or do you think there is a lot of variation based on things like cultural and religious differences? If different cultures do have different value priorities, how important do you think it is for the health system to reflect those differences?

4. Should people from different cultures be able to decide how and by what means their health needs will be met, or should health care services be the same for everyone?

APPENDIX 3

DELIBERATIVE INFORMATION

Figure A

Comparative levels of satisfaction with health system*

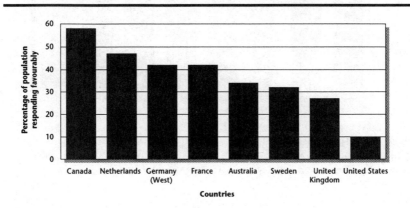

Source: *Satisfaction with Health Systems in 10 Nations,* Blendon et al. 1990.

* On the survey, the question was worded as follows: "On the whole, the health care system works pretty well, and only minor changes are necessary to make it work better."

Figure B

Total health expenditure as a percentage of total domestic expenditure

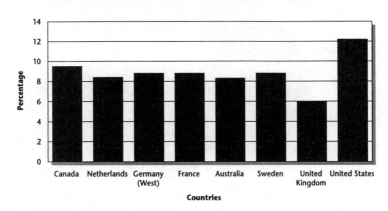

Source: OECD Health Systems, 1993.

Figure C

Cost satisfaction index*

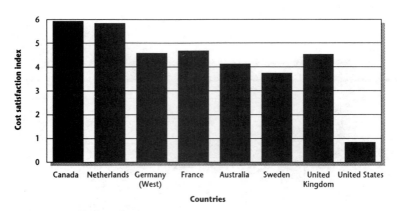

Source: OECD Health Data. 1993.

* Cost satisfaction index is the percentage of population indicating satisfaction with their health system (figure A) divided by the percentage of total domestic expenditure it takes up (figure B).

Figure D

Government spending

Governments spent $355 billion in 1993–1994
(approximately $12,340 for every man, woman, and child in Canada)

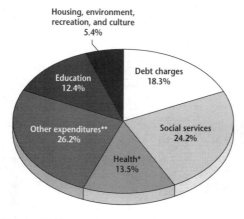

Source: Statistics Canada. 1995.

* Health includes health services and administration, research, public health, etc.

** Other expenditures include protection of persons and property, transportation and communications, resource conservation, etc.

Figure E

How money was spent on health care in 1975 and 1993

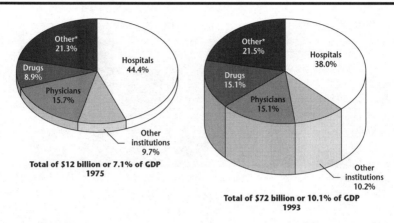

Source: Health Canada. 1994.

* Other includes other health professionals, capital expenditures, health research, and public health.

Figure F

Money spent on health relative to the economy

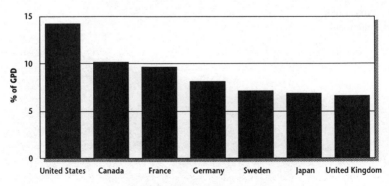

Health expenditures as % of GDP, 1993

Source: OECD Health Data. 1993.

Figure G

Average length of life, various countries

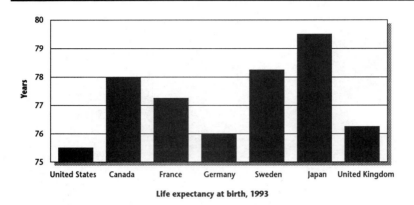

Life expectancy at birth, 1993

Source: OECD Health Data. 1993.

Figure H

Where health care funding comes from

% distribution of health expenditures by sector of finance 1993

- In 1993, public health expenditures (by all levels of government) represented 71.9% of total health expenditures in Canada.
- Private health expenditures accounted for 28.1%.

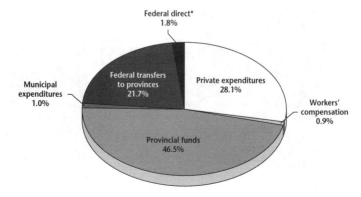

Source: Health Canada. 1994.

* Federal direct includes health services for Aboriginal peoples, veterans, armed services personnel, research, etc.

APPENDIX 4

SURVEY QUESTIONNAIRE

Quantitative Component for Research on Canadian Values in Relation to Health

1. **Listed below are a number of statements.** Please rate the degree to which you agree or disagree with each statement using a 7-point scale where 1 means you strongly disagree, 7 means you strongly agree, and the midpoint 4 means you neither agree nor disagree.

	STRONGLY DISAGREE		NEITHER			STRONGLY AGREE	
a. *I think that the health care system is more about values than economics*	1	2	3	4	5	6	7
b. *I have more confidence today that the health care system will take care of me than I did five years ago*	1	2	3	4	5	6	7
c. *Individuals should be allowed to pay to get quicker access to health care services*	1	2	3	4	5	6	7

2. **There are a number of values or ultimate goals that can define our health care system.** Please rate how important each of the following values should be in shaping the health care system, using a 7-point scale where 1 means not at all important, 7 means extremely important, and the midpoint means moderately important.

	NOT AT ALL IMPORTANT		MODERATELY IMPORTANT			EXTREMELY IMPORTANT	
a. *Equality of access*	1	2	3	4	5	6	7
b. *Freedom of choice*	1	2	3	4	5	6	7
c. *Efficiency*	1	2	3	4	5	6	7
d. *Flexibility*	1	2	3	4	5	6	7
e. *Performance/results*	1	2	3	4	5	6	7
f. *Compassion*	1	2	3	4	5	6	7
g. *Prevention*	1	2	3	4	5	6	7

3. Which one of the following aspects of health care is of greatest importance to
    you? [Please make only one selection.]

    Quality of health care service   1

    Costs of health care system to country   2

    Health of the Canadian population   3

    Equal access to health care for all Canadians   4

4. Now we have a few final questions for statistical purposes only. In what year
    were you born?

    $\underline{|\ 1\ |\ 9\ |\ \ \ |\ \ \ |}$

5. What is the highest level of schooling that you have completed?

    Public/elementary school or less (grade 8)   1

    Some high school   2

    Graduated from high school (grade 12/13)   3

    Vocational/technical college or CEGEP   4

    Trade certification   5

    Some university   6

    Bachelor's degree   7

    Professional certification   8

    Graduate degree   9

6. Are you...?

    Male   1

    Female   2

APPENDIX 5

VERBATIM COMMENTS

- A universal first-class distribution of health care. Perceived to be envied by the world.
- Good system, going broke slowly.
- Canada's health care system is a decentralized (provinces) good system accessible to every citizen.
- Canada's health care provides care for all citizens. The care is probably the best in the world.
- Allows all citizens to have access to medical facilities and doctors regardless of cost and regardless of who the citizen is.
- In my opinion, Canada's health care system is one of our greatest assets. This doesn't mean, however, that it is without flaws. I think the idea of health care is very important but it may need to be reworked or improved.
- Canadian health care is available to anyone who needs or wants it at no personal cost whatsoever. It's one of the best plans worldwide.
- Available to everyone who lives in Canada (some form).
- Canada's health care system is a government-run program that attempts to provide free/inexpensive medical services to the general population. With regard to services, they include both reactive and proactive aspects of medicine, with the emphasis on reaction.
- Canada's health care system guarantees free access to medical care, professionals, and facilities to all Canadians.
- The Canadian health care system is a well-structured system that sees that all people are eligible to receive care.
- I would describe the health care system as a universal system providing equal access to everyone.
- The health system is not cost effective or health effective. It is overstrained, understaffed, and the myth of its availability is undone by its ineffectiveness.
- Comprehensive, high-quality socialized health care system.
- It's about having freedom as a Canadian. Not having to worry about cost and liability. A definite plus for Canadians.
- Health care system is universally accessible and generally effective—but it is overbuilt, costs are hidden, and too much focus on large, high-tech institutions with high overheads.
- The Canadian health care system is, in my opinion, simply the best of its kind in the world

- Is one of the best systems Canada has.

- Accessible to all, rich or poor, and equal to all as not based on a fee structure but a monthly "OHIP" premium.

- The Canadian health care system is—or should be—fair, open, and accessible to all. It is also affordable for all.

- In a state of flux between universality and an unknown destination. At its best it is the single greatest most beneficial difference between us and our southern neighbours.

- Deteriorating—government involvement gets more specialized with specialists such as doctors being elected who soon lose their focus on care and focus on cost. There is a dichotomy between cost and service; they are not mutually exclusive.

- There used to be everything—now everything is being cut, sometimes I understand from the media and friends, to the detriment of patients. I am concerned with the care of the elderly, in particular.

- System is going in a backward direction falsely thinking it is going forward. Patients are being neglected and sent home too early, being told home care is better.

- Well I think too many nurses are being laid off. Not enough of one on one or one on two. Not enough coverage for welfare system.

- Universal and thorough. A bit slow but very comprehensive or inclusive.

- Canadian health care system is a public system which is primarily undergoing some major changes.

- I think we have one of the best health care systems in the world. If you have a problem you can go directly to your doctor or a hospital without worrying if you have insurance or not because they will look after you.

- One of the best in the world—envy of many nations. About to suffer significantly from fiscal restraint.

- Fairly good, no real national direction, facing problems with funding cuts and bleak economic forecasts.

- Universally available to everyone but becoming overextended, needs to be better controlled.

- Universal health care system that for the most part provides for everyone equally, but has become too expensive to continue in its present form.

- As I see health care in Canada today: Health care for everyone in Canada at reasonable cost and available in all remote regions—having the use of top-notch doctors, nurses, and hospitals.

- A federal government system for universal health care. I think it is coordinated with the various provincial governments.

- The clinic facilities are a major asset, medicine availability. The doctors at the clinic very helpful. The operational hours are also excellent. No need for an appointment is good.

- The need of medical services when you are working at minimal wage—your medical expenses could be astronomical with no assistance if you do not have a medical plan with the company you are employed by.
- Health care in Canada today is generous—all-comprehensive, adequate. Reasonable in cost for what you get.
- I think that the health care in Canada is superior to most places in the world, but could be improved on.
- I think the standard of our health care is going downhill due to lack of staff and rooms in hospitals.
- The health care system is in a crisis. In need of a shake-up to make sure we are getting the best system for the money. But I do think despite the problems we do have a good system.
- A comprehensive government plan to cover all major medical needs of citizens of Canada. Major medical expenses are covered in almost every situation.
- Seems to be going down the drain right now—has been good for many years— till they started all the cutbacks.
- In general the health care system is good.
- Social welfare system with standards set by the federal government.
- The health care system is ideally a system whereby people have access to medical services regardless of economic status.
- The health care system in my opinion is a very good system compared to other parts of the world.
- Canadian health care is an inexpensive medical program that is available to most Canadians. We have excellent facilities and very good medical coverage.
- In Canada we are fortunate to have universal health care, provided equally to all. This system contributes to the fact we have one of the highest rates of taxation in the world.
- A not so efficient means to allow most citizens access to medical attention in the form of doctors, hospitals, etc. It's a good system in that we (Canadians) do not need to worry too much about how to pay for health care, which can be expensive.
- Health care in Canada is for everybody.
- I think we are fortunate to have our health care system. Don't have to worry about large costs if something happens to you.
- Our health care system is adequate as I know it. My care in hospital is excellent. We have ready access to specialists.
- The health care system has deteriorated dramatically.
- The quality of health care in Alberta has been declining steadily under Ralph Klein's rule. Each month we are progressing towards a two-tier system in which those that can pay have access to private services, quicker.

- Our health care system is set up to accommodate the needs of the sick and healthy. It used to cost us very little; now because of years of abuse from patients, doctors, and governments, it is in a state of change.
- Health care very essential for the society.
- Health care in Alberta is being developed to a high degree of effectiveness; however, it is in a state of transition. Cuts are not effective.
- In the past, we have had the best health care system. With a great change in technology (transplants, etc.) we live too long, help many hopeless cases, etc. We can no longer provide the same care. At this time, we are basically out of control.
- A health care system that is available to all and provides a very respectable level of care.
- The health care system (in Alberta) is generally very good with the exception of the present state of economics. People within the system are requiring more funding while taxpayers are saying enough is enough.
- Our health care system is set up to accommodate all Albertans regardless of financial standing.
- Health care in Alberta, while having high standards, is declining and appears to be becoming obscure.
- The Alberta health care system is undergoing an Americanization. That is, it is going to hell in a handbasket.
- A good system that is undergoing some radical but perhaps too quick changes. It is an efficient and fair way to deliver health services.
- Our health care is lacking confidence in the abilities to keep the general population healthy.
- Saskatchewan is unique in its health care for our province in that it states that all people are entitled to health care. It is universal.
- Saskatchewan has historically been the backbone and designer of "Medicare" in the health care area. Open access to all citizens for health.
- The health care in Canada is quite satisfactory. Personal experience I've always received what I needed.
- Not enough First Nations medical staff to meet the needs of First Nations people. Everyone deserves proper medical care.
- Health care in Saskatchewan is an all-round medical care for individuals. Doctor and hospital visits are reasonably accessible, doctors anyways.
- I have been very fortunate to be healthy but do see some deficiencies in the overall system.
- The health care system in Canada is comprised of two parts by acute care or hospital services and community health initiatives. One half cares for the ill, the other is focused on education and prevention of disease/illness.

- There is great difficulty in securing a family physician but, nevertheless, it seems that there is "adequate" health care.

- Health system in Saskatchewan is a federally funded program which helps individuals in need regardless of economic, social, or racial background.

- Health care in Saskatchewan is rapidly deteriorating.

- Health care in Saskatchewan is about people caring for people at a reasonable cost compared to health care in the States.

- Health care is a wellness medical system for individuals.

- Health care in Saskatchewan thus far is covering people's basic needs, no more no less. The cutbacks in health care are affecting the ones who cannot afford to comply with the high cost.

- Health care in Saskatchewan is a universal system of medical treatment that covers the residents of the province from cradle to grave. It is a key element of the social fabric of our prairie lifestyle.

- Health care in Saskatchewan is government operated. It is universally available.

- An excellent system that is being handicapped by government cutbacks, and restraint.

- Health care in Saskatchewan is a rapidly declining system where care in the past has not been based on age, financial status, etc. More and more we are digressing to a state where dollars buy care.

- Our health care system is much better than the United States.

Best Three Things about the Health Care System

Universal
Free
No complaints of quality

All people

Accessible to every citizen
Quality

Accessible to everyone
Technically very good
Facilities are adequate

Free access to all doctors
Timely
Treats people with dignity

(Reasonably) nondiscriminatory
Fair—for *everyone* not just those who can afford it

Noncostly to user
Available to anyone
Best anywhere

Easily accessible
High quality of care
Basic care to everyone

Accessible
Prevention oriented
Community clinics

Available to everyone
Choice of doctors and specialty care people

Covers almost everything medical necessary to keep us healthy and well
Universal to everyone
It is covered by our tax dollars. It is something that we would stand up for.

Quality
Access
Commitment

No hospital bills
Easy access to medical help
Free (almost)

Quick and universal access
Professional and skilled help
High success rate

Equality of access
Quality of service
Value for money

Medical care
Hospital system

Fair to all, no preferences
No need to worry if ever sick to have to borrow or mortgage home

No user fees
Few waits for doctors or tests

The ability of anybody, regardless of economic stature, to get help
A level of care that is superior to that of most of the world
Access across the country

Accessibility
Emergency care
Doctors/patients relations

Well-educated and knowledgeable people (doctors, nurses)
Up-to-date equipment for tests
With medical plans + MSI, don't have to pay often for services (tests, doctor's visits, etc.)

Equal access
Paid by taxes
Up-to-date technology

MSI coverage

Universal
No limits

It's available theoretically to all citizens at no cost
Obviously one of the best in the world
Open access

Excellent doctors, nurses, etc.
Excellent facilities
No need for insurance

Accessibility
Professionalism
Compassion

No cost to get care
Fairly good quality care
Seems rather uniform

Available to everyone
No excessive hospital bills (like the U.S.)
Same level (quality) of care everywhere

A system which makes the best of a gigantic task
Everyone has access to basic services based on need, not ability to pay

Universality
Quality
Accessibility

Everybody included
Clinics

Universal—everybody eligible to participate
Free choice of primary physicians

Supportive
Includes: physio, ambulance, drugs
Freedom of choice

Everyone is looked after in the system
The choice of doctors is not limited

Available to all
No need for worry over paying
Universal in whole country
Rich and poor treated alike

Universality
Availability
Cost to the patient

Hospitals are free

In general, it is completely paid for
Good facilities and medical services

It is there when needed
Keeps medical issues more or less in the open

Many doctors
Many health care programs
Advanced technology in health care

Accessible to most people
Low cost
High levels of competence

Universality
One of, if not the highest, standards of health care as it relates to the implementation
of state-of-the-art medical knowledge and practice
Easy and generally immediate access

Not expensive
Easy access (i.e., drop in, lots of doctors' offices, etc.)
Very convenient (but that's not very important)

Easily accessible
Quite efficient

Good medical plan—low cost
Extra services—choice physio./chiro.
Low costs for people not working

Very good specialists
Adequate beds at hospitals
Emergency service is excellent

We have hospitals

Dedication of staff that have not yet been laid off
Modern facilities

Cost
Service
Flexibility

It gives us confidence
It gives us unity
It gives us peace of mind

Accessible
Highly trained

Equal opportunity (i.e., for welfare recipients, poor)
Can still choose physician

Is accessible when needed
Provides some basic level for all
Some services don't require up-front payment

Relatively inexpensive
High quality
Readily accessible

Caters to all
Subsidies available

State-of-the-art technology
Highly skilled professionals

Wonderful training programs
Fantastic facilities

Good modern facilities
Accessible
Competent health care providers

Facilities in larger centres
Emergency care at facilities
Support for senior citizens and disabled

It is accessible by everyone regardless of race or money
The quality of health care has always been good
There are now boards that can be approached that ordinary people can appeal
to. These boards are lay boards.

Universality of care
Historically the highest ratio of beds per population
Now on the direction of preventiveness model

Service now, pay later
OH Reserve (health committee)

No cost for medical services to Treaty Indians, most of whom could not afford
medical care if not provided
Dental services
Eyeglasses paid for

That everyone is taken care of
Medical clinics are fairly accessible

No direct cost to the user
Access at all times
Accessing new equipment free

The dedication of the workers
Caring
Availability

Universality
Comprehensiveness
Government funded
Quality service

Quality of health providers
Quality of institutions
Cheap drugs

Universal
Widely available
Affordable

Equal to all
No extra fees
Government controlled

Health care is available to everyone
Diagnostic tests are accessible

It is not very costly for us
Everyone is allowed care if they have a health care
The waiting period for operations is not that long as far as I know

Worst Three Things about the Health Care System

Too costly for our tax base
Delays are tedious and possibly dangerous
Fraudulent use by nonCanadians is an issue
Research falling behind

Anyone can use it for any little thing
Costs taxpayers major bucks

Patients sent home too soon
Hospitals not doctored from 8:00 a.m. to 12:00 p.m.
Too much life support especially for over 75s and newborns

Not fraud resistant
Impersonal
Not enough attention on prevention
Role of family doctor too little

Allows noncitizens to use health care paid for by Canadians which might dilute
health care for Canadian citizens

Cost
Abused by many people including noncitizens

It's losing money—perhaps waste from within
Waiting lists
Public

Not enough support (i.e., equip./personnel)
Easily defrauded by those not entitled
Not controlled well enough at both ends—patients/doctor

Expensive to operate
Opportunities south of the border drew medical workers trained in Canada
Can be too bureaucratic

Sometimes too much red tape
Too many channels to go through

Too expensive
No caps on doctors salaries
No cutoffs for heart surgery

Costs too much at present
Too much red tape
May be too much to keep up

Ineffective in health results
Ineffectiveness in economic terms
Understaffed

Funding problems
Mismanagement macrolevels
Sustainability/potential for erosion

Can't afford to give free care for everyone
Very expensive
Not organized, not known what the cost

Emphasis on equipment
Hidden costs
Emphasis on large institutions

It may not survive the current political (fiscal) climate

Bureaucratic
Slow at times (waiting list)
Technology more behind U.S.A.

High drug prices
Governments reducing funding
Duplication of services

Drug costs for people with ongoing problems
The breakdown of federal standards and possibly different directions taken by different provinces

Waiting for tests, operations, etc.
Cuts in beds
Cutting down number of nurses

Reform implemented before systems in place
Overlog of patients
Outpatient service a scam

Too many layoffs
Letting elderly people leave hospital after a couple of days when they should stay longer

Slow
Expensive
Noneducational

System was used for political purposes in the past
Not very efficient—too bureaucratic

Expensive in form of taxes
Lengthy wait for surgery if many with same problem

Open for abuse by citizens
Lengthy waits for emergency care
Rising costs for those without medical plans

Trouble keeping excellent people
No national control
Overcrowding

Too expensive
Subject to misuse
Lack of direction and awareness of costs and over capacity

Very political
Abuse

Problems of waiting lists for such things as heart bypass operations
Problems of queue jumping when operations are backlogged
Relatively poor control of costs

Too generous to immigrants
Doesn't include dental

Waiting for surgery
Cutbacks on types of prescriptions

Long waiting lists

Appears admin. costs are growing
Often provincial governments try to modify system

Length of time for waiting for treatment
Could be increased to perhaps eye care, etc.
Should not have to go outside for treatment
Overused by both patients and doctors

Waiting lists for surgery seem too long
Changing medication for no-name brands

Too long waiting list for operations
Different fees for across Canada
Too much waste   .

Essential surgery may have long waiting lists
In B.C. seniors have to pay for coverage

It is in the hands of people who want it to collapse
Too much dependence on drugs
It is breaking down

Government toying to reduce health care benefits
Doctors billing patients for certain
Waste
People abusing the system
Not enough preventive medicine

Due to low population vs. large geographic areas, specialists and specialty resources
generally are distant
Bureaucracy

Not personable
Not a good diagnostic and healing system
A bit slow, waits for important stuff, etc.

Sometimes waiting is too long
In hospital, very little stay after the operation
Employees of hospital should not go on strike: it should be made essential
service

Transplants-wait
Overcrowding, delays
Emergency departments

Not enough doctors go to the small towns of B.C.—more incentive for them
Too much abuse of the emergency department of the hospital
Treating preventable illnesses in excess

Alberta health care doesn't cover very much
Hospitals are quite empty

Two tier
Waiting lists
Government involvement

Abuse (doctors/patients/government)

Uncontrollable
Selfish doctors
Costs too much money

Bloated administration
Overlapping services

Too long waiting for tests (e.g., MRI, etc.), surgeries
Loss of best physicians
System can still be abused by malingerers, lonely persons

Easily abused
Too much administration
Costs too much

Present state of turmoil
Heading toward two-tier system

Long waiting lists to see specialists

Diminished service
Inadequate institutional care
Receding quality control

Our cuts supplying the world (esp. U.S.) with top-quality professionals
Have way too many facilities across the province (former government's
purchasing election!)

Waiting lists
Hospitals are not the best places to get well
Lack of coverage on some services leave some people unprotected

Support for preventative health
Too easily used (overused)
Overbilling on other health care professionals

Saskatchewan's health programs are declining in quality
Health's workforce i.e., nurses, hospital staff, etc. is a shrinking workforce. They
are leaving the province.

Rural areas here lost their clinics and small hospitals which works hardship on
our agrarian population

Economics have driven quality caregivers out of province
Rural/northern have limited access to care
Right-wing drive to begin private care facilities

Overcharging on prescriptions of First Nations people
Poor public relations towards First Nations people especially in emergency rooms
Types of services being offered in dental health

Waiting lists are too long for operations
Indian bands should not care over their own medical concerns

Waiting periods
Lack of hospital accommodation
Shortage of staff at all levels in hospitals

Physicians who are exceptional are not here due to lack of funding

The best doctors leave due to $
Lack of specialists
Long waiting list

Not enough good doctors
Not enough acute care in small communities
Not enough health care dollars

Extensive wait lists
User fees
Understaffed

If a single parent is trying to make ends meet, they struggle with a sick child
It's beginning to be the rich man's luxury
As for aging people, they have enormous costs to face monthly

Waiting lists
No rural doctors
Cutbacks

Government debt threatens quality
Rules are driving good doctors elsewhere
Politicians can effect with poor policies

Waiting list
Funding cutbacks
Doctors leaving

Shortage of beds
Lower calibre of doctors
Lacking good specialists
Waiting lists for elective surgery

As soon as our doctors and nurses graduate a lot of them are lured to work in the U.S.
The people in rural Saskatchewan have a tough time getting to a hospital (long distance)
It is costing our government far too much money (it should be looked at more carefully) as in patented drugs, etc.

The Feasibility of a National Canadian Advisory Committee on Ethics: Points to Consider*

THÉRÈSE LEROUX, B.Sc., Ph.D, L.L.B.
SONIA LE BRIS, L.L.M.
BARTHA MARIA KNOPPERS, Ph.D.
WITH THE COLLABORATION OF
LOUIS-NICOLAS FORTIN AND JULIE MONTREUIL

Centre de recherche en droit public
Université de Montréal

SUMMARY

Extraordinary developments in medical research, medicine, and biotechnology have created the need for legal and other kinds of regulatory interventions. A myriad of policy considerations – ethical, philosophical, social, and legal – emerge from these new developments. The creation of a national consultative body concerned with ethics constitutes an alternative. Canada has not yet established a national ethics structure, despite the research of the Law Reform Commission of Canada, which drew some conclusions in 1990 about the feasibility of indeed the need for, such a body and issued certain recommendations on its form.

As the federal government transfers responsibilities to provincial governments and health care is progressively privatized, account must be taken of the experience of other countries, of the areas of intervention of ethics structures, of their efficacy and their social impact, as well as the functions they can perform. It is also

---

* This text is the translation of "Éléments de réflexion sur l'opportunité d'un comité consultatif national d'éthique canadien."
Information used in this text is complete as of December 1996.

necessary to consider the Canadian situation and to determine whether Canada can accommodate a national ethics structure and, if so, what kind of structure using what mode of operation.

This comparative study of national consultative ethics structures, the experience of other countries, and the various existing models; the survey of the Canadian bioethics landscape through the examination of a range of ethics bodies, their foundation and their organization; and the comparison of international experiences with the Canadian reality, lead to a number of conclusions.

The reflection on the feasibility and usefulness of a national body must take into account the Canadian constitutional context, which is based on the distribution of powers. Although the provinces are granted exclusive jurisdiction over health care services, the federal Parliament could legislate on certain areas of public health, probably including biomedical ethics.

Each model for ethical reflection has advantages and disadvantages. Even if the status quo allows for great flexibility and the expression of a plurality of ideas, we still have a complex, heterogeneous system marked by a lack of coordination and poor distribution of information. The national ethics committee – centralized, permanent, and autonomous – is supposed to ensure continuity and coherence, but has proved to be a disappointing experience in federal countries such as Australia. National ethics boards, with more flexible structures, are created as they are needed and permit a rapid and thorough assessment of the problem being studied, but reflection is fragmented. Finally, the model of the permanent conference of ethics committees recently adopted in Europe is flexible and less likely to raise constitutional problems, but may prove difficult to organize and cumbersome to operate.

There is certainly room to improve on the current situation by setting up a Canadian institute for bioethics information and coordination. Such an institute would be responsible for gathering, managing, and distributing information and would meet an observed need—responding to the fragmentation of and exponential growth in ethical reflection. Whatever form the ethics body takes, the extent of its mandate will have to be considered as well as its link to the empowering authority, its composition, the method of appointing members, and the resources available to it.

TABLE OF CONTENTS

> *The ethical dimension is affirmed anew, and we must increase the debate on these most fundamental subjects that touch on the concept of humanity and society. Beginning with what we, the scientists, say about the laws of nature, it is up to us to do our duty and decide, as a function of a certain concept of life and being human, what to do to continue the debate in philosophical and ethical terms, so that our conscience may progress as much as science progresses.*[1,**]

INTRODUCTION

Within the state, public policy is usually set through "adjustment" among the executive, the legislature, and pressure or other concerned groups. Extraordinary developments in medical research, medicine, and biotechnology have created the need for legal and other kinds of regulatory interventions. Jurists face the demands of researchers and practitioners and are aware of the risks. Often confronted as well with highly specific situations and with public opinion, they vacillate between fear and hope, while decision makers, who have little idea of how to intervene, also try to find their ways through the impasse. A myriad of policy considerations—ethical, philosophical, social, and legal—emerge from these new developments. The alternative of a national consultative body concerned with ethics can be found at the intersection of these considerations: the continuing fragmentation of the state, the necessary appraisal of federal-provincial reality and the severity of the problems associated with bioethics.

Of relatively recent origin, bodies of this type tend to multiply under the same names, but not necessarily for the same reasons, as international ethics committees or, at the local level, as clinical ethics committees or research ethics committees.[2] In all cases, these committees are responding to a protean demand from all disciplines, as well as from the public, to find, by means of discussion, a better understanding for acting and intervening in the "material" or "stuff" of life. Canada has not escaped this questioning and is already involved in various ways[3] without having decided, for the moment, to establish a national ethics institution, despite the research of the Law Reform Commission of Canada, which drew some conclusions in 1990 about the feasibility of (versus the need for) such a body and issued certain recommendations on its form.[4]

Six years after the report of the Law Reform Commission of Canada, as the federal government transfers responsibilities to provincial governments and health care is progressively privatized, the question of founding a national, consultative ethics structure comes to the fore again.[5] It is reflection on this subject that the National Forum on Health has entrusted to us. In

---

** Notes are found before the appendices.

this way, it hopes to be in a position to "recommend to government, means of action that take account of the values of the population and are motivated by solid proof." In this regard, the Forum, aware of the pluralism and the multiformed ethics structures in Canada, wanted (a) to be informed about experience in other countries, their areas of intervention, their efficacy and their social impact, as well as the functions that they perform; (b) to map the predominant Canadian situation; and (c) to know whether Canada can accommodate a national ethics structure and, if so, what kind of structure; using what models?

To respond to these various issues, our study proceeds on three levels. First of all, after demonstrating the internationalization of medical ethics ("Preliminary"), we provide a comparative study of national consultative ethics structures, established with the benefit of other countries' experience, allowing us to identify the various existing models (part 1). Then, in order to better survey the Canadian bioethics landscape, we address the range of Canadian ethics bodies and present their bases and their organization (part 2). Finally, in light of the lessons learned from international experiences in the face of the Canadian reality, we present conclusions on possible alternatives for the establishment of a Canadian consultative ethics body (part 3).

PRELIMINARY: INTERNATIONAL AND SUPRANATIONAL INITIATIVES

> Everyone has the right to enjoy the fruits of scientific progress and its applications. Noting how certain advances, especially in the biomedical and life sciences as well as in information technology, can have terrible consequences for the integrity and dignity of the individual, and for the exercise of individual rights, the World Conference on Human Rights appeals to the nations to cooperate to ensure that personal rights and dignity are broadly respected in this area, in the universal interest.[6]

As attested by this declaration of the World Conference on Human Rights, the link between ethics and human rights needs to be stronger, and to be officially imposed on ethics at the international level. This seems logical since the ethics of life sciences and health frequently concern fundamental, wide-ranging questions that arise with similar intensity not only across the developed nations, but also in developing nations.

That there is no such thing as an international organization specifically devoted to bioethics does not indicate a lack of interest on the part of the great international health and social development organizations and agencies. Far from it—in a United Nations initiative, various international organizations and agencies are launching committees to examine general and specific ethics issues. This is the case, for example, with the ethics committee of the Human Genome Organization (HUGO),[7] which works to promote and foster understanding of the social, legal, and ethical issues linked to the HUGO project. It is also the case with the International Ethics Committee on AIDS.[8] At the same time, international organizations such as the World Medical Association (WMA),[9] the World Health Organization (WHO),[10] and the Council for International Organizations of Medical Sciences (CIOMS)[11] have provided principles and issued rules of conduct in their respective areas.[12]

The complete inventory of international activities is of little relevance to the question of whether Canada should establish a national consultative ethics body. On the other hand, a quick overview of three international organizations that are innovative in both form and spirit seems appropriate. It would show that the political, economic, and cultural context of each country does not necessarily preclude the establishment of a forum for thought and discussion as long as the structure is flexible, the political willingness to sit down together is real, and discussion is conducted harmoniously. The first of these examples—UNESCO's International Bioethics Committee (IBC)—is genuinely international. The other two are regional: the European Commission's group of experts on biotechnology, and the permanent committee on bioethics of the Council of Europe, which gave rise to the Permanent Conference of European Ethics Committees.[13]

Section 1 – UNESCO's International Bioethics Committee

Bioethics is not new to UNESCO—the organization's involvement in the area began in 1970.[14] Several things explain this involvement. First, UNESCO's experience allows the organization to ensure that a cross-cultural debate takes place in consultation with other international and regional organizations.[15] In addition, according to certain authors,

> ... in a field in which basic knowledge about human beings raises ethical, social, cultural and legal questions, UNESCO has a duty to bring the developing countries into this debate and to prevent flagrant inequities from forming between the countries of the North and those of the South.[16]

Finally, UNESCO's involvement guarantees that knowledge will be shared internationally. Developed in this triple context, the IBC represents, without a doubt, the most innovative structure or program put in place to attain these objectives.[17]

In 1989, a resolution adopted by the UNESCO General Conference has invited its Director General to

> ... study ways of establishing a permanent consultation on information exchange and experimental data on contemporary science and technology ethics boards to make UNESCO a world documentation and information

centre on this question at a time when decisive progress is being made in the life sciences and, in particular, in their medical application.[18]

In 1992, UNESCO's Director General assigned Noëlle Lenoir to define an intellectual basis and a practical framework for developing the concept of the human genome. In 1993, this mission took shape as the UNESCO General Conference created the International Bioethics Committee (IBC) in a resolution concerning the preparation of an international instrument to protect the human genome.[19]

Established on September 15, 1993, this multidisciplinary committee now has more than 50 members from 35 countries, chosen from the world's specialists in biology, science, genetics, medicine, law, and philosophy.[20]

Located at UNESCO headquarters, the IBC operates on a very limited budget, except for the annual meetings of the IBC and of the Legal Commission, which is the productive arm of the IBC. In short, UNESCO pays the IBC's operating costs, including, apart from the IBC general secretariat, travel and lodging costs for members, who receive no other remuneration.

The IBC is a consultative body with a triple role. First of all, it is a forum; it also takes on a teaching role; and finally, it fills a legal function as author of an international instrument.[21] As well, the IBC constructively examines bioethical questions, especially those associated with situations in which genetic advances can contribute to improvements to the well-being of individuals and to reductions in the world's inequities. Its current highest priority is the development of a Universal Declaration on the Human Genome and Human Rights, which the IBC hopes the UNESCO General Assembly will adopt by 1998.

Section 2 – European Ethics Boards

In Europe, two regional organizations are active in bioethics: the Council of Europe[22] and the European Union (EU) (formerly known as the European Community).[23] Some authors[24] say that the Council of Europe is weak in political will,[25] and that the EU lacks the authority to harmonize efforts that touch on fundamental liberties.[26] Nevertheless, the EU and the Council of Europe are predominant in the internationalization of bioethics and are fora for discussion on ethics. Although they both have various internal ethics boards,[27] we will deal with those whose role currently most closely resembles that of a national ethics committee. These are the Group of Advisers on the Ethical Implications of Biotechnology (GAEB) and the Steering Committee on Bioethics (CDBI) of the Council of Europe, which we will present in succession.

The Group of Advisers on the Ethical Implications of Biotechnology (GAEB)

The European Commission formed the GAEB on November 20, 1991.[28] Operating independently of the Commission's services, notably of the General Directorate for Research and Development, the GAEB reports directly to the President of the Commission and is located in the same building as the General Secretariat.[29]

Originally composed of six councillors, the GAEB now numbers nine members working in the areas of biomedical sciences, law, philosophy and theology, with a good mix of expertise, as its members include two jurists, two geneticists, three philosophers, a biologist, and a physician. In addition to these permanent members, who have a renewable two-year mandate, external experts are chosen for specific topics. Each GAEB member serves *ad personam*.[30] The European Commission pays the GAEB's operational costs.[31] Meeting bimonthly, the members receive no remuneration, but receive travel and lodging expenses on the scale established by the European Commission.

The GAEB has a threefold mission: first, to identify and define bioethical questions raised by biotechnology; second, to evaluate, from an ethical point of view, the impact of the activities of the EU in the area of biotechnology; and, finally, to advise the Commission in the exercise of its powers concerning the ethical aspects of biotechnology while ensuring that the public is clearly informed.[32] We should point out that the GAEB is strictly consultative (its advice is not binding on the Commission) and independent (it practices total freedom of opinion for the group as a whole, for its members, and for its governing body). As a rule, the European Commission requests advice from the GAEB on specific questions, but the GAEB also examines issues on its own initiative.[33]

The Steering Committee on Bioethics (CDBI)

The Committee of Ministers of the Council of Europe created the CDBI in the early 1980s, when bioethical inquiry was in full expansion and concerns about developments in genetic engineering were particularly pressing.[34] Following adoption by the Parliamentary Assembly of the Council of Europe of a resolution on genetic engineering that emphasized the need for broader ethical study, the Committee of Ministers instituted the *Comité ad hoc d'experts sur la génétique* (CAHGE) [the ad hoc committee of experts on genetics] which, in 1985, became the Ad Hoc Committee of Experts on Bioethics (CAHBI). This committee, in turn, finally became the Steering Committee on Bioethics (CDBI) in March 1992.[35]

Comprising about 60 members nominated by the member states of the Council of Europe, generally government experts from various fields (two or three representatives from each country), the CDBI has evolved as national ethics committees have been created and members have been invited to join the national delegations.[36] Generally meeting semiannually, the CDBI is divided into specialized working groups that meet more frequently. The Directorate of Legal Affairs of the Council of Europe provides the CDBI with a secretariat and pays its operating costs.[37] Most CDBI members are public servants who do not receive remuneration for their service, but they are paid travel and lodging expenses.

The work of the CDBI is meant principally to "provide states with harmonized documents responding to the challenges raised by the prodigious growth of the biomedical sciences"[38] and to promote information exchanges with professionals and the public. While the CDBI encourages states to define their own bioethics regulations, it also thought it necessary "to affirm, in the form of an international governing document, a Convention, a certain number of fundamental principles."[39] Accordingly, in 1992, the Council of Ministers gave the committee of experts the task of developing a convention on biomedicine.[40] Once completed, this convention will include a limited number of general principles, the more specific aspects being dealt with in additional protocols.[41]

In rapidly concluding this topic of the "internationalization of ethics,"[42] it is appropriate to note that the model of creation and composition used for the IBC and the GAEB differs from that used for the CDBI. In the case of the CDBI, the members are nominated by governments, with the result that they have no real room to manoeuvre in discussion since, above all, they represent their nations. Consequently, this type of committee sometimes becomes very political, as when it wrote the Draft European Convention on Human Rights and Biomedicine. Members of the IBC and the GAEB are chosen *ad personam* for their expertise; therefore, they act completely independently and are not responsible to their countries.

With respect to the impact of discussions, recommendations and proposals, it is evident that the very structure of an ethics body is significant. For example, in the case of the CDBI, once the members have agreed on a proposal and transmitted it to the Committee of Ministers, which comprises the foreign affairs ministers of the member countries, the document almost always receives the seal of the Committee of Ministers and is distributed in the relevant countries, although it is not binding on the governments.[43] In the case of the IBC and the GAEB, the distribution of opinions given and their reception on the national level can be much more unpredictable since the states do not consider themselves bound at all, even morally, by positions adopted by people, however prominent, who sit in a purely individual capacity.

Nevertheless, it is true that, independent of how it is structured, the debate takes place, the public is informed, and thought evolves. It is even truer that, at the national level, now is the time to act, and that numerous groups of varying forms and purposes are joining the debate on ethics.

PART I – A COMPARATIVE SURVEY OF NATIONAL ETHICS BODIES

The phenomenon of reflection on ethics, which some have termed a "call for ethics,"[44] first appeared in the 1960s in most of the Western countries; since then, it has been frequently called the medical revolution.[45] Ethics boards existed before, but they were either internal to the medical profession or frustrated by the confusion of boards representing the profession.[46] Numerous bodies tried, little by little, to define certain fundamental principles, especially in the field of life sciences and health.[47] First, there were research ethics committees; then, in the 1970s, clinical ethics committees (also called hospital ethics committees) appeared; and, finally, in the 1980s, ethics committees were assigned to study social questions.[48] Among the committees of this last type we find the national ethics boards.

Whatever their structure, functional design or mission, these national ethics bodies are found in various countries and develop according to the pressing issues of the day. A brief comparative survey will establish how closely the Canadian situation resembles the situation abroad.

The first objective of a comparative survey is to map, as faithfully as possible, the national ethics bodies, whatever their structure. Already, in 1991, as part of the First International Round Table on Ethics Committees, a preliminary comparative study of the state of national ethics boards in Europe,[49] Canada, and the United States was completed, and was followed up and confirmed in 1993 by a U.S. Office of Technology Assessment study.[50] The updating of these studies, thanks to the reexamination of these national ethics bodies' constitutions (where they existed) and to the work of some foreign correspondents, allows us today to confirm and refine the conclusions of the 1991 study.[51] Our various conclusions revolve around two axes: the makeup and organization of national ethics bodies (section 1), and the mission and activities of these national ethics bodies (section 2).

Section 1 – Composition and Organization of National Ethics Bodies

By definition, there can be no organization without infrastructure. Getting some idea of the architecture that is adopted, and of its functioning and logistics (both administrative and financial) is, therefore, essential for determining which model offers the most advantages. In the domain of national ethics bodies, there are four alternatives, which can be grouped into two categories: on the one hand, national ethics committees based on the French model, which was the first of its kind; and, on the other hand, those we have grouped under the more generic designation of national ethics boards, which, for the purposes of our study, will include all national authorities other than the national ethics committees.

National Committee or National Board?

A first premise must be set out before we try to describe the prevailing situation of national ethical structures: we are speaking of a phenomenon peculiar to Western countries, especially Latin or Nordic countries. Once this premise has been enunciated, we see that many countries have a national ethics structure of some kind.[52] This demonstrates the critical nature of the problems associated with biomedical advances and the increasing demand from the medical and scientific communities, the public, and public authorities for the erection of certain frameworks, and for the beginning of ethical reflection on a national scale.[53]

Two trends predominate at the moment with regard to the structure of national ethics forums. While some countries have chosen to establish a *national committee that is specific, independent and permanent,* other countries have opted for a multiplicity of boards that seem to be ad hoc, *ad tempus,* or *ratione materiae.*[54] An interesting and notable phenomenon is that the existence of a national ethics committee does not in any way hinder the emergence of other national authorities equally involved in ethical reflection,[55] which permits us to reject certain criticisms associating the presence of such a committee with the genesis of a monolithic system of ethical thought.[56] In concrete terms, what this means for Canada is that the establishment of a national ethics committee would not in itself put in question the role of the Medical Research Council or the National Council on Bioethics in Human Research.

National Ethics Committees

If we look at the countries that have opted for a national ethics committee corresponding to the definition we have just given,[57] we can reach at four principal conclusions.

First conclusion – It is essentially those countries with a Latin or Nordic heritage that have adopted the concept of a national ethics committee.[58] France was the first to choose this option,[59] followed by several other countries.[60] This choice is undoubtedly justified by the appropriateness of this type of structure in the institutional, legal, and cultural context of these countries.[61] Thus, for example, it appears that most of the countries that adopted the concept of national ethics committees, or those that foresee doing so, are unitary, homogeneous, usually fairly small states.[62] Are countries with a federated or confederated structure thus excluded de facto? Two cases,[63] those of Belgium and Australia, seem interesting for Canada. However, before we briefly analyze the situation in these countries, we would state that two reasons seem to justify establishing such structures in federated countries: the need to coordinate expertise, and "the extreme political sensitization of opinion with regard to certain biomedical issues."[64]

With regard to the two known attempts, we note that while the attempt is laudable the results are misleading. Thus, the Australian Health Ethics Committee (AHEC) is, to an extent, a reincarnation, in a fundamentally different form, of the National Bioethics Advisory Committee (NBCC), established in 1988 as an autonomous, multidisciplinary body.[65] Challenged on its overliberal position on surrogate motherhood, the NBCC was finally dissolved in 1992,[66] simultaneous with the legislated restructuring of the National Health and Medical Research Council (NHMRC).[67]

As part of this restructuring, the Australian Health Ethics Committee was established as one of the committees of the NHMRC. Composed of 20 members, the Australian Health Ethics Committee has a mission to carry out studies and to advise on ethical, legal, and social issues related to public health, medical practice, and research on human beings. It takes part in developing rules of conduct in the field of health, notably with respect to the law on privacy. It must also promote debate on issues related to health ethics.[68] Since regulation of medicine and research is a constitutional responsibility of governments at the state level, activity in the area of ethics is a major preoccupation of the states and territories.

Belgium's national advisory committee on ethics came into existence in the form of a cooperative accord, thanks to a political understanding between the state and the Flemish, French, and German communities.[69] The committee seems to have numerous operational problems, however; the nomination of members seems to have been especially political.[70]

There are certainly lessons to be learned from these two experiences, inasmuch as the distribution of skills and the structural, cultural, and linguistic context resembles the Canadian situation in many ways. However, more precise information is needed before a true analysis of the deeper reasons for the apparent failure of these two attempts can be made. It will also be important to follow developments in Switzerland, which are still in their earliest stages.

A second conclusion on national ethics committees – These committees are recent (they were created between 1983 and 1995),[71] and others are envisioned but not yet established.[72] This can be explained fairly easily. As it happens, committees often accompany the development of medically assisted reproduction and genetic medicine, which, more than any other biomedical advances, have underscored not only the limits to the state's power to intervene, but also the necessity for individual and collective reflection on social choices that involve current as well as future generations.

Third conclusion – The various countries with national ethics committees use relatively uniform terms.[73] The French National Ethics Advisory Committee for the Life and Health Sciences, the first of its kind, has been taken up, although with modifications or refinements that are often far from anodyne. Thus, in a general way, these countries have accented the advisory character of the committee by inserting the qualifier "advisory" in their name.[74] This qualification is hardly neutral; in fact, it signifies two possibilities that should be kept distinct.

> First of all, it shows that from now on, a new institution will insert itself into the process of reflection, and perhaps even of decision-making, an institution which one hopes will become an essential, if not mandatory passageway. Furthermore it means that the contribution of the Committee to the debate does not bind the one who asks for it; but by the same token, the committee, since it is not bound by the decision on the issue, can always change its opinion.[75]

The committee is advisory, in this second sense, because it has no decision-making or coercive power: "It is a place for confrontation, for dialogue, for reflection and for advice."[76]

Generally, regardless of the political structure of the country (whether it is a unitary or a federal state), the term "national" is used to describe these ethical bodies.[77] We could not obtain any information on whether the use of this term provoked reactions in federal countries. It does seem evident, however, given the attachment of the Canadian provinces to their jurisdiction over health, that the use of such a term in Canada could provoke resistance and perhaps even jeopardize the viability of such a structure. In this respect, it would surely be more appropriate to speak of an "interprovincial ethics committee" or a "pan-Canadian ethics committee."

Most countries, as it happens, have opted for the term "committee" or "council,"[78] undoubtedly in response to cultural preferences.[79] The titles of many committees indicate that their fields of investigation are limited to the life sciences and health—that is, to medical ethics, which is vast enough.[80] It is worth noting, however, that Norway retained the reference to bio-technology in the title of its national council.[81]

A last important characteristic of these national ethics committees derives from the fact that most were established by the executive arm of government;[82] the rest were created by the legislature.[83] This institutionalization is important because it gives the ethical body legitimacy as much in the public opinion as in the medical and scientific community, a legitimacy that ad hoc national ethics boards do not necessarily enjoy. As Ian Kennedy rightly points out, "if you can prove a legal basis and some kind of *imprimatur* on general policy, they have to listen to you; they can't throw you out of the game right at the start."[84] It is true, however, that some other kinds of boards also occasionally benefit from this legitimacy because they were established by public authorities. Even so, this does not mean they exhibit the characteristics of a real national ethics committee (namely, permanence or a general mandate) but rather that they simply seem worthy of respect.[85] The best examples are the various commissions established since 1978 in the United States.[86]

Institutionalization implies oversight. In most cases, this authority is vested in the Minister of Health, the Minister of Social Affairs,[87] or his equivalent; more rarely in the Minister of Research;[88] and only exceptionally in other ministers, notably those of education[89] or justice.[90] We think ministers of health should be responsible for these areas, since it is the ethical aspects of life and health that are specifically, if not uniquely, targeted. As to the frequent subordination of these committees to ministers of social affairs, this could perhaps result from "the sociosanitary element" in medical ethics, which is a "discipline promoting and protecting the person."[91] Sometimes, national ethics committees depend not on one or even several ministries, but on superior entities such as the privy council[92] or the head of state.[93] This option has the advantage of helping to prevent ministerial quarrels over issues that certainly relate primarily to health, but that also have elements which are social, legal, and economic.

To summarize, three criteria seem to distinguish national ethics committees from national ethics boards. The first derives from the institutional or noninstitutional character of the national ethics bodies, depending on whether they have been created by acts of government or by legislative texts. The second relates to the authority of oversight. National committees are nearly always accountable to the government for their activities,[94] in contrast to national boards, which are completely independent of public authorities. (This does not mean, however, that the boards have no obligation to report to the professional, private, or political authorities that established them.) The third criterion relates to the field of expertise, which, in national committees, must embrace the ethics of medical research and its applications in a universal way, whereas national boards often have a more limited and detailed mandate.

National Ethics Boards

While national committees are emerging in some countries, in other countries ethical reflection takes place within many different institutions that vary as much in form as in spirit.[95] These national ethics boards are created either *ratione materiae* to study a specific ethical issue brought up by the appearance of a new technique[96] or *ratione temporis* to study all the ethical issues current in a specific period of time.[97] Sometimes, national boards are directed within the framework of their mission or practice toward a specific ethical issue.[98] This most often applies to medical and scientific organizations,[99] more rarely to legal and social organizations.[100]

It is important to note that this involvement of professional organizations in the domain of ethics also persists in countries with national committees, which demonstrates that committees have no prerogative over medical ethics.[101] Contrary to conventional wisdom, the presence of an ethics committee does not necessarily undermine any other forum of reflection; indeed, other fora may inspire the committee, which in turn may influence them. These other national boards, however, are more often concerned with applied ethics than with reflections on universal ethics.[102]

In conclusion, we can only acknowledge the prevalence of two trends— national committee and national board—and note that this dichotomy is not about to disappear, since it originates partly in considerations that are undoubtedly as cultural as they are historic and political. This diversity does not, in itself, seem to constitute a problem because, although their constitutions are totally different, the internal organization of national committees and national boards reveals that they share common goals and methods.

Composition, Assignment, and Remuneration

Having established the heterogeneity of national ethics bodies, we must study their composition, their methods for choosing members, and the presence or absence of remuneration[103], to see whether the difference in form influences their modes of operation.

Composition

The principal characteristic of the composition[104] of both national com- mittees and national boards is the multidisciplinarity[105] of these different bodies, including those that, at their inception, were essentially medical. This "intrusion" of nonscientists and nonphysicians into ethics bodies is interesting from several points of view. First of all, it supports the idea that scientists and practitioners are not always equipped to evaluate independently all aspects of their actions[106] and that, these days, it is no longer possible either to give them *carte blanche* or to let them face alone the possible con- sequences of new medical developments. Next, this multidisciplinarity is characteristic of ethical reflection itself, which by nature cannot be restricted to a single field of expertise, be it scientific, legal, philosophical or other, but must be situated at the crossroads of all these domains. Finally, the domain of ethics involves, not an oration, but a conversation. Indeed, the more diverse the experiences and points of view, the more enriching the exchange.[107]

One reservation must be noted with regard to multidisciplinarity, which, although it tends to be general, is not expressed in the same way in various countries and on various boards. Sometimes there is a true balance between scientists and nonscientists;[108] sometimes, however, the scientific and medical community is overrepresented compared with disciplines derived from the human sciences.[109] More and more, however, the pure sciences are less dominant as society increasingly demands the right to participate in the debate.[110]

Certain segments of society are still too often excluded or under-represented on national ethics committees as well as on national ethics boards: these are the public and the media. On this point, however, it is worth noting and applauding the efforts made by some countries.[111] The presence of a lay person on a committee has various advantages, of which the most notable are that it permits the committee to gauge public under-standing of scientific developments, and that it allows the committee to test the comprehensibility of the information and recommendations it makes public. With respect to this last concern, a person familiar with commu-nications and the media would be a valuable committee member; scientists often have difficulty conveying information about developments in medicine to the media. Media representation on ethics committees is, however, far from being universal at the moment.[112]

One point that seems more controversial concerns the composition of national ethics committees that include political representatives or parlia-mentarians (the question does not arise for boards, which are not established by a political authority). The likelihood that a committee will include political figures seems to depend heavily on national custom and on the esteem in which politics is held. Thus, for example, in Sweden, half the members are parliamentarians representing the main political movements of the nation. They sit on the committee apparently untroubled by their political alliances. This comfortable relationship is a product of Swedish tradition, in which, before any legislation is proposed, parliamentary commissions consult experts. In Denmark, on the other hand, whenever a parliamentary com-mission is formed to follow up on the work of the Danish Ethics Council, the two bodies are completely separate, although the Danish Parliament appoints eight members to the council. The Danish council works in total autonomy and shares its conclusions with the parliamentary commission, although no member of Parliament sits on the council for fear that parliamentarians would try to impose political values and considerations that might bias the debate.[113] In other countries, such as France, Italy and Norway, parliamentarians attend by virtue of constitutional statutes,[114] but only *sua spontanae*, as they may attend only with the consent of the com-mittee itself.[115] This divergence of point of view may seem, a priori, over-whelming if one considers that national ethics committees are only consultative bodies. However, on examination, the presence of parliamen-tarians can, in the medium term, either nullify or enhance the credibility of a board. This depends not only on how politics is viewed, but also on the councillor mandate in the exercise of public authority. Nevertheless, many think that an ethics committee should never be an antechamber of Parliament.[116]

For lack of data, we could not determine the balance between men and women,[117] nor were we able to determine the representation by age group, on the various committees and boards listed. These elements are, nevertheless, important because all the sociological studies show that men and women often have different sensitivities regarding social questions, a phenomenon that becomes more striking with age.

The desire to include this or that category of person inevitably comes up against an imperative that cannot be ignored: the size of the national committee or national board, which, if the body is to be efficient and effective, cannot be disproportionate. Thus, independent of the type of structure adopted, the number of people making up national committees and national ethics boards fluctuates between 10,[118] 20,[119] and 40[120] members. A smaller group may be more flexible regarding operational, procedural, and organizational matters. On the other hand, small groups do not represent all faiths, all cultures, and all minorities; it is a challenge to choose members so that no group feels excluded.[121] In fact, the important thing is to ensure that the expertise of the committee is broad, complementary, and balanced. It is also essential to ensure that individual members have four specific aptitudes. First, they must be able to acquire a degree of knowledge of health problems and issues. Second, they must demonstrate a good capacity for analysis. Third, they must be sensitive to and aware of the public.[122] Finally, they must know how to communicate, not only with a knowledgeable audience, but also with the public at large. A larger group can be more representative, but also entails a heavier burden of administration and planning.

To accommodate both representativeness and functionality, committees or boards that have opted for a fairly large group (more than 30), could provide themselves with technical sections and subcommittees. These could be charged with doing the initial spadework on a given problem to facilitate the plenary discussion.[123] Neither is the better solution; to be precise, it really depends on choices related to national customs and preferences. No matter how many people are members of the ethics groups, it is not their number that is important, but how they are assigned.

Assignment

The method of choosing and appointing members of boards and ethics committees must be examined with particular attention because it indicates the extent, real or imagined, of the room to manoeuvre and the degree of independence an ethics body truly enjoys relative to the administrative, professional, or private entities that created it. In fact, it is interesting that, regardless of structure, no ethics body has elected members; all are nominated,[124] exclusively or mostly, by the initiating authority, which is often the oversight authority. Depending on the country, this nomination may be made either after consultation with or at the discretion of the oversight authority.

It might seem that this power to nominate is only to be expected of an organization that establishes and funds an ethics body. The infiltration of the committee or board with one school of thought by nominating, for example, members who represent the beliefs of the governing authority, is to be avoided. This position, which is not a priori inconceivable, would do considerable harm to the credibility of the national ethics body and would obliterate the moral authority of the recommendations it might make, thus destroying the original goal. On the contrary, appointments founded exclusively on expertise and experience should be much more objective. Certainly, many countries appear to be convinced of this.

Remuneration

Setting up a new structure typically generates some costs, which depend on a number of variables, notably whether the members are remunerated. This aspect is often mentioned but rarely clarified because the meaning of the term "remuneration" varies from one country to another.[125] That said, it seems that no country pays a salary to the members of its national ethics committee or national ethics board. This is surely justified by the fact that, with some exceptions, all committee and board members meet only at intervals and continue to pursue their professional careers.

In the absence of salaries, a daily attendance stipend is, in some countries, disbursed to members.[126] However, most of the time, only expenses may be reimbursed, whether they be the costs of travelling, representation, or conference registrations. We think that this lack of emoluments for members of committees and ethics boards could have one of two explanations. It could be a question, first of all, of altruism on the part of the members, who might agree to meet solely for reasons of personal interest and conviction. Looking at it more pragmatically, aside from the desire to save public or private funds, this nonremuneration of members of national ethics bodies could be a way to avoid making "ethics professionals" of the members of national ethics committees and boards, and to avoid making "ethics workplaces" of national bodies, to emphasize instead their aspect as fora. This attitude is part of the logic of citizenship and democracy, in which ethics are *res communis,* not a matter for specialists.[127]

Parallel to the sitting members, the national ethics committee or board must have a solid administrative and financial management structure to be able to function in a continuous and effective fashion.

Administrative and Financial Logistics

Whatever their size and structure, national ethics bodies require certain minimum human, material, and financial resources. The comparative study[128] reveals disparities of personnel, premises, and budget that are related more to the nature of national ethics bodies than to circumstances peculiar to the countries in which they operate.

Personnel

From a reading of the texts and the responses received, we see that the administrative staff of a committee is often limited—two to five people as a rule, some, if not all, employed part time.[129] In addition, administrative personnel are often seconded to an ethics body from the overseeing authority. This slenderness of staff may explain the difficulties that committees and boards sometimes encounter in productivity and in the dissemination of their opinions.

Administrative staff seem to be mostly executive assistants and directors[130] supplemented by a few academic specialists in ethics, health, or research.[131] Experts on contract are regularly added to this core to respond to urgent situations or to produce documents and study reports.[132] The openness of the permanent secretariat to the outside world offsets its smallness and gives it access to experts as needed. This broadens the horizons of the ethics structure, reduces the risk of inertia, and ensures a greater pluralism of ideas.

Premises

A national ethics body has either its own premises,[133] or its headquarters in the offices of its oversight authority or of a host organization specified by the founding agreements.[134] The comparative study of countries indicates that the solution adopted is not related to the type of structure (national committee or national board) but usually results from discretionary choices made by the initiating authority. Thus, an ethics group established by a public authority will not necessarily be headquartered with the public authority.

The installation of the committee or board in the offices of the initiating authority is, nevertheless, not an effective measure of the dependence of the national ethics body, as many internal and financial contingencies may enter into consideration. A more reliable criterion—although still not irrefutable—is the allocated budget: its nature, origin, destination, and amount.

Budget

Not surprisingly, just as staff and premises are either specific to a national ethics body or dependent on its governing authority, the budget may also be either proper to the ethics body or inserted in the budgetary line of the minister or the professional oversight authority, whether associated or private. With the exception of the Nuffield Foundation,[135] which relies solely on private funds, all the national ethics committees and boards studied are financed essentially by public funds.[136] These funds are allocated either by giving the ethics body its own budget[137] or by giving it specific credits within the global budget of the oversight authority.[138] In the case of national ethics committees, this allocation of public funds is a direct, not to say logical, consequence of their attachment to a public administrative entity. In the case of national boards with an *ad tempus* mandate, the budget is established either on an annual basis or as a lump sum for the duration of the mandate, and the ethics board is entrusted with managing it as best it can.

There is always a link among the nature of the group's offices, its personnel, and its budget. This relationship is easy to understand: as soon as a body is provided with its own budget, its sphere for planning and action increases, but it must take responsibility for its operating costs. A budget included in that of another administrative authority, public or professional, is generally dedicated to specific actions, while material aspects are directly covered in the global budget of that governing authority.

Comparatively speaking, the allocation of an independent budget to an ethics body has the advantage of allowing more flexible management, while the management of a budget included in that of another organization is always subject to innumerable formalities and controls. This aspect can result in sluggishness and can impede the smooth functioning of the national ethics committee or board.

Indeed, in the framework of an autonomous budget, the power of decision and action of the national ethics body is necessarily greater, since the choices have been delegated to it. Controls exist, but are applied a posteriori, when the report is presented, most often on an annual basis. If, on the other hand, the budget is included in that of another organization, the controls are applied a priori. In extreme cases, this can result in veto politics that interfere with the proper functioning of the national ethics structure and limit the body's freedom of action. In practice, this risk will depend a great deal on the legislation governing the use of public funds in each country. The requirements may be more or less constraining in different cases. Only a study of the legislation, within the objectives of the research, would allow us to determine the solution most often adopted.

The size of the budget typically allocated is hard to estimate because too few of the countries[139] gave us sufficiently precise information on this point. Nevertheless, one must remember that to establish a national ethics body, whatever its structure, without giving it an adequate budget is a pointless exercise, because the ethics body will not have the means to support its goals. One must, therefore, pay close attention to the budget, for it makes a difference. The budget will or will not allow the ethics body to hire qualified staff in sufficient numbers, will or will not allow recourse to the services of outside experts, and will or will not permit the dissemination of opinions or recommendations under optimal conditions.

With missions and desired actions as a starting point, it would be a good idea to proceed to serious and realistic budget estimates so that a budget that will be both reasonable and most suited to the group's objectives can be calculated. Although we are in an era of restricted public spending, there is still a risk that these estimates could be as tight as possible and short term, when it would be better to invest in the long term. We should not lose sight of the fact that, although the creation of an ethics board *ratione temporis* or *ratione materiae* may seem more economical at first, the cost of the infrastructure for each new commission and the consultants who must be called in to compensate for the groups' limited mandates will ultimately be greater than the cost of a permanent group. And the effectiveness of these individual commissions will be difficult to assess as no follow-up procedures will be in place.

The budget should not, however, be judged out of context. In fact, although some organizations do not a priori have large budgets, they nevertheless benefit from both logistical and communications support from their oversight authorities.[140] Criteria for international comparisons must, therefore, embrace not only the financial data but also the advantages in human or material resources that the ethics body can exploit. In fact, countries attempting to rationalize their expenses and consolidate public and parapublic administrative authorities may find this intermediate solution attractive.

Finally, some budget allocation trends should be illustrated. As a general rule, the bulk of the budget is dedicated to covering the national ethics committee's operating costs,[141] whether it be to pay the staff, the daily stipends or members' expenses, or the rent for office space. At the same time, part of the budget is often dedicated to research work, the organization of conferences, the establishment of a centre of documentation, and so on.[142] The budget, then, is allocated in many ways, since spending often depends on the priorities of the committee or the board.

In concluding this first section on the establishment and organization of national ethics committees and boards, let us note that a constitution that is fundamentally antinomian does not in any way modify the internal organization of the national structure adopted. On a daily basis, the same problems are encountered, the same dangers have to be avoided. Distinctions between committees and boards, when they exist, relate far more to internal contingencies or options than to association with one or the other of the two types of structure mentioned. It is often the same for matters related to the mission and activities of these committees or boards with national influence.

Section 2 – Missions and Activities of the National Ethics Bodies

Although new medical and scientific advances are a source of hope and joy, they also inspire reservations and anxiety, since people seem to be increasing their control over their lives and their environment.[143] Far from being an epiphenomenon, this knowledge of human life advances from day to day, and obliges us to make new social choices and to undertake new responsibilities. Without consensus on and significant analysis of what is at stake, legislative intervention does not always seem to be the ideal solution. At the same time, social conscience is beginning to regain its normative function, in or through the various national ethics bodies. These bodies, however, must not in any way replace the lawmaker, the judge, or the theologian; these bodies must, above all, be assigned the mission of promoting and disseminating their thoughts on the issues associated with biomedical developments so that individuals can make decisions and arrive at the most informed choices possible.[144] In this regard, the national ethics bodies should be involved in activities that are as much advisory, educational, and informational as judgmental.

The Missions of the National Ethics Committees and National Ethics Boards

As a general rule, the scope of the mission and the great number of action priorities allocated to national ethics bodies are often their most striking characteristics. As for mandates, although they also aim to predict the social stakes related to medicine and medical research, they still vary in form and can be multiple, specific or, on the contrary, general.

Mandate

Although it is true that, a priori, national committees may seem to be charged with a broader mission than national boards (justified by the *rationae materiae* or *ad tempus* nature of the latter), this distinction is not as clear-cut as it appears. It is true that not all national committees have de facto and *in se* a general mandate on issues of medical ethics, whereas some national boards tend to have a fairly extensive mandate. Thus, depending on the case, national ethics committees are sometimes called upon to discuss the collective ethical, social, and legal implications of biomedical advances,[145] whereas, at other times, their mandate is limited to the strictly ethical, social, or legal consequences of biomedical research.[146] Generally, this interest in the issues at stake in medical research corresponds more to the mandates assigned to national ethics boards,[147] even if there are some exceptions to note.[148]

While national ethics structures often mean to take an interest in the ethical, legal, and social implications of medical research, a comparison between that mandate and the themes that are in fact dealt with or envisioned tends to demonstrate that the mandate broadens to a reflection on the practice of medicine itself. This is the result of the critical nature of the problems, the demand for a framing of the issues, and legislators' silence. In fact, because every medical act has its unwanted side effects and every therapy is, in a sense, an experiment, and because the lapse of time between the development of a therapy and its clinical application is becoming shorter and shorter, the whole field of health and medicine is definitely concerned. This also corresponds to a collective awareness of and a reaction against the paternalistic tradition in medicine.

As the mandate (whatever it may be) nevertheless remains fairly exhaustive, certain priorities are finally established. Thus, even though the original goal of these national ethics committees and boards was promotion of and respect for human dignity, the actual choices made to assure this promotion vary from country to country. This, once again, supports the idea that differences are essentially a matter of cultural, historical, and political contingencies and are not usually associated with the type of structure (national committee or national board) put in place.

Priorities

As they should be, priorities are linked closely to the assigned mandate. Thus, when national ethics bodies have a mandate to study the implications of medical research, one finds this preoccupation at the front and centre in their statement of priorities.[149] When the mandate is more general, an internal hierarchy establishes itself. Sometimes actions take priority and sometimes research in particular fields is promoted to first rank. This allocation is not necessarily neutral. To favour certain activities means favouring the informational, educational, and evaluative functions of the national ethics structure adopted. Giving the advantage to research means promoting the deliberative and advisory functions of this structure. Eventually, however, a kind of osmosis develops between the two.

An attentive reading of priorities allows us to note that, in certain countries (luckily a minority), the first goal of the national ethics board is to contribute to the development of legal norms.[150] This function invites certain questions because the advisory role of the body finds itself de facto usurped by a hidden normative function.[151] The choice of structure and its title should, therefore, be determined judiciously to avoid confusion between ethics and law, or between ethics and deontology.

Another significant aspect relates to the determination of priorities. Disparities are evident as much in the mode of seizure of the ethics structure as in the development of its priorities for action.

Thus, in most countries, priorities are determined by the ethics body itself,[152] either directly by the chairman or by the members as a group. This option, which recognizes that national ethics committees or boards have discretionary power to determine the actions they will favour, is a significant index of their autonomy and their independence from the governing authority; one might otherwise have reason to fear dependency.

Nevertheless, although some national ethics boards that are internal to other organizations do determine their own action priorities, they do so necessarily as a function of the preoccupations of the organization they represent. At the same time, other national boards and committees could be influenced in their choices by the demands of pressure groups. Indeed, the boundary is sometimes unclear between what constitutes a real social concern and what is related to a quest for power that would be legitimated by the seal—and, to a certain extent, the reputation—of the national ethics body. This risk of pressure is inevitable; one could almost say it is proper in a democracy. Even so, it is through its ability to resist these pressures that the ethics structure will increase its credibility and impact, and justify its existence.

Another interesting way to get an index of the room for manoeuvre available to the ethics structure is by determining its mode of seizure, that is, by determining who is calling for ethics.[153]

On this point, national ethics boards are less prolific than national committees.[154] This relative silence could be explained by the nature of this type of national ethics body. The mandate of a board created for specific ends or for a limited time is usually detailed by the initiating institution in the board's founding articles. The board is established with a specific goal by a specific institution that presents it with a predetermined mandate, which consequently allows no room for seizure by other authorities, except in certain cases set out with limitations in the mandate.

With national boards of a professional nature, indications of the mode of seizure are also not necessarily set out; perhaps it is taken as a given that the rules of seizure of the other authorities of the professional body will apply.

In any case, given the diversity of types of national ethics boards established around the world, one notices a great variety of holders of power of seizure, a variety that corresponds to the specificity of each national ethics board in each country. In fact, we could be speaking of government, of certain administrative authorities, of groups of health and medical professionals, of patients and their families, or of local committees.[155]

As the national ethics committees, they show both diversity and coherence[156]—diversity in the titular holders of the power of seizure, since we could be speaking of the government, of the parliament, of political or professional groups, of local or regional ethics committees, as well as particular groups such as patients' associations; coherence, because this relative liberty of seizure can be found in almost all countries that have such committees. This openness is fundamental since it is the essence of ethics itself, which, as we have already said, is not a decree but rather a debate nourished by exchanges among individuals of various allegiances and conditions.

Finally, by comparing the information obtained regarding seizure and the determination of priorities among various national committees, one conclusion is inevitable. If the government is most often in a position to take control of the national committee, the latter, once under control, is still free to fulfil or not the formulated request. There is, on this point, no equivalence between modes of seizure and the determination of priorities for action. There does not seem to be the same elasticity when it is a question of a national board *ad tempus* or *ratione materiae* because such a board almost always has an established mandate from which it cannot really stray. The possibility that the national ethics structure will be "seized" should be considered a normal check, given its creation and financial management by the public authorities. At the same time, the freedom accorded to the ethics body to manage its own priorities should be interpreted as a logical corollary to its apolitical, "nonlegal" and "nonscientific" character.

These comments having been made, all that remains is this: to put its priorities into operation, the national ethics structure must gear up for action.

Activities of the National Ethics Boards and Committees

As we have seen over the course of the preceding analysis, the mandate of ethics bodies is large, the action priorities are diverse, and the goals are fundamental. This is the context in which the national ethics structure must adapt its actions. These are quite various, since the ethics body must simultaneously provide advice and recommendations, impart information, engage in communication and counselling, organize education and training, and see to the ethical and scientific evaluation of its research.[157]

Advisory Activity

This activity constitutes, in fact, the Gordian knot of the action of national committees and boards.[158] It responds to a pressing need: recent biomedical advances are shaking up the law, leaving individuals perplexed and imposing new choices; traditional reference points are rapidly becoming obsolete,[159] judicial responses more nebulous,[160] and uncertainty greater.[161]

In this context, the national ethics bodies have a kind of deliberative function. When we say deliberative we imply advisory, and this constitutes an important characteristic of all these national ethics structures. None has decision-making or repressive power; the accent is always on their character as *agora*, places for meeting and discussion. Thus, through the opinions and recommendations it offers, the national ethics structure nourishes general reflection, opens new avenues, and establishes new reference points based on fundamental discussion and research.[162]

This deliberative and advisory function of national committees and boards does not make them "supreme arbiters of ethical questions"[163] because their discourse must avoid being purely casuistic; on the contrary, it should attempt to be unitary and conceptual. Some see in the lack of sanctioning power a limit to the impact of the values and principles the ethics bodies seek to promote. Even so, it is through their reputation, competence, and objectivity that ethics bodies will acquire legitimacy and moral authority. Better still, this pure guidance, transmitted through the opinions of the ethics bodies, is fundamental because it substitutes empowerment, which is more and more valued, for coercion, which is always resented.

With respect to this mission of deliberation, the permanent character of national ethics bodies could be determining, or at the very least desirable. In fact, ethics are not immutable. On the contrary, ethics evolve in time and space, in the face of scientific advances that never cease to push back the frontiers of the possible, of knowledge, and of thought. Because they are constantly in renewal, techniques and technologies change the parameters of traditional responses that are often set in legislation, the fruit of yesterday's consensus. Since they have the opportunity to undertake a timely follow-up, not only of a given technology, but also of the questions that go with it, national ethics bodies can issue recommendations and opinions that correspond to the current state of knowledge and keep pace with the evolution of that knowledge. As time goes by, ethics bodies can, if necessary, modify their positions to integrate new scientific data and a new consensus in society so as to maintain a forward outlook on biomedical developments.[164]

Indeed, although in some domains reflection seems to happen *a posteriori*,[165] much discussion is now expected before developments occur, particularly in the domain of genetics and its branches. This evolution is interesting because it shows that national ethics bodies are effectively places for consultation and thought and not places for legitimation, obliged to issue opinions quickly to avoid being bypassed by technologies and practices already widespread. This does not mean that the actions of national ethics bodies are oriented only toward the future, for it is better to evaluate a practice *a posteriori* than not to evaluate it at all. In fact, ethics committees must be, on the one hand, catalysts for discussion of the social and ethical issues generated by current practice and, on the other, innovators by anticipating issues associated with technologies or practices that may still be at the experimental stage but close to a breakthrough.

It is worth noting that the themes dealt with, or soon to be dealt with, generally correspond to current preoccupations, questions, and choices.[166] This can be interpreted in two ways. Perhaps the ethics structures are acting as the voice of the people and are discussing the themes that preoccupy the public; in doing so, they function as intermediaries between the lay person, the scientist, and the politician.[167] Or it could be that these ethics structures, by pronouncing on this or that medical technique or aspect of research, are stimulating an awareness in society and making of this new theme a major public preoccupation. The truth probably lies between these two propositions, in the interdependence of these phenomena.

This interaction, however, can be effective only if national ethics bodies are in a position to discern public opinion and give the public the means to express itself. Indeed, on this point, the experiences mentioned often reveal gaps. All too often, the public still does not have a voice. As a case in point, most of the countries queried claim to do research on public perceptions[168] but, paradoxically, we see that they rarely have the means to do so, and that a certain confusion reigns in some people's minds between information and expression. Awareness of public opinion does not come from press releases, exhibitions, or radio or television programs, which merely convey information. To give the public a way to express its point of view means, in reality, to allow it to speak, to integrate it into working groups, to let it participate in conference debates and round tables, and to organize public hearings.[169] This is a difficult challenge, for it implies a willingness on the part of the members of the national ethics boards and committees to make their discourse comprehensible and transparent, without falling into popularization and reductionism.

To express a point of view, one must have knowledge and, therefore, access to information. It is essential to the work of national ethics committees and boards that they circulate as much information as possible on biomedical advances, the choices that are emerging, the answers being defined, the doubts that come up. In general, they do this very well.[170] This information should target the public, not just scientists and politicians. To guarantee the accessibility of this information to the greatest number, a judicious way to proceed would be to publish and distribute the study documents, the opinions and recommendations rendered, and the proceedings of the conferences organized.

This publication activity seems to be accomplished in most countries by either national ethics committees or national authorities, although, for the latter, the target readers are more often health professionals. Given the limited administrative and financial structures these national ethics bodies often have at their disposal,[171] publication is sometimes difficult to manage, and distribution, for lack of sufficient means, is often too limited to reach entire sectors and populations. In addition, this undertaking is, in itself, particularly delicate, since, to be interesting and reliable, the information must be precise, recent, and complete. It is important, therefore, that excessively long publication delays not be allowed to slow distribution and render the information meaningless, if not actually obsolete. This unfortunate state of affairs could surely be avoided if the national ethics structures worked with dedicated, consistent publication budgets that were specific and significant. This would also make it possible to create a basic documentary archive that would be very useful for the educational and training activities the national ethics structures are trying to initiate.

Educational Activity

While the public certainly has a pressing need for education, it is far from being the only beginner in the field of medical ethics. The scientific community, as well as governments, elected officials, and various administrators, also need direction and ethical signposts to improve their understanding of their responsibilities and the implications of their actions. One of the key roles for national ethics committees and national ethics authorities is to see to this information and education.

With regard to public authorities, this task is, in one sense, a test of the independence of the national body, since politicians find themselves in the role of mandatory. This is perhaps truer for national ethics committees[172] than for national ethics boards, even if some, in fact, play a fairly similar role.[173] In any case, it is particularly important that the ethics body take its function as "educator" seriously, because it is in the halls of councils and legislatures that, at a given moment, sooner or later, decisions will be made, laws ratified, and standards imposed.[174] If this framework is not to be discredited before it is voted on, out of date before it comes into force, or forgotten before it is applied, elected officials must be aware of the stakes, the divisions and agreements in society, and the values and principles involved. The national ethics body, which is a meeting place and central element for reflection and discussion, should be able to put the legislature in touch with the pulse of society, showing it the ins and outs of the possible choices without sinking into Manicheism or dogmatism.

This role of the intermediary who tries to bring together two extremes—public authorities and public opinion—by educating them and making them aware of specific problems that have been identified but not solved, is a new step in the promotion of human rights.[175] As Philippe Lazar stated:

> The debate about ethics, far from being a sort of dike put up by society to contain the rising tide of science and its applications in order to resist the permanent disruption of its habits and the established order, could, on the contrary, be an extraordinary means of communication and exchange between the public, its representatives and researchers.[176]

This education is also taking place in the medical and scientific communities,[177] which, let us not forget, were the instigators of these national ethics bodies.[178] This is particularly true when the national ethics board is of a professional nature. This remains true for other forms of national ethics structures as well, as soon as they have a well-established policy of disseminating their thoughts and opinions. From now on, it is undeniable that the medical and scientific community needs to know the boundaries within which it can legitimately evolve, to know the issues provoked by its discoveries and practices, and, finally, to be made aware of its new responsibilities. Indeed, the national ethics committee or board may validly and effectively assume this role by bringing together medical and scientific knowledge and other forms of knowledge, whether they be legal, philosophical, social, ethical, economic, or historical.

What is more, a consensus is emerging: we can no longer "believe that we can derive moral and political lessons from science, [because that would be] taking a device for discovery and making it a machine for dictating behaviour."[179] Everyone, including scientists themselves, agrees that we cannot leave to scientists the responsibility entailed by their actions and the sole power to decide on the validity of the goals they pursue. On the contrary, given what is at stake, the choices have become social choices, and the responsibility a shared one.

However, if this education of the various parties is to be effective, it must be accompanied by some kind of training in medical ethics. The national bodies have much to gain from initiating and fostering such teaching, especially at the university level but also at the level of high schools. On this point, some countries have shown initiative by participating in the development of teaching materials[180] and by involving themselves in training practitioners as well as the public authorities and the public itself.[181] The means used to arrive at this goal are not always clearly defined. They should stand out more in the future since this activity, which is relatively recent, seems to be intensifying.

A certain vigilance would seem to be in order however, since national ethics committees cannot and should not replace professional and other deontological bodies. It is clear that many of them do more than stimulate thought on the ethical implications of the sciences of life and health. They contribute to the redefinition of the duties and obligations of practitioners, and impinge on the field of deontology. Elsewhere, this tendency seems to be reinforced by the activities of ethical and scientific evaluation of research that are sometimes assigned to them.

Evaluative Activity

This activity, when it exists, puts the national ethics committees and boards in the role originally assigned in the 1960s to local and regional committees—an echo of the requirements set out by the Helsinki Declaration. Vesting such power of ethical and scientific evaluation of research in national ethics bodies could a priori give the impression that they are charged with supervising the activity of local and regional committees, that they evaluate protocols themselves, and that they act as an appeal board against the opinions rendered by these committees of inferior territorial jurisdiction.

In reality, and despite exceptions,[182] local and regional committees are rarely subordinate to national ethics committees or boards. The local and regional committees consult them in difficult cases, collaborate with them, but are never obliged to account to them for their activities.[183] Nevertheless, it seems clear that, given the expertise and competence of the members of the national bodies, the opinions they may be led to formulate are very likely to be sought and applied.

The fact that the national ethics structure is also not usually an appeal board[184] is also very significant and reinforces the dominant activities of consultation and information. To make it a "court of appeal" or a "superior court" would have made it an authority over science in general, and we have already mentioned the disadvantages of such a function. In fact, the activity of ethical and scientific evaluation as it is exercised by national ethics bodies consists of defining general principles for conduct that are likely to guide the new fields of medical research and their applications.[185] This evaluation function is, in a way, the direct continuation of its consultative and advisory functions.

In concluding this second part, one could say that, if distinctions occasionally appear between the actions taken by the national ethics boards and the national ethics committees, these differences are minor compared to the general harmony that emerges from the goals pursued, the means put into effect, and the domains explored. These distinctions, when they exist, result less from the founding principles of the national committee or national board than from internal or statutory contingencies, or cultural, economic, social, and other considerations.

Finally, created in a climate of uncertainty in the face of the tremendous explosion of the biomedical and genetic sciences, the national ethics bodies exert themselves well or badly—and more often well than badly—in response to the growing demand for ethics coming from public authorities, the medical and scientific communities, and from the general public.

Whether they are committees or boards, these national ethics bodies find themselves being assigned very broad mandates, of varied natures and goals, while often being given fairly limited human and financial resources.

Characterized by the multiplicity of their actions, their purely advisory nature, and the moral authority associated with their opinions and recommendations, these national ethics structures have undeniably become the stage for thought and discussion on the values and principles society should promote, the choices it should make, and the responsibilities it should affirm. This balance achieved, national ethics bodies still must define the Canadian bioethical landscape, so that we can decide, in the light of foreign experiences, whether we really can accommodate a Canadian national ethics committee.

PART II – OVERVIEW OF THE CANADIAN SITUATION

Any review of the appropriateness of establishing a Canadian Advisory Committee on Ethics, and the concomitant definition of its structure and mandate, first requires an overview of the current situation in Canada. We set about this task by contacting the deans of every medical faculty in Canada, as well as every provincial and territorial health ministry and department. As expected, the documents received showed that the ethical thinking engendered and intensified by recent developments in health has been channelled into two types of local structures, namely research ethics boards (REBs) and clinical ethics committees (CECs). A review of the documents received also revealed the significant role played by other discussion fora at the regional and provincial levels. As any future national body would have to deal with this complex reality, it seems appropriate to include in our description of the current situation in Canada the regional, provincial, and territorial ethics bodies and the Canada-wide ethics bodies. Let us begin with local ethics bodies.

Section 1 – Local Ethics Bodies in Canada

For the purposes of this report, the local level includes hospitals and extended care facilities, or research centres and universities. In such institutions, one generally finds bodies responsible for reviewing ethical problems raised by medical practices (clinical ethics committees), or research protocols for human research (research ethics boards). Like some other authors,[186] we found distinctions not only between these two types of local authorities, which was to be expected, but also among the various bodies. Beyond these differences, it nevertheless remains important to recognize the similarities, one of which is fundamental: their common objective to protect human dignity and rights. A review of the structure and organization of these bodies, as well as of their mandates and actions, will highlight both the differences and similarities among local ethics bodies.

Structure and Organization of Local Ethics Bodies in Canada

The first step in examining local structures will involve a review of the origins of the two major categories of local ethics bodies—research ethics boards and clinical ethics committees—followed by some comments concerning the various names applied to them. Then, in the next section, we shall review the composition of the bodies, along with ways to assign and remunerate members. We will conclude with a section on administrative and financial logistics. The administrative and financial logistics information, combined with the information obtained in section 2, will provide an index of the level of independence enjoyed by these fora for ethical thought.

Research Ethics Boards and Clinical Ethics Committees

We note at the outset that research ethics boards are more readily identifiable than clinical ethics committees. Indeed, the former are generally associated with universities, which usually have policies on human experimentation that determine the mandate, composition, and operation of their research ethics boards. We have used the documented policies of each university to prepare tables that set out the information that we have compiled, and these tables are found in appendix 3 of this report.

Research Ethics Boards

The first thing that becomes clear from a glance at university policies is that they all have the same objective—the protection of subjects used in research—but their approaches for achieving this vary. Some universities have adopted a succinct document that emphasizes a description of the structures established, whereas others describe their policies in detail, with guidelines that members of research ethics boards should follow when appraising protocols submitted to the board.

Although most universities refer to the guidelines issued by the Medical Research Council of Canada,[187] it is interesting to note the many different ways in which research ethics boards operate.[188] From the very outset, one can see that, depending on the size of the university, there may be one or several research ethics boards. Some universities have, therefore, established a liaison committee to coordinate the work of the research ethics boards at the various hospitals and research centres affiliated with the university, some of which, moreover, may have more than one research ethics board. On the other hand, some hospitals combine their efforts and submit their research protocols to a joint board, a practice that is sometimes followed because there are not enough protocols to justify the establishment of a board at each hospital, and sometimes because clinical trials are carried out on a multicentre basis. There are, therefore, many different structures.

Local ethics bodies vary not only in number, but also in name; this is particularly striking as the various names refer to the concept defined by the Medical Research Council of Canada. The name usually involves the term "ethics," accompanied by either "committee" or "board."[189] In some cases, research specifically on humans is referred to, clearly identifying the committee's area of responsibility. However, some institutions use a laconic name that leaves room for interpretation, such as "Screening Committee," "Joint Medical Ethics Committee" or "Ethics Committee."[190] In their defence, we recall that research ethics boards were established before official clinical ethics committees began to appear. As early as 1966, the Medical Research Council of Canada was asking for local ethical assessments before financing research projects,[191] but clinical ethics committees did not begin to proliferate[192] until the 1980s. University institutions did not deem it worthwhile, over the years, to change the names of their research ethics boards, probably because of the influence of existing practices. The use of the qualifier "déontologique" in French, or the expression "use of human subjects in research" in English, is no doubt also inherited from the era when the institutional policy was adopted. Indeed, some of these policies go back to the late 1970s or the early 1980s, and seem not to have been updated recently.

Whenever they were instituted, institutional policies stipulate that the oversight authority for the research ethics board of an institution be either the president or rector (of a university) or the board of directors (of a hospital).[193] There is usually a process to ensure that information, often an annual report, be sent to the senior authorities of the institution.

Clinical Ethics Committees

It is very difficult to list clinical ethics committees, partly because they were often established on the initiative of professional associations in hospitals and extended care facilities. Yet, as early as 1985, the Canadian Hospital Association[194] asked the Hospital Accreditation Council to consider requiring hospitals to have ethics committees.[195] In the 1992 edition of its standards, intended for a variety of institutions, including those with a short life span, the Canadian Council on Health Services Accreditation advocated the establishment of such committees.[196] This position definitely had something to do with the appearance of clinical ethics committees in hospitals, although the current process (1995) of accreditation visits does not specifically require such committees.[197] The impact of provincial hospital associations[198] and health ministries[199] must not be forgotten, as they too recommended the establishment of such committees.

There have already been four major studies[200] of clinical ethics committees, including the 1989 study by Janet Storch and Glenn Griener, who surveyed 70 clinical ethics committees in English-language hospitals with 300 or more beds.[201] As with research ethics boards, the names assigned to clinical ethics committees vary considerably.[202]

The Quebec study established a correlation between a hospital's size and whether it had a clinical ethics committee.[203] Some hospitals have a single local structure that combines the functions of a research ethics board and a clinical ethics committee.[204]

It is interesting to note that, in the papers that advocate the establishment of clinical ethics committees, readers are told how important it is to choose the oversight authority carefully.[205] This involves setting out the advantages and disadvantages of reporting to the hospital board of trustees or to a body such as the hospital's medical, dental, or pharmaceutical board. According to the study by Laval University's Groupe de recherche en éthique médicale (GREM),[206] the latter alternative was preferred by clinical ethics committees.

The reporting structure of an ethics committee is important, but its composition and the assignment of its members also have a key impact on its direction and its work.

Composition, Assignment, and Remuneration

An examination of an ethics body's composition, along with assignment and remuneration of members, often makes it possible to determine whether it exists simply to meet certain administrative requirements and, hence, is in danger of performing no more than a hollow role, or whether it can indeed perform its important function of deliberating on ethical matters. These parameters are crucial if the ethics body is to be credible and survive. These factors are a valuable source of information about how ethics bodies operate. A comparison of the two types of local ethics bodies will show that there are certain similarities between them.

Composition

Both for research ethics boards[207] and clinical ethics committees,[208] multi-disciplinarity is a sought-after characteristic that is apparent from the available data. It is equally clear, however, that members from the scientific and medical fields predominate over other areas of activity on both types of body. Clinical ethics committees often have a member trained in theology, philosophy or ethics, sometimes the chaplain.[209] Of those who are not part of the medical and scientific community, legal experts are most often sought to contribute to the work of the research or clinical ethics committee. Indeed, the legal expert is often one of the few committee members who is not part of the institution in question. Representation from the public is low, so low. Yet, six of the nine university policies that specify the composition of the research ethics board specifically require a member from the community.[210] At any rate, given the dynamics inherent in teamwork, a single community representative with no authority is unlikely to make much impact in a group of 10 to 12 members. And, although the need to designate a community member on local ethics bodies is revealing, the methods for selecting such persons are even more revealing.

Assignment

A reading of the university policies shows that members of research ethics boards are usually appointed, not elected. In some instances, appointments are made after consultation with deans or upon deans' recommendations.[211] Some key selection criteria are: the field in which the person works, followed by expertise in either the area of endeavour pursued by the institution or the type of research being reviewed in the protocol.

The surveys conducted by GREM and by Janet Storch indicate that members of clinical ethics committees are appointed by the authorities they report to, and are often selected by nomination.[212]

Remuneration

None of the university policies reviewed referred to the remuneration of members of research ethics boards. As Janet Storch says, members of these boards receive "little reward beyond academic satisfaction."[213] This also applies to members of clinical ethics committees, as authors of studies on such committees have never received any particular form of recompense.

Administrative and Financial Logistics

Even with the best of intentions, research ethics boards, like clinical ethics committees, cannot function effectively without administrative and financial support.

University policies on research involving human subjects say nothing about it but, at the very least, clerical support is essential. Generally speaking, the authority that established the research ethics board provides such support, usually by seconding someone for a specified period, often part time.

As for office space, apart from space required for the clerical staff, the ethics bodies do not usually have an office set aside solely for their activities, no matter how often they meet.

With respect to budgets, we note that a recent Quebec report asked research centers to be more generous in covering the costs inevitably involved in monitoring the research protocols carried out in the institution.[214]

So local ethics bodies are largely dependent on the oversight authority for their infrastructure. What needs to be determined is the influence of this situation on their activities.

Mission and Activities of Local Ethics Bodies

Everyone agrees that the purpose of local ethics bodies is to protect the dignity and rights of patients and research participants; it is, in other words, to ensure compliance with certain values. Broad ethical principles, such as human sanctity, individual right to exercise free will, charity, justice, and privacy, underpin the work of these bodies. Research ethics boards and clinical ethics committees are guided by the same ideals. However, their activities vary according to their respective missions.

Mission

Describing the mission of local ethics bodies amounts to examining their official mandate. As a rule, the mandate of a research ethics board is more clearly set out than the mandate of a clinical ethics committee. A research ethics board usually concentrates on ensuring that general ethical rules are applied to the types of research being carried out in the institution,[215] focusing on a specific area of activity, but a clinical ethics committee is required to deal with a host of situations arising from recent developments in medicine. The complexity of clinical ethics committees stems from this explosion of developments and from the variety of activities that may confront them.

Activities

In general, local ethics bodies focus on three major activities, namely consultation, education, and evaluation. These activities are not exclusive, but are shaped by the mandate assigned to the ethics body. Indeed, some committees or boards may act in all three areas to varying degrees, whereas others will be confined to one form of action.

Consultation

For research ethics boards, neither consultation, nor the advisory function, are predominant. In rare instances, a university will specifically assign this function.[216] Under these circumstances, a research ethics board can provide a service to members of the university community who may want to submit a research protocol and who wish to have further information; such a function, however, is related much more to the educational activity. The board may also serve as an agency that can suggest to the university authorities ways of amending the institutional policy. Proposed amendments would stem from the experience the board acquired in carrying out its primary function, which is to evaluate research protocols.

Clinical ethics committees, on the other hand, spend most of their time on consultation. They formulate opinions on a variety of medical practices in which ethical problems arise. These may appear at the individual level, such as problems within the doctor-patient relationship, or affect a whole population, such as the systematic screening for HIV or access to genetic tests. For the latter, the intervention of the clinical ethics committee would in all likelihood be requested by the hospital authorities; the opinions issued by the committee could be transformed into institutional policies if the authorities approved them. Otherwise, the opinions would have no coercive power; they would be intended as tools to help decision makers think about problems. Case-by-case recourse to a clinical ethics committee, often initiated by a health professional,[217] remains optional, as does the implementation of the opinion eventually put forward.[218]

Education

The second function of local ethics bodies is educational. This activity too, is more commonly found in clinical ethics committees than in research ethics boards. The importance of this function is clearly revealed in studies that assume clinical ethics committees are responsible for informing the various health care stakeholders about the ethical dimensions of decisions.[219] This task may take the form of conferences or seminars organized by the committees for all staff. Topics on which the committees have spent some time deliberating, or that are the focus of an institutional policy, will then be discussed.

Evaluation

This type of activity falls essentially within the purview of research ethics boards, which evaluate research projects to ensure that researchers respect the rights of subjects. Research ethics boards do not adopt standards and priorities to decide whether studies are appropriate, necessary, or desirable.[221] They have no such mandate. Research ethics boards review research protocols in the order in which they are received and do not necessarily compare them with protocols received before. In the event of any similarities, they may, of course, investigate the impact of the new protocol on the target population. Although approval by a research ethics board is necessary, it does not necessarily mean that financing from a granting agency will be automatic. Also, a research ethics board cannot assume that a protocol it had authorized and is currently under review by a granting agency, conflicts with a protocol the ethics board is examining. Each research protocol is reviewed independently.

The major Canadian granting agencies (the Medical Research Council of Canada [MRC], the Social Sciences and Humanities Research Council of Canada [SSHRC], and the Natural Sciences and Engineering Research Council [NSERC]), along with the provincial granting agencies and many foundations, require approval by a research ethics board. The Health Protection Branch of Health Canada also requires that an ethics board appraise any protocol to be used in developing drugs.[222] The pharmaceutical industry is, therefore, covered by this measure, which involves control by a research ethics board.

A research ethics board may accept, refuse or, more often than not, ask for changes to the protocol that has been submitted.[223] The decision is taken by consensus or by a vote of members.[224] Some universities have introduced an appeal mechanism to deal with cases in which the researcher is not satisfied with the research ethics board's decision.[225]

Under the Civil Code of Quebec, the decision authority of the research ethics board designated by the Minister of Health and Social Services is mitigated when the board reviews a research protocol that involves children or an adult with disabilities. After reviewing a file, the chair of the designated ethics board must hand down the board's decision in the form of a notice to the Minister; it is the Minister who issues the required authorization. Quebec legislation sets out criteria to guide research ethics boards in their decisions.[226]

Although we may consider it laudable that research ethics boards are enshrined in legislation with respect to research protocols involving "vulnerable" populations no matter what the source of funding, we must recognize at the same time that the board's authority is also restricted by the legislation.

Local medical ethics bodies, whether research ethics boards or clinical ethics committees, make an active contribution to the discussion process because they act as catalysts in the review of bioethical disputes. However, ethics matters are not confined to this area. Indeed, many professional bodies and associations have felt the need to establish an ethics body to help their members deal with the ethical problems that arise in their everyday work. Likewise, some provincial ministries have deemed it appropriate to establish advisory structures to advise them in policy formulation. These provincial and territorial deliberative bodies are discussed in the next section.

Section 2 – Provincial and Territorial Ethics Bodies

There are no provincial federations of local ethics committees and little communication among the committees.[227] There is, no doubt, some relationship between this and the committees' lack of uniformity. Provincial or territorial fora for ethical discussion are another matter. Ethical debate is sometimes organized by professional associations and corporations, sometimes by government commissions, councils or committees and, much more recently, by networks formed specifically to stimulate ethical reflection. There may be many fora and models, but the objective is the same: to suggest solutions to increasingly complex ethical problems generated by developments in the health sector.

Professional Bodies

The professional bodies of the medical field make a real contribution to discussions generated by ethical conflicts. Aware of their role in guaranteeing the quality of services delivered to the public, they make an effort to inform their members about the ethical dimensions of the situations they have to deal with. To do this, a professional body may print a regular feature in its journal[228] or discuss a controversial subject at its annual convention.[229] A professional code of ethics is often the cornerstone of positions taken by a professional body. Among the bodies that contribute to ethical reflections are the provincial hospital associations, some of which have published documents specifically addressing local ethics bodies with a view to making their presence felt in health institutions.[230] They do this to inform their members about these realities and to offer them an alternative way of dealing with ethical dilemmas they encounter in their institutions.

In addition to federations based on professional training, the workplace or interests shared by members, there are other ethics fora, such as the various research centres and groups.[231] Through their publications and the seminars, symposia, and meetings they organize or participate in, such centres and groups contribute to ethical discussions and supply information to persons concerned about the issues.

The large number of these bodies is, no doubt, one reason why it is difficult to gather information about them. At the moment, creating an exhaustive list of professional bodies that have ethics committees or subcommittees, whether standing or ad hoc, with a limited or broad mandate, would be a major undertaking.

Parallel to these various ethics fora, the initiative of establishing a working group to examine an ethical problem is also something that governments do. Such groups can take various forms.

Bodies Linked Directly to Provincial Governments

Bodies directly linked to provincial governments are grouped around two departments: health and justice. The law reform commissions usually confront the ethical concerns of justice departments.[232] Yet, law reform commissions cannot ignore the ethical dimension when they analyze such issues as living wills,[233] AIDS screening,[234] or the protection of persons with disabilities.[235] The fact remains, however, that the existence of law reform commissions does not automatically mean that governments will be aware of the ethical dimensions of their policies. Some law reform commissions do not consider health sector problems, focusing their efforts instead on areas such as business law. Most regrettable, as well, is the decision of the Province of Ontario to shut down its law reform commission.

A government that wishes to be well informed about ethical issues in the biomedical sector must obviously establish bodies that are closely linked to its health ministry. Some of these bodies are specifically established to promote medical research to improve public health.[236] Provincial funding agencies do not usually have research ethics boards to evaluate projects submitted for funding; this is left to the ethics board of the university concerned. However, these agencies may have internal committees that advise on policies to be adopted to set guidelines for certain activities (e.g., research using children), to correct wrongful conduct (such as conflicts of interest), and to harmonize their rules with the rules of similar agencies. Such committees, when tied specifically to funding agencies, are concerned both with protecting people who participate in research and with the scientific integrity of the investigators carrying out the research.

In the area of human research, we note the existence in Quebec of a provincial ethics committee established by the Minister of Health and Social Services pursuant to the Civil Code of Quebec.[237] The mandate of this committee is to evaluate research projects that meet two conditions: they must involve either minors or persons with disabilities who have reached the age of majority, and they must be carried out in an institution that lacks an ethics committee designated by the Minister. If the committee's opinion is favourable, it is forwarded to the Minister, who decides whether to authorize the research project. The committee is not attached to a university or hospital, and it covers private sector projects involving subjects who are minors or persons with disabilities who have reached the age of majority, because the source of project funding does not affect the committee's jurisdiction. It has no links with local ethics bodies. The provincial ethics committee meetings, whose frequency is a function of the number of research protocols to be reviewed, are held in the offices of the Fonds de la recherche en santé du Québec.

As research on humans is not the only area of activity that can generate ethical problems, the ministries of health find it appropriate to create commissions, councils, or committees to advise them. Some of these are formed for only a short time to address specific questions, and others eventually become permanent bodies where serious reflection on such issues is carried out. Some of these committees have an explicit mission regarding the ethical dimension of the issues submitted to them,[238] whereas this is not necessarily the case in the requests forwarded by the ministry to other committees. In the latter situation, several councils and committees may coexist.[239] This generates confusion with respect to roles and mandates, to say nothing of the fragmentation of ethical concerns among the many councils or committees established to provide advice on health policies. Their membership is varied, as are their mandates, even though the ultimate objectives converge toward the same ideal, which is to provide people with the best possible care.

In view of the multiplicity of fora for ethical discussion, and in response to the isolation felt by members of various local ethics bodies, a new structure intended to encourage contact and exchange has recently appeared—the ethics network.

Institutional Ethics Networks

Two Canadian provinces, Alberta and Quebec, have institutional ethics networks.[240] The first network appeared in 1994 in Quebec, established with a grant from the Fonds de la recherche en santé du Québec to encourage practitioners and researchers to work closely with social sciences and humanities professionals to "recognize, identify, analyze and address the institutional ethics issues and problems that exist in Quebec's health services."[241] The network comprises a coordination centre and six subject units: institutional ethics in medicine and surgery, institutional ethics in pediatrics, institutional ethics in psychiatry, institutional ethics in oncology and palliative care, institutional ethics in genetics, and the foundations of institutional ethics. The subject units are multidisciplinary and include varying numbers of experts, as many as 36 in some cases. The missions of the network are essentially advisory and educational. However, the organization of the network implies a coordination mission as well.

The Alberta Provincial Health Ethics Network was established in 1996. This multidisciplinary provincial agency under the authority of the Department of Health has a 12-person board.[242] Its extremely broad mandate combines coordination, information, education, and leadership with deliberative and advisory functions. It operates as an ethics consulting agency and facilitates the transmission of information and discussion on ethical dilemmas in health care.

Although the Quebec and Alberta ethics networks have similar names and missions, the manner in which they were established and the way in which they operate are quite different. For example, the Quebec network is a bottom-up organization that owes its existence to researchers who obtained a grant to establish it, whereas the Alberta network is a creature of government. The mandate of the Alberta network is also broader than that of the Quebec network.[243]

A closer look shows that the Alberta Provincial Health Ethics Network resembles the British Columbia Advisory Committee on Ethical Issues in Health Care.[244] Both come under the authority of the Department or Ministry of Health. In addition, the same number of persons is closely involved in implementing their mandates. However, they have different procedures for referral. In Alberta, a health professional may request an opinion from the Provincial Health Ethics Network, which functions as an ethics advisory agency for those without access to ethics resources. This does not appear to be possible in British Columbia, because health professionals and the Advisory Committee on Ethical Issues in Health Care do not interact directly.

Our account shows that bodies at both the local and provincial levels are many and varied; hence, no doubt, the inevitable observation concerning the lack of communication among them, whatever their level. And yet the ethical problems of the biomedical sector display similarities that would certainly benefit from a richer exchange of information and resources. Local and provincial bodies do not seem capable of meeting the need for communication and coordination. What of federal bodies?

Section 3 – Pan-Canadian Ethics Bodies

The national dynamic for stimulating ethical reflection is comparable to that at the local and provincial levels; for example, the development plan for structures dedicated to discussing ethical issues is similar. Both provincially and nationally, no associations of ethics bodies operate at lower levels. Furthermore, regional or provincial ethics bodies do not link local and national ethics bodies. Local ethics bodies, like provincial ethics bodies, are isolated. As a result, the examination of ethical problems takes many and complex routes.

Leading the national ethics debate are Canadian professional associations and agencies directly linked to the federal government, and another well-known participant involved in human research, the National Council on Bioethics in Human Research. Again, we must recognize that diversity and multiplicity are characteristic of the preferred fora for ethical reflection.

Canadian Associations

According to the director of the department of ethics of the Canadian Medical Association,[245] the CMA is the only Canadian professional association to have a permanent ethics committee, the creation of which is provided for in the CMA's bylaws.[246] In addition, some of its member associations, for example the Canadian Psychiatric Association, have created their own ethics committees. Therefore, as part of the current revision of the CMA's code of ethics,[247] the department of ethics is preparing a directory of ethics committees in the various sectors.

The Royal College of Physicians and Surgeons of Canada and the College of Family Physicians of Canada also promote awareness of the ethical problems doctors encounter in their practices. The CFPC assigned its ethics committee to study the ethical implications of health sector reforms.[248] The biomedical ethics committee of the RCPSC initiated the inclusion of bioethics education in resident training programs, a significant change.[249]

Doctors are not the only health professionals who are becoming concerned about general and specific ethical issues in their areas of practice. The Canadian Nurses Association chose to create ad hoc committees to meet specific needs. The reports produced by these working groups, or resulting documents, are distributed to members.[250] As observed at the regional and provincial levels, the annual meetings of Canadian professional associations also encourage members to discuss problems related to ethics in their analyses.

With respect to health institutions, the Canadian Hospital Association and the Catholic Health Association of Canada aim to stimulate ethical reflection using (among other methods) their publications.[251]

In addition, there has been a groundswell of associations of individuals wishing to share their interest in ethical questions, including the Canadian Bioethics Society, now in its eighth year of operation. It is a multidisciplinary society, and its 500 members[252] include health professionals, ethicists, legal scholars, and members of ethics committees from across Canada. The CBS organizes an annual public conference to promote discussion on a theme corresponding to immediate concerns in the health sector.

Moreover, since 1994, some individuals have had access to a new communications method to share perspectives on ethical problems. Exchanges are now possible on a network managed by the Centre of Applied Ethics at the University of British Columbia (BIOETHNET). Network start-up was funded by a SSHRC grant to facilitate research on ethics by its members. It is not intended for undergraduate students, or the public in general, or as a consultation service for health professionals.[253]

The goal of this brief overview, which is far from complete, is to illustrate the range and continuing emergence of national associations and fora for discussion on ethics. Such interest in the ethical nature of issues resulting from biomedical advances is not exclusive to these associations; agencies directly linked to the federal government also share this interest.

Agencies Directly Linked to the Federal Government

Until now, when the Canadian government was confronted with ethical problems resulting from or exacerbated by scientific advances, it chose to create working groups on the model of a national ethics body defined in the first part of this document. In response to growth in new reproductive technologies, the government created the Royal Commission on New Reproductive Technologies.[254] Confronted with the AIDS epidemic, in 1987 it created, among others, the Federal Centre for AIDS, with its offices and working groups.[255] In response to legal problems related to euthanasia and assisted suicide,[256] the Senate of Canada mandated a special committee to examine the issue.[257] This is an ad hoc and fragmented approach because problems are addressed piecemeal, as the need for specific reflection is acknowledged. One can only wonder at the consequences of such an approach. However, problems associated with research involving human subjects are given more consistent consideration by the funding agencies.

We have selected two of these diverse federal agencies—the Medical Research Council of Canada (MRC) and the National Research Council of Canada (NRC)—to demonstrate that, although they have similar missions (i.e., to promote scientific development through techniques such as experimentation on human subjects), their difference lies in their approach to ensuring respect for ethical values.

We chose the MRC because it is the main federal agency responsible for promoting and supporting health sciences research and because it is a leader in the development of the guidelines currently used when examining the ethics of research projects involving human subjects.[258] As already mentioned in the description of local ethics bodies, ethical considerations have long been a concern of the MRC.[259] These concerns gave rise to the guidelines used by the research ethics boards responsible for studying the ethics of projects seeking MRC funding. The MRC does not evaluate the projects itself, but abides by the decision of local bodies, a reason why providing guidance in their project analysis process is so important. The Council also has a standing committee to recommend changes to its guidelines that take into account new advances and problems resulting from those advances.[260] In 1994, with two other Canadian funding agencies, SSHRC and NSERC, the MRC agreed to produce joint guidelines applicable to all projects involving research on human subjects funded by any of the three agencies. A working group was formed for this purpose and produced a preliminary report[261] that is currently under consultation. In summary, the MRC recommends active participation by the scientific community and promotes respect for ethical values through a devolution of responsibility to local ethics bodies, i.e., research ethics boards.

To establish a parallel,[262] we chose the NRC, which has a mandate to support research into new technologies that may improve Canadians' quality of life. Pursuant to its policy, any activity conducted or financed by the NRC, including projects funded by the Industrial Research Assistance Program (IRAP) must meet the same strict ethical standards that the NRC has defined for itself.[263] If an NRC project is approved by or conducted in the NRC laboratories, and is deemed in advance to be scientifically valid, the NRC's Ethics Committee for Research on Human Subjects evaluates the project. Even if the project has been reviewed by a local ethics body, it is reevaluated by the NRC's ethics committee.[264] However, this is not done automatically for IRAP when technical and financial support is asked for.[265] In that situation, the local ethics-in-research committee may play an important role.

Thus, the primary interest of the MRC and the NRC is to protect research subjects by requiring that researchers respect the dignity and rights of any individual who participates in their projects. Even if the ultimate objective is the same, the preferred method for attaining that objective is not, despite the considerable contribution of local ethics-in-research committees.

National Council on Bioethics in Human Research

As we have just seen, the MRC plays an important part in developing standards for research involving human subjects. It also had a determining role in the creation of the National Council on Bioethics in Human Research (NCBHR). The need for this agency became apparent during amendments to the 1978 version of the MRC guidelines.[266] It required the application of the new guidelines[267] for all projects involving human subjects, and a uniform interpretation and implementation of those guidelines across Canada. However, because the MRC was funding barely 50 percent of medical research at that time, it seemed more appropriate that the Royal College of Physicians and Surgeons of Canada (RCPSC) take the lead, because most research projects using human subjects are clinical studies.[268] For this reason, in 1989, the RCPSC established the NCBHR at the request of the MRC and with funding from the MRC and Health and Welfare Canada.[269] Its primary mission is to maintain high ethical standards in biomedical research involving human subjects. To attain this objective, the NCBHR must interpret and promote guidelines related to ethics; advise researchers, funding agencies, and research ethics boards; and, finally, inform health professionals and the public about the ethics of biomedical research.[270] Concretely, in addition to organizing workshops on issues relevant to research ethics boards,[271] publishing reports[272] and a newsletter, the NCBHR provides a consulting service that evaluates research ethics boards. From 1990 to 1993, the NCBHR toured all Canadian faculties of medicine;[273] the analysis of the data gathered was published in a report presented at a workshop and distributed in a special edition of the *NCBHR Communiqué*,[274] in which the NCBHR makes recommendations for improving the functioning of research ethics boards.

Initially, in 1989, the NCBHR comprised 12 representatives from key clinical research organizations and four members of the general public.[275] The RCPSC appointed five members, two from its Research Committee and three from its Biomedical Ethics Committee. In addition, the Canadian Medical Association (CMA), the Association of Canadian Medical Colleges, the College of Family Physicians of Canada (CFPC), the Canadian Nurses Association, the Canadian Society for Clinical Investigation, and Health and Welfare Canada each had a seat on the NCBHR. The President of the MRC or his delegate served as an ex officio member.[276] By 1992, in the second edition of the brochure describing the NCBRHC, under the heading "Members," a member of the community has been added and the MRC is no longer shown separately from the other agencies.[277] Another difference between the two versions concerns the method of appointing those individuals: in 1992, the participation of a NCBHR Nominating Committee[278] was expressly mentioned, which was not the case in the previous version of the brochure.

In 1993, the NCBHR was externally evaluated. In the evaluation report, completed in 1994, the committee recommended expanding the NCBHR mandate to include social sciences and health research.[279] In June 1995, an NCBHR resolution was adopted to that end. This revised mandate resulted in changes to the composition of the NCBHR; for example, SSHRC and NSERC are now represented. When its mandate was revised, an NCBHR Coordinating Committee was created.[280]

The widening of the mandate and the accompanying revision of guidelines applicable to research on human subjects is significant.[281] In addition, the new attributes of the NCBHR[282] give more formal recognition to its role as a link between research ethics boards.[283] However, this role as a catalyst is limited to the research sector and, probably, to universities.

This overview of local, regional, provincial, and national ethics bodies illustrates the exponential growth in reflection on ethics in Canada. The fora for discussion are many, complex, and often unable to communicate with similar or complementary structures. This state of affairs results in a dissipation of energy through duplication of effort and fragmentation of analysis because the limited mandate prevents ethics bodies from developing a global vision. In our conclusion, we will present the various methods available for coordinating ethical reflection in Canada, taking into account the specifics of the Canadian situation and the experience of other countries.

PART III – CONCLUSION

This reflection on the relevance of creating a national ethics agency is part of a growing international awareness of the problems caused by advances in life sciences and health. That said, and having presented the experiences of other countries and described the existing bodies in Canada, it is still premature to recommend the establishment of a national ethics body without first examining the capacity to implement any such recommendation. Over and above the purely institutional aspect, the feasibility and usefulness of a national biomedical ethics agency cannot be examined without a review of the restrictions arising from the Canadian constitutional context. We then summarize the advantages and disadvantages of the various existing alternatives for meeting the need for coordination of the growth in ethical reflection. Finally, in order to promote the discussion of ethics in Canada, we highlight the critical points to which particular attention must be paid, regardless of the model selected.

Section 1 – A Canadian Reality: Our Political System

In a country like Canada, the existence and, above all, the effectiveness of a national ethics body are influenced by the legitimacy of the powers granted to the initiating authority. As a result, it is essential to examine Canadian constitutional law and how it allocates jurisdiction. Sections 91 and 92 of the Constitution Act, 1867[284] list the areas of jurisdiction granted to Parliament and the provincial legislatures.

Biomedical ethics, like other new areas of study, are obviously not subject to the specific provisions of the Constitution of 1867 or amendments to it. They are related to the area of public health, however, and they challenge it, hence the relevance of examining where jurisdiction for biomedical ethics lies.[285]

Provincial Jurisdiction

First, subsection 92(7) of the Constitution Act, 1867 grants the provinces exclusive jurisdiction over health care services (the establishment, maintenance, and management of hospitals, asylums, charities, and eleemosynary institutions).

This jurisdiction, together with that stated in subsection 92(16) of the Constitutional Act, 1867, which involves all matters of a merely local or private nature, explains why general jurisdiction over health has traditionally devolved to the provinces.[286] Several decisions have recognized provincial jurisdiction over health, although the act addresses the local aspect of health.[287]

Federal Jurisdiction

Even so, provincial jurisdiction over health does not exclude the possibility of the federal Parliament having recourse to powers granted it under the Constitution to legislate on certain areas of public health, probably including biomedical ethics.

Such federal intervention, although certainly limited, could be based on the general power of the federal Parliament to make laws for the peace, order and good government, be accessory to the powers stipulated in section 91 of the Constitution Act, 1867, or even arise from spending powers.

Peace, Order and Good Government[288]

The opening paragraph to section 91 of the Constitution Act, 1867[289] grants the federal Parliament residual jurisdiction.[290] Thus, the federal Parliament has emergency powers, but the resulting intervention may be only temporary and, therefore, not suited to an issue such as biomedical ethics.

The federal Parliament can also use the theory of "national dimensions". This approach would, no doubt, be more suitable, because, as pointed out by professors Brun and Tremblay, "widely applied, this could even allow the federal Parliament to interfere in provincial jurisdiction at will if it deems that an issue has national scope; it could then grant itself jurisdiction that it can exercise on a permanent basis, contrary to the definition of emergency powers."[291] However, if this theory is to apply, the issues involved must exceed local or provincial scope and fundamentally "concern the country as a whole."[292] To qualify as such, an issue must meet the criteria stated by Justice Le Dain in *R. v. Crown Zellerbach Canada Ltd.*, that is, "a singleness, distinctiveness and indivisibility that clearly distinguishes it from matters of provincial concern and a scale of impact on provincial jurisdiction that is reconcilable with the fundamental distribution of legislative power under the Constitution."[293] But does biomedical ethics meet all these criteria?

Exclusive Federal Jurisdiction

The approximately 30 categories of issues listed in section 91 of the Constitution Act, 1867 fall within exclusive federal jurisdiction. Some of them could probably serve as bases for possible federal legislative measures in the area of health, including bioethics. For example, one has only to think of federal jurisdiction in the areas of criminal law (subsection 91[27]), trade and commerce (subsection 92[2]), or taxation (subsection 91[3]).

Protection of the public has already been recognized as one of the "customary objectives" of criminal law, and this power may be exercised to protect the public against a "harmful or undesirable effect."[294] Such jurisdiction over criminal law also gives the federal control over pharmaceutical products[295] and led to the Food and Drugs Act[296] and the Narcotics Control Act.[297] Recently, in *RJR-MacDonald Inc. v. Canada (AG)*, Justice La Forest pointed out that

> the scope of the federal power to create criminal legislation with respect to health matters is broad, and is circumscribed only by the requirements that the legislation must contain a prohibition accompanied by a penal sanction and must be directed at a legitimate public health evil. If a given piece of federal legislation contains these features, and if that legislation is not otherwise a "colourable" intrusion upon provincial jurisdiction, then it is valid as criminal law.[298]

Federal jurisdiction over the regulation of trade and commerce, unlike jurisdiction in the area of criminal law, is generally subject to restrictive interpretation. Although the courts recognize that Parliament can regulate interprovincial and international trade and exchanges that affect Canada as a whole, it is still not authorized to regulate the operations of a particular industry or area of trade.[299] Nevertheless, it is possible to envisage federal regulations addressing the interprovincial and international aspects of biomedical ethics issues, such as the commercial aspects of research involving human subjects or the trade in tissues and organs.

With respect to federal jurisdiction in the area of taxation, it should be pointed out that this could serve as a basis for a program of tax incentives to encourage individuals and companies involved in research on human subjects to respect standards or guidelines. Such an approach was recommended to the Royal Commission on New Reproductive Technologies.[300]

Other Areas of Jurisdiction and Powers

Other areas of federal jurisdiction, such as spending power and the prerogative to enter into international treaties, although not explicitly stated in the areas of jurisdiction listed in section 91 of the Constitution Act, 1867, would also merit consideration. It should be remembered that federal spending power,[301] defined as Parliament's authority to "pay certain amounts to individuals, organizations and governments, the purposes over which Parliament does not necessarily have legislative powers,"[302] allow the federal Parliament to implement programs in areas of provincial jurisdiction.[303]

At a time when the feasibility and usefulness of a national advisory body on biomedical ethics is being examined, the constitutional implications of such a project cannot be ignored, particularly with respect to the sharing of legislative powers by Parliament and the provincial legislatures. Although merely granting powers for joint action and deliberation to such a body is not in itself a threat to the provinces' regulatory powers, the logical consequences of such a process must still be taken into consideration. What will happen to "recommendations" arising from the agency's work, particularly when they involve the adoption of new measures, sometimes legislative, in unexplored areas?

Over and above constitutional considerations, it must be acknowledged that ethical reflection calls upon fundamental values that all Canadians share.[304] In addition, discussions on ethics do not necessarily result in legislative intervention. However, because cooperation and joint action foster productive discussion, such an attitude should be promoted. We will look at the various models experimented with in other countries and summarize each of them to identify the one most likely to satisfy these expectations.

Section 2 – Summary of Models Observed

It must be admitted at the outset that no model is perfect and each has advantages and disadvantages that we have outlined in a diagram to facilitate comparison.[305]

Even if the status quo allows for great flexibility and consideration of local characteristics and the expression of the plurality of ideas, we still have a complex, heterogeneous system marked by a lack of coordination, poor distribution of information, and a sectorial approach that is often reactive.

Another approach is the national ethics committee, a centralized forum for discussion. At first glance, it may seem ideal because it allows for ongoing reflection and the establishment of consistent positions, largely the result of the permanence, autonomy, and greater legitimacy that arise from its institutionalization. However, given the context of the Canadian Constitution and the disappointing experience of federal countries such as Australia, it does not appear to be the ideal formula.

National ethics boards, with more flexible structures, have the advantage of being created as they are needed. Their mandates, for a specific issue or period, permit a faster, more thorough assessment of the problem being studied, but ethical reflection is fragmented, ad hoc, and can even lead to the issuing of varying opinions by concomitant national ethics bodies.

Finally, what is it about the model of the permanent conference of ethics committees that was recently adopted in Europe? Again, this is a flexible system that, being solely an assembly of committees, is less likely to raise constitutional problems. It also has the advantage of promoting participation, encouraging the exchange of information, and stimulating the search for consensus. However, its effectiveness and permanence require a level of organization that may be difficult to ensure. In addition, due to the multiplicity and diversity of current ethics bodies, it would be difficult to appoint—and, in some cases, justify—representatives to such a permanent ethics committee. Perhaps this model can only be established later, once the essential preliminary step of coordinating existing bodies has been taken.

In these circumstances, there is no doubt a place for improving on the current situation and setting up a Canadian institute for bioethics information and coordination. Such an institute, responsible for gathering, managing, and distributing information, would meet an observed need in Canada: responding to the fragmentation of and explosive growth in ethical reflection. In addition to such a role, the institute could be given a mandate to advise the prime minister, to whom it would be responsible, on the need to conduct studies on specific subjects. This recommendation could result from the compilation of documents stating that a need exists, or from a list of subjects determined by the Federal-Provincial-Territorial Conference of Deputy Ministers of Health. It could even be possible to extend the institute's mandate to include a coordination role to structure specific studies. Following a call for proposals, the proposals submitted by teams composed of representatives from two or more provinces would be peer evaluated. In addition, the institute would be required to make public the results of such studies in order to promote the distribution of information. Thus, the institute could, based on the extent of its mandate, (1) centralize existing information, (2) stimulate reflection on ethical problems and, finally, (3) oversee studies on specific themes.

Whatever form the ethics body takes, and independent of the model selected, there are certain overriding parameters.

Section 3 – Elements Critical to the Smooth Functioning of a National Ethics Committee

These elements fall into five categories: the nature of the mandate, the link to the initiating authority, composition, the method of appointing members, and available resources.

First, before selecting any form for an ethics body, the extent of its mandate must be determined. Should clinical and research ethics be combined? As we have seen, these two areas of application are often studied by separate bodies. Nevertheless, the move from science to medical practice is accelerating and the gap between the two is narrowing. Clarity is, therefore, an essential prerequisite to fulfilment of a mandate.

Similarly, the link to the initiating authority is a determining factor in accomplishing the mandate. It must be well established and ensure that it grants the autonomy necessary to prevent biased reflection.

We come now to the composition of the body. Who participates in the work? Should representativeness or expertise take precedence? The first may lead to a large organization in which, despite efforts to the contrary, all groups are not always present. The second risks ossifying ethical reflection, particularly if there is no mechanism for renewing the membership, and may also affect the method of member selection.

In a democratic and pluralistic society such as ours, should members be elected or appointed? These are not trivial questions, since the composition and method of appointing members have, in some countries (e.g., Belgium), produced problems with implementing the committee.

Finally, the functioning of an ethics body also depends on the resources available to it. Lacking resources, the ethics body will be unable to fulfil its mandate. Even willing participants cannot perform their duties without the necessary support.

This is a brief summary of the factors to consider when evaluating the creation of a national ethics consulting agency. We believe that the status quo does not meet the need for ethical reflection on problems arising from advances in health and the life sciences. None of the models examined corresponds perfectly to Canadian reality; hence our suggestion that the current situation be improved by implementing a Canadian institute for bioethics information and coordination.

It cannot be denied that ethics is part of prudent decision making, and it is therefore important to acknowledge that, like any prudent decision, it "is not exempt from debate because (it) is ultimately the result of research involving trial and error, hesitation, discussion and argument."[306] Hence, the importance of an information and coordination infrastructure that allows such debate to take place.

Thérèse Leroux, *B.Sc., Ph.D., L.L.B., is an associate professor in the Faculty of Law and a researcher at the Centre de recherche en droit public at the University of Montreal. Her work focuses, among other subjects, on the legal and ethical perspectives of testing new drugs on humans, on xenotransplantation, and on public protection regarding biotechnology products. She is a member of hospital, university, institutional, and provincial clinical and research ethics boards. Ms. Leroux also serves on the National Council on Bioethics in Human Research and on the Canadian Council on Animal Care.*

Sonia Le Bris, *L.L.M., is a researcher at the Centre de recherche en droit public at the University of Montreal. She specializes in comparative medical law and, for almost ten years, has been interested in the issues surrounding reproductive medicine, in alternative methods of biotechnology regulation and, more recently, in the relationships between ethics, deontology, and law. Ms. Le Bris worked as a consultant for the Council of Europe, the European Commission, and the Canadian Human Genome Project. She teaches medical law, health law, and alternative methods of biotechnology regulation. In 1993, she was the author of the first comparative study on national ethics bodies, sponsored by the Council of Europe.*

Bartha Maria Knoppers, *Ph.D., is counsel to the firm of McMaster Meighen, a professor in the Faculty of Law at the University of Montreal, and a senior researcher at the Centre de recherche en droit public. She has served as an expert to committees of the World Health Organization and the National Institutes of Health. She is currently chair of the International Ethics Committee of the Human Genome Project, and a member of the International Bioethics Committee of UNESCO. In 1995, Dr. Knoppers became chair of Social Issues Committee of the American Society of Human Genetics and, in 1996, chair of the Organizing Committee of the First International Conference on DNA Sampling Human Genetic Research: Ethical, Legal and Policy Aspects, held in Montreal.*

Acknowledgements

The authors are grateful for the collaboration of all those who responded to our requests for information. The data gathered in this way helped us improve the quality of the report we produced.

We also express our sincere gratitude to Cécile Dubeau for the efforts of the secretariat, and to Édith-Geneviève Giasson, Marie-Angèle Grimaud and Jean-François Noël, who assisted in the production of this report.

NOTES*

1. Jacques DELORS, opening address at the conference "Droits de l'homme et Communauté européenne: vers 1992 et au-delà" [Human Rights and the European Community: Toward 1992 and Beyond], Strasbourg. November 20–21, 1989. [translation]

2. Christian BYK and Gérard MÉMETEAU, *Le droit des comités d'éthique*, Collection médecine et droit (Paris: Éditions Alexandre Lacassagne and Éditions Eska, 1996); Sonia LE BRIS, *Les instances nationales d'éthique* (Strasbourg: Les Éditions du Conseil de l'Europe, 1993); OFFICE OF TECHNOLOGY ASSESSMENT, *Biomedical Ethics in U.S. Public Policy* (Washington, D.C.: U.S. Government Printing Office, 1993).

3. For example, the 1987 Group of Seven Summit included an international bioethics symposium on the topic "Towards an International Ethic for Research with Human Beings." See also various guidelines of the Medical Research Council of Canada (MRC), the work of the National Council on Bioethics in Human Research (NCBHR), and the work of the Royal Commission on New Reproductive Technologies.

4. LAW REFORM COMMISSION OF CANADA, *Toward a Canadian Advisory Council on Biomedical Ethics—Study Paper* (Ottawa: Law Reform Commission of Canada, 1990).

5. CANADIAN BAR ASSOCIATION, *What's Law Got to Do with It? Health Care Reform in Canada* (Ottawa: Canadian Bar Association, 1994).

6. UNITED NATIONS, WORLD CONFERENCE ON HUMAN RIGHTS, "Declaration and Program of Action," Vienna, June 14–25, 1993, Part I, ss. 11, par. 3. Cited in COMITÉ INTERNATIONAL DE BIOÉTHIQUE DE L'UNESCO, *Actes 1995*, vol. 1, p. 6.

7. For more information, please refer to tables 1A, 1B, and 1C in the appendices.

8. And more specifically, Ethics and Research, Ethics and Information, Ethics and Socio-Economic Aspects. For a succinct presentation of the work of this International Ethics Committee on AIDS, see Christian BYK and Gérard MÉMETEAU, *Le droit des comités d'éthique*. Collection médecine et droit. Paris: Éditions Alexandre Lacassagne and Éditions Eska, 1996, 291–292.

9. To be convinced of the "ethics activity" of the World Medical Association, one has but to consult the collection of the declarations it has adopted since its creation, in WORLD MEDICAL ASSOCIATION, *Handbook of Declarations* (Ferney-Voltaire, France: World Medical Association, September 1995).

10. The World Health Organization entrusts to its working groups the task of developing ideas about specific subjects that raise ethical or legal issues within its various programs. This was notably the case with genetic developments. For an example of this concept, see D. WERTZ, J. FLETCHER and K. BERG, *Guidelines*

---

* Sources are complete as of December 31, 1996.

on Ethical Issues in Medical Genetics and the Provision of Genetic Services (Geneva: Hereditary Diseases Programme, World Health Organization, 1995).

11. For a list of CIOMS activities related to bioethics, see Z. BANKOWSKI, "Éthique et santé," *Forum mondial de la santé* 16 (1995), 125–130.

12. For a more general presentation of the role of international organizations in health, see Sonia LE BRIS, "Les organisations internationales et la médecine moderne: promotion ou protection des droits de la personne?" *Médecine moderne et droits de la personne*, ed. Lucie LAMARCHE (Ste-Foy: Laval University Press), p. 17.

13. COUNCIL OF EUROPE, *Proceedings of the Standing Conference of European Ethics Committees* (Strasbourg: Directorate of Legal Affairs, 1994) Doc. CDBI/CPCNE, Acte 1.

14. UNESCO, "L'UNESCO et la bioéthique." Internal document, October 26, 1992.

15. Christian BYK and Gérard MÉMETEAU, *Le droit des comités d'éthique*, Collection médecine et droit (Paris: Éditions Alexandre Lacassagne and Éditions Eska, 1996), 289.

16. Christian BYK and Gérard MÉMETEAU, *Le droit des comités d'éthique*, Collection médecine et droit (Paris: Éditions Alexandre Lacassagne and Éditions Eska, 1996), 289. [translation]

17. N. LENOIR, "Les États et le droit de la bioéthique," *Revue de droit sanitaire et social* 31 (2): 257–270 (1995).

18. UNESCO, Resolution 25 C/5.2, para. 1(a), 1989; see also 24 C/13.1 and 25 C/7.3.

19. UNESCO, General Conference, 27th session, 1993. Doc. 27 C/45, p. 9.

The General Conference,

Bearing in mind the Universal Declaration of Human Rights, the International Covenants on Human Rights and international conventions for the protection of human rights, in particular the United Nations Convention on the Elimination of all Forms of Discrimination against Women and the United Nations Convention on the Rights of the Child,

Recalling 24 C/Resolution 13.1, 25 C/Resolution 5.2 and 25 C/Resolution 7.3 urging the Organization to promote and develop ethical studies, and the actions arising out of them, on the consequences of scientific and technological progress in the biomedical field, within the framework of respect for human rights and freedoms,

Recognizing the need to ensure the participation of all in the advances of the biomedical and life sciences and in the resultant benefits, with due regard for the freedom, dignity and identity of the human person,

Aware of the increasing scale, at the international level, of the ethical debate on progress in the control of the human genome, and of the essentially cultural and educational dimension of bioethics, which is in line with the purposes of the Organization,

Having examined the 'Study submitted by the Director-General concerning the possibility of drawing up an international instrument for the protection of the human genome' (27 C/45),

1. Approves the establishment by the Director-General of the International Bioethics Committee;

2. Invites the Director-General to continue in 1994–1995 the preparation of an international instrument on the protection of the human genome and to report to the General Conference at its twenty-eight session on the implementation of this resolution.

20. N. LENOIR, "Les États et le droit de la bioéthique," *Revue de droit sanitaire et sociale* 31(2): 257–270 (1995).

21. N. LENOIR, "Les États et le droit de la bioéthique," *Revue de droit sanitaire et social* 31(2): 257–270 (1995).

22. For a summary description of the COUNCIL OF EUROPE, see Council of Europe, *Le Conseil de l'Europe: activités et réalisations* (Strasbourg: Public Relations Service, 1996). For a history of the involvement of the Council of Europe in bioethics, see A. ROGERS and D. DURAND DE BOUSINGEN, *Une bioéthique pour l'Europe* (Strasbourg: Les éditions du Conseil de l'Europe, 1995), 219–225.

23. For a summary description of the EU, see Jean RIDEAU, *Droit institutionnel de l'Union et des communautés européennes* (Paris: L.G.D.J., 1994).

24. Christian BYK and Gérard MÉMETEAU, *Le droit des comités d'éthique*, Collection médecine et droit (Paris: Éditions Alexandre Lacassagne and Éditions Eska, 1996), 278.

25. We must qualify the comments of Byk and Mémeteau. The Council of Europe is essentially a forum for discussion and considerations to promote harmonization of legislation. It does not have the same powers and prerogatives as the European Union, in the sense that the states remain entirely free to choose whether to follow the recommendations of the two executive bodies of the Council of Europe, namely, its Committee of Ministers and its Parliamentary Assembly. On the other hand, and precisely because the functions of the Council of Europe are based on unrestrained discussion and the complete freedom of states, it is a privileged, avant-garde forum for discussing particularly delicate and controversial subjects, such as bioethics. For information on the work of the Council of Europe on bioethics, see the document produced by the Directorate of Legal Affairs, *Texts of the Council of Europe on Bioethical matters*, (Strasbourg: Directorate of Legal Affairs, 1993).

26. On this point too, Byk and Mémeteau seem categorical. The power of the European Union is certainly limited in the area of health; nevertheless, for the first time, under article 129 of the Treaty of Maastricht, its authority is recognized in the area of public health, as part of the EU's mission to contribute to the creation of a high level of health protection. The EU's power is not absolute, however; it is limited to coordination and does not extend to regulation. This means, in effect, that there is no obligation to harmonize laws and regulations in the area of health or, therefore, of bioethics. See Sonia LE BRIS, "Les organisations internationales et la médecine moderne: promotion ou protection des droits de la personne?" in *Médecine moderne et droits de la personne*, ed. Lucie LAMARCHE (Sainte-Foy: Laval University Press), p. 17. Also, in the context of the European Union, a fourth program of community action for research, technological development, and demonstration (1994–1998), medical ethics is one of the action themes of the biomedicine and health program (Doc. COM [94] 68 final, Brussels, March 30, 1994, p. 271).

27. For a presentation of the European Commission's various activities in bioethics, see EUROPEAN COMMISSION, GENERAL SECRETARIAT, *Activités de la Commission européenne en matière de bioéthique* (Brussels, 1994).

28. EUROPEAN COMMISSION COMMUNICATION, "Promoting the Competitive Environment for the Industrial Activities based on Bioethics within the Community" (sec. [91] 629 final) (Brussels, 1994).

29. Christian BYK and Gérard MÉMETEAU, *Le droit des comités d'éthique*, Collection médecine et droit, (Paris: Éditions Alexandre Lacassagne and Éditions Eska, 1996), 288.

30. EUROPEAN COMMISSION, *Group of Advisers to the European Commission on the Ethical Implications of Biotechnology* (Luxembourg: Office for Official Publications of the European Communities, 1996), 9.

31. EUROPEAN COMMISSION, *Group of Advisers to the European Commission on the Ethical Implications of Biotechnology* (Luxembourg: Office for Official Publications of the European Communities, 1996), 12.

32. EUROPEAN COMMISSION, *Group of Advisers to the European Commission on the Ethical Implications of Biotechnology* (Luxembourg: Office for Official Publications of the European Communities, 1996), 8.

33. EUROPEAN COMMISSION, *Group of Advisers to the European Commission on the Ethical Implications of Biotechnology* (Luxembourg: Office for Official Publications of the European Communities, 1996), 10. Since its creation in 1991, the GAEB has rendered six opinions bearing on the ethical implications of biotechnologies, and several other opinions are currently in preparation. Apart from advice on specific questions raised by biotechnology, the GAEB has developed a series of ethical principles based on its case-by-case method of working. Generally, the GAEB tries to emphasize an ethic of responsibility "based on respect for the fundamental rights of Europe's citizens." More specifically, the group emphasizes ethical principles such as human dignity; freedom of opinion and scientific work (but limited by the preceding principle); the assessment of risks and results of biotechnological progress; the public's right to safe products and services of decent quality; the safeguarding biological diversity; and the right of the public to be clearly and fully informed. One notes also the importance the group gives to the socioeconomic context of the European Commission's activities. In effect, if ethics is to be integral to the politics and development of the sectors concerned, one must also insist on "the need for genuine ethics teaching." As to whether it is appropriate to legislate with respect to the questions under study, the GAEB treats that aspect in "the light of ethical imperatives linked to Community responsibilities, with due account being taken of the subsidiarity principle."

34. A. ROGERS and D. DURAND DE BOUSINGEN, *Une bioéthique pour l'Europe* (Strasbourg: Les éditions du Conseil de l'Europe, 1995), 221.

35. A. ROGERS and D. DURAND DE BOUSINGEN, *Une bioéthique pour l'Europe* (Strasbourg: Les éditions du Conseil de l'Europe, 1995), 223. The distinction between an ad hoc committee and a steering committee, according to the statutes of the Council of Europe, is neither neutral nor devoid of meaning, as the status of a steering committee gives it a permanent character and additional powers. In a way, this gives it greater legitimacy.

36. Christian BYK and Gérard MÉMETEAU, *Le droit des comités d'éthique*, Collection médecine et droit (Paris: Éditions Alexandre Lacassagne and Éditions Eska, 1996), 279.

37. Christian BYK and Gérard MÉMETEAU, *Le droit des comités d'éthique*, Collection médecine et droit (Paris: Éditions Alexandre Lacassagne and Éditions Eska, 1996), 279.

38. Christian BYK and Gérard MÉMETEAU, *Le droit des comités d'éthique*, Collection médecine et droit (Paris: Éditions Alexandre Lacassagne and Éditions Eska, 1996), 280. [translation]

39. Christian BYK and Gérard MÉMETEAU, *Le droit des comités d'éthique*, Collection médecine et droit (Paris: Éditions Alexandre Lacassagne and Éditions Eska, 1996), 280. [translation]

40. COUNCIL OF EUROPE, "Draft Convention for the Protection of Human Rights and Dignity of the Human Being with Regard to the Application of Biology and Medicine: Convention on Human Rights and Biomedicine." Strasbourg: June 1996, CDBI (96) 26.

41. A. ROGERS and D. DURAND DE BOUSINGEN, *Une bioéthique pour l'Europe* (Strasbourg: Les éditions du Conseil de l'Europe, 1995), 223.

42. N. LENOIR, "Les États et le droit de la bioéthique," *Revue de droit sanitaire et social* 31(2):257–274 (1995). [translation]

43. The recommendations adopted by the Committee of Ministers as proposed by the CDBI are addressed to the governments of the member states but have no binding authority, unlike conventions, which are binding on states when they have ratified them. In this regard, if the Draft Convention on Human Rights and Biomedicine is adopted, it will become binding on those countries that have ratified it and incorporated it in their internal law.

44. G. BALADIER, "La demande d'éthique," *Cahiers internationaux de sociologie* 88 (1990): 11. [translation]

45. F.A. ISAMBERT, "Révolution biologique ou réveil éthique," *Science, technologie et société* 11 (1986): 9.

46. Christian BYK and Gérard MÉMETEAU, *Le droit des comités d'éthique*, Collection médecine et droit (Paris: Éditions Alexandre Lacassagne and Éditions Eska, 1996), 44.

47. We must note that this call for ethics also appeared in new sectors such as the environment, communications, business, etc. A contemporary philosopher interested in this phenomenon called it the "waltz of ethics." See Alain ETCHEGOYEN, *La valse des éthiques* (Paris: Éd. François Bourin, 1991), especially the section on ethics committees on pages 203–219.

48. Christian BYK and Gérard MÉMETEAU, *Le droit des comités d'éthique*, Collection médecine et droit (Paris: Éditions Alexandre Lacassagne and Éditions Eska, 1996), 45.

49. Sonia LE BRIS, *Les instances nationales d'éthique*, (Strasbourg: Les Éditions du Conseil de l'Europe, 1993).

50. OFFICE OF TECHNOLOGY ASSESSMENT, *Biomedical Ethics in U.S. Public Policy* (Washington, D.C.: U.S. Government Printing Office, 1993).

51. The analysis and conclusions presented in 1991 are still valid; this study is simply an update of the previous study, dated May 31, 1996. The organization and certain passages of the 1991 study have been kept *in extenso*, especially with regard to the missions of national ethics bodies, although we found it necessary to recast most of the rest of the report in the interest of clarity and precision.

52. Australia, Belgium, Canada, Cyprus, the Czech Republic, Denmark, Finland, France, Germany, the Holy See, Malta, Mexico, Norway, the Netherlands, the Philippines, Poland, Portugal, Romania, Spain, Sweden, Switzerland, Tunisia, Turkey, the United Kingdom, and the United States.

53. Christian BYK and Gérard MÉMETEAU, *Le droit des comités d'éthique*, Collection médecine et droit (Paris: Éditions Alexandre Lacassagne and Éditions Eska, 1996), 48; Philippe LAZAR, *L'éthique biomédicale en question* (Paris: Liana Levi, 1996), 27.

54. See table 2C in appendix 2.

55. Compare table 2B with column 3 in table 2C.

56. Christian BYK and Gérard MÉMETEAU, *Le droit des comités d'éthique*, Collection médecine et droit (Paris: Éditions Alexandre Lacassagne and Éditions Eska, 1996), 262.

57. Namely, an independent, permanent committee specially founded to deal with ethical issues in the fields of health and medicine, including medical research. For a list of these countries, see table 2B in appendix 2.

58. Christian BYK, "Les instances de l'éthique en droit comparé," *Cahiers internationaux de sociologie* 88 (1990): 230.

59. We note that, since 1974, INSERM (Institut national de la santé et de la recherche médicale) has had the first committee responsible for giving advice on ethical questions arising from medical research, instituting a kind of self-regulation through peer review. Following the example of the Organisation d'une colloque national de la recherche, the French national ethics committee was founded to "permit serene reflection on ethical and technological choices" [translation]; J. P. CHEVÈNEMENT, "Des principes résolument universels," *Autrement* 93 (1987): 72. Interestingly, the establishment of a national consultation group on research intended at first to replace the National Order of Doctors, which the socialist government of François Mitterand hoped to abolish, as Mitterand promised in his presidential program of 1981. The National Order of Doctors survived in the end, and the national ethics committee found itself in the game without having to displace it. See Christian BYK and Gérard MÉMETEAU, *Le droit des comités d'éthique*, Collection médecine et droit (Paris: Éditions Alexandre Lacassagne and Éditions Eska, 1996), 55.

60. Belgium, Denmark, Finland, Italy, Luxembourg, Malta, Mexico, Norway, the Netherlands, Portugal, Sweden, and Tunisia; see table 2B in appendix 2.

61. Christian BYK, "Les instances de l'éthique en droit comparé," *Cahiers internationaux de sociologie* 88 (1990): 226–227.

62. Belgium, Denmark, Finland, France, Italy, Luxembourg, Malta, Norway, Spain, Sweden, and Tunisia; see table 2B in appendix 2.

63. We note that Switzerland's current draft legislation on human reproduction also anticipates the creation of a national ethics committee (personal communication, Dominique Sprumont, University of Neufchâtel).

64. Christian BYK, "Les instances de l'éthique en droit comparé," *Cahiers internationaux de sociologie* 88 (1990): 230. [translation]

65. OFFICE OF TECHNOLOGY ASSESSMENT, *Biomedical Ethics in U.S. Public Policy* (Washington, D.C.: U.S. Government Printing Office, 1993), 44: "The NBCC was established in 1988 by the joint Meeting of Federal and State Ministers of

Health and Social Welfare. NBCC's role was to advise the Ministers, and it was composed of professionals from a number of fields… While the NBCC's work provoked much public discussion,… the Federal and State Ministers of Health and Social Welfare withdrew their support."

66. See Christian BYK and Gérard MÉMETEAU, *Le droit des comités d'éthique*, Collection médecine et droit (Paris: Éditions Alexandre Lacassagne and Éditions Eska, 1996), 275.

67. *National Health and Medical Research Council Act 1992*, Bill 225 of 1992, reproduced in NATIONAL HEALTH AND MEDICAL RESEARCH COUNCIL, *Functions, Composition and Membership of the Council and Its Committee Structure for the Triennium 1994–1996* (Canberra: National Health and Medical Research Council, 1995).

68. NATIONAL HEALTH AND MEDICAL RESEARCH COUNCIL, *Functions, Composition and Membership of the Council and Its Committee Structure for the Triennium 1994–1996* (Canberra: National Health and Medical Research Council, 1995).

69. *International Journal of Bioethics* at p. 60; Christian BYK and Gérard MÉMETEAU, *Le droit des comités d'éthique*, Collection médecine et droit (Paris: Éditions Alexandre Lacassagne and Éditions Eska, 1996), 266.

70. Marie-Thérèse MEULDERS-KLEIN, Louvain-la-Neuve, Belgium, personal communication.

71. See table 2B in appendix 2.

72. This is the case for Spain, where the discussion has continued for years without ever reaching a conclusion. It is also the case for Switzerland and Poland. Regarding the situation in Poland, see Z. CHLAP, "L'activité des comités d'éthique en Pologne," in *Proceedings of the Standing Conference of European Ethics Committees*, COUNCIL OF EUROPE (Strasbourg: Directorate of Legal Affairs, 1994).

73. See table 2B in appendix 2.

74. The term "advisory" appears in the titles of the Belgian, Finnish, French, Luxembourgeois, Maltese and Dutch committees; see table 2B in appendix 2.

75. Christian BYK and Gérard MÉMETEAU, *Le droit des comités d'éthique*, Collection médecine et droit (Paris: Éditions Alexandre Lacassagne and Éditions Eska, 1996), 140. [translation]

76. D. THOUVENIN, "Les comités d'éthiques en France," in *Bioéthique et droits de l'Homme* by F. FURKEL and H. JUNG (Berlin: Carl Hymanns Verlag, K.G., 1993), 113. [translation]

77. Thus, with the exception of Denmark and Finland, all countries use the term "national." In Denmark, one refers to the Danish Council on Ethics; in Finland, to the Advisory Board on Ethics in Research. See table 2B in appendix 2.

78. The two terms are not altogether etymologically synonymous, even if, these days, there is frequently more recourse to the one than to the other. The word "council," from the Latin *concilium*, carries the connotation of deliberation, of a structure intended to govern behaviour. It means an assembly that has a composition determined in advance and is designed to deliberate and advise. The word "committee" comes from the Latin *comitia*, the commons, indicating the Roman popular assembly. It means a group of people chosen to deal with specific business

and to give advice. On the face of it, the council is more elitist than the committee. For a definition of "committee," see Christian BYK and Gérard MÉMETEAU, *Le droits des comités d'éthique,* Collection médicine et droit (Paris: Éditions Alexandre Lacassagne and Éditions Eska, 1996), 105–106.

79. For example, the term "council" would surely be more appropriate to the customs of Canada. See LAW REFORM COMMISSION OF CANADA, "Toward a Canadian Advisory Council on Biomedical Ethics—Study Paper (Ottawa: Law Reform Commission of Canada, 1990).

80. Often, national ethics committees "are less concerned with research than with its applications and their consequences for the individual and, by implication, for the social group to which the individual belongs." D. THOUVENIN, "Les comités d'éthiques en France," in *Bioéthique et droits de l'Homme* by F. FURKEL and H. JUNG (Berlin: Carl Hymanns Verlag, K.G., 1993), 113.

81. In fact, Norway has a separate National Committee on Ethics in Medical Research.

82. Belgium, Finland, the Holy See, Italy, Luxembourg, Malta, Mexico, the Netherlands, Norway, Sweden, and Tunisia; see table 2B in appendix 2.

83. Denmark and Portugal; see table 2B in appendix 2.

84. Ian KENNEDY, "Influence des comités d'éthique sur la législation," in *Proceedings of the Standing Conference of European Ethics Committees,* Council of Europe (Strasbourg: Directorate of Legal Affairs, 1994). [translation]

85. M. TURNER-WARWICK, "Conseils aux autorités et au système de santé," in *Proceedings of the Standing Conference of European Ethics Committees,* COUNCIL OF EUROPE (Strasbourg: Directorate of Legal Affairs, 1994).

86. For a synthesis of the American situation, see OFFICE OF TECHNOLOGY ASSESSMENT, *Biomedical Ethics in U.S. Public Policy,* (Washington, D.C.: U.S. Government Printing Office, 1993), 7–13.

87. Denmark, France, Malta, Tunisia; see table 2D in appendix 2.

88. France and Norway; see table 2D in appendix 2.

89. Norway; see table 2D in appendix 2.

90. LAW REFORM COMMISSION OF CANADA, "Toward a Canadian Advisory Council on Biomedical Ethics—Study Paper (Ottawa: Law Reform Commission of Canada, 1990).

91. LAW REFORM COMMISSION OF CANADA, "Toward a Canadian Advisory Council on Biomedical Ethics—Study Paper (Ottawa: Law Reform Commission of Canada, 1990).

92. Italy, Portugal, and Sweden; see table 2D in appendix 2.

93. For example, in the United States; see table 2D in appendix 2.

94. With the exception of Denmark, where it is directly accountable to Parliament; see table 2D in appendix 2. For a study of the Danish system, see especially, L. N. NIELSEN, "La mise en place des comités d'éthique," in *Proceedings of the Standing Conference of European Ethics Committees,* COUNCIL OF EUROPE (Strasbourg, Directorate of Legal Affairs, 1994).

95. See table 2C in appendix 2.

96. This was the case in the United States with the President's Commission for the Study of Ethical Problems in Medicine and Biomedical and Behavioral Research

from 1980 to 1983; in Great Britain with the Warnock Commission on Fertilization and Human Embryology, the Polkingthorne Commission on the use of fetal tissue, and the Clothier Commission on genetic therapy; in Germany with the Benda Commission on the analysis of the genome; in Canada with the Royal Commission on New Reproductive Technologies, to name only some of the best known.

97. In fact, commissions created *ratione materiae* are often also *ratione temporis*. This was the case with both British commissions, the Warnock Commission and the Clothier Commission. It was also true in the United States of the National Commission for the Protection of Human Subjects of Biomedical and Behavioral Research (1974–1978) and of the President's Commission for the Study of Ethical Problems in Medicine and Biomedical and Behavioral Research (1978–1983).

98. For example, this is the case with the ethics commissions of the colleges of physicians and surgeons.

99. See Belgium, Canada, Cyprus, Finland, Germany, Romania, Switzerland, Turkey, the United Kingdom, and the United States; see column 3 in table 2C.

100. Christian BYK, "Les instances de l'éthique en droit comparé," *Cahiers internationaux de sociologie* 88 (1990), 226–227. It was, for example, the case with the Canadian Law Reform Commission, which has since disappeared. We note in this regard the draft Bill C-9 on the creation of a Canadian Law Commission (adopted but not promulgated), which would have such a general mandate it would have difficulty deciding whether to intervene in medical ethics issues.

101. In this respect, compare table 2B with column 3 in table 2C in appendix 2.

102. M. TURNER-WARWICK, "Conseils aux autorités et au système de santé," in *Proceedings of the Standing Conference of European Ethics Committees*, Council of Europe (Strasbourg: Directorate of Legal Affairs, 1994).

103. See table 2D in appendix 2.

104. See table 2D in appendix 2.

105. With the exception of Cyprus and the Czech Republic; see table 2D in appendix 2.

106. Christian BYK and Gérard MÉMETEAU, *Le droit des comités d'éthique*, Collection médecine et droit (Paris: Éditions Alexandre Lacassagne and Éditions Eska, 1996), 97.

107. Philippe LUCAS, "Lier ou délier? L'expérience du Comité national d'éthique," *Cahiers internationaux de sociologie* 88 (1990): 243.

108. As is the case, for example, in Australia, Denmark, and Sweden; see table 2D in appendix 2.

109. As is the case, for example, in the Czech Republic, France, and Switzerland; see table 2D in appendix 2.

110. Philippe LUCAS, "Lier ou délier? L'expérience du Comité national d'éthique," *Cahiers internationaux de sociologie* 88 (1990): 243.

111. Thus, for example, Canada, Norway—for the National Committee on Ethics in Medical Research—and the Netherlands; see table 2D in appendix 2. As for involving the public however, Denmark has tried the greatest number of initiatives; see A. ROGERS and D. DURAND DE BOUSINGEN, *Une bioéthique pour l'Europe* (Strasbourg: Les éditions du Conseil de l'Europe, 1995), 227 and following.

112. In fact, only the Nuffield Foundation and the Comité éthique français seem to have members from the news media.

113. COUNCIL OF EUROPE, *Proceedings of the Standing Conference of European Ethics Committees* (Strasbourg: Directorate of Legal Affairs, 1994) (intervention by Mrs. Nielsen).

114. As is the case in France, where the two legislative houses, namely, the National Assembly and the Senate, have the power to appoint a member; see table 2D in appendix 2.

115. As is the case in Norway and was, at one time, the case in Italy; *Proceedings of the Standing Conference of European Ethics Committees*, COUNCIL OF EUROPE (Strasbourg: Directorate of Legal Affairs, 1994) (interventions by Svein Christoffersen and Giovanni Berlinguer).

116. For example, Philippe LAZAR, *L'éthique biomédicale en question* (Paris: Liana Levi, 1995), 23.

117. In the founding articles of the Danish Council, there is an explicit requirement for parity between men and women; table 2D in appendix 2.

118. Canada (17), Denmark (17), Finland (10), Germany (9), Luxembourg (15), the Netherlands (10), Norway (12), Switzerland (17), Tunisia (14), Turkey (9), the United Kingdom (15); see table 2D in appendix 2.

119. Australia (20), the Holy See (21), Malta (21), Portugal (20), Sweden (20); see table 2D in appendix 2.

120. Belgium (35), France (40), Italy (40); see table 2D in appendix 2.

121. For a critique of this requirement for representativeness, which seems to preoccupy all newly established boards, see Ian KENNEDY, "Influence des comités d'éthique sur la législation," in *Proceedings of the Standing Conference of European Ethics Committees*, COUNCIL OF EUROPE (Strasbourg: Directorate of Legal Affairs, 1994). Kennedy thinks it impossible to achieve a balanced representation because there is always someone who does not agree with the point of view under consideration. According to him, the important thing is the aptitudes of the members, not the interests they may represent.

122. Ian KENNEDY, "Influence des comités d'éthique sur la législation," in *Proceedings of the Standing Conference of European Ethics Committees*, COUNCIL OF EUROPE (Strasbourg: Directorate of Legal Affairs, 1994).

123. Like, for example, the Czech Republic, Denmark, France, Italy, and the Netherlands; see COUNCIL OF EUROPE, *Proceedings of the Standing Conference of European Ethics Committees* (Strasbourg: Directorate of Legal Affairs, 1994).

124. See table 2D, column 4, in appendix 2, except Mexico, where the members are volunteers.

125. See table 2D, column 5, in appendix 2.

126. See Italy, Luxembourg, Norway, Sweden, Turkey, and the United States, in table 2D in appendix 2.

127. COMITÉ CONSULTATIF NATIONAL D'ÉTHIQUE POUR LES SCIENCES DE LA VIE ET DE LA SANTÉ, *Recherche biomédicale et respect de la personne humaine* (Paris: La Documentation Française, 1988), 67.

128. See table 2D, columns 6, 7 and 8, in appendix 2.

129. Luxembourg, Norway, the Netherlands, and Sweden; see table 2D in appendix 2.

130. Canada, Denmark, Finland, France, Italy, Luxembourg, Norway, Portugal, and Switzerland; see table 2D in appendix 2.

131. Canada, Denmark, the Holy See, Luxembourg, the Netherlands, and Sweden; see table 2D in appendix 2.

132. Canada and Italy; see table 2D in appendix 2.

133. Canada, France, the Holy See, Italy, Luxembourg, Norway, Sweden, and the United Kingdom; see table 2D in appendix 2.

134. Cyprus, the Czech Republic Finland, Germany, Malta, the Netherlands, Poland, Portugal, Romania, and Switzerland; see table 2D in appendix 2.

135. See the United Kingdom, table 2D in appendix 2. The Mexican committee also seems to operate on donations.

136. Canada, Denmark, Finland, the Holy See, Luxembourg, Malta, Norway, Sweden, and the United Kingdom; see table 2D in appendix 2.

137. Canada, France, Malta, Norway, Sweden, and the United Kingdom; see table 2D in appendix 2.

138. Cyprus, the Czech Republic, France, Germany, Italy, the Netherlands, Poland, Portugal, Switzerland, and Turkey; see table 2D in appendix 2.

139. Canada, France, Malta, Norway, Sweden, and the United Kingdom; see table 2D in appendix 2.

140. For example, this is the case when the national ethics committee or the national ethics board receives staff on secondment from its parent institution, or when it has access to staff or facilities of that same oversight authority. See Canada, the Czech Republic, Finland, France, Germany, Luxembourg, Malta, the Netherlands, Poland, Portugal, Switzerland, and Turkey.

141. Canada, Denmark, Finland, Germany, the Holy See, Italy, Luxembourg, Mexico, Norway, the Netherlands, Portugal, Sweden, Turkey, the United Kingdom, and the United States; see table 2D in appendix 2.

142. Canada, Denmark, Finland, France, Germany, Italy, Luxembourg, Malta, the Netherlands, Norway, Portugal, the United Kingdom, and the United States; see table 2D in appendix 2.

143. D. LECOURT, *Contre la peur – de la science à l'éthique, une aventure infinie* (Paris: Hachette, 1990); F. LENOIR, *Le temps de la responsabilité* (Paris: Fayard, 1991).

144. Philippe LAZAR, *L'éthique biomédicale en question* (Paris: Liana Levi, 1995), 53.

145. Greece, Luxembourg, Malta, Portugal, and Sweden; see table 2E in appendix 2.

146. Denmark, Finland, France, the Netherlands, and Norway; see table 2E in appendix 2.

147. Canada, Norway, Poland, and the United Kingdom; see table 2E in appendix 2.

148. National boards with broad mandates: the Holy See and Switzerland; *contra* national boards with specific mandates: Cyprus, the Czech Republic, Germany, Turkey, and the United States; see table 2E in appendix 2.

149. Canada, the Czech Republic, Norway, and the United States; see table 2E in appendix 2.

150. The Czech Republic and Poland; see table 2E in appendix 2.

151. In this regard, advice is not always presented and recommendations are not always formulated in a straightforward fashion. For a discussion of the analogy of form between opinions of the French national ethics committee and the presentation of case law, see Dominique THOUVENIN, "Les comités d'éthique en France," in *Bioéthique et droits de l'Homme,* by F. FURKEL and H. JUNG (Berlin, Carl Hymanns Verlag, K.G., 1993), 116.

152. Canada, Denmark, France, Norway, Romania, Spain, Switzerland, the United Kingdom and the United States; see table 2E in appendix 2.

153. An allusion to Baladier's expression when he speaks of the call for ethics; see G. BALADIER, "La demande d'éthique" *Cahiers internationaux de sociologie* 88 at page 11.

154. The Czech Republic, the Holy See, Poland, Romania, Switzerland, and Turkey have indicated their mode of seizure; see table 2D in appendix 2.

155. See table 2D in appendix 2.

156. See table 2D in appendix 2.

157. For another kind of typology of the missions of national ethics bodies, see Christian BYK and Gérard MÉMETEAU, *Le droit des comités d'éthique,* Collection médecine et droit (Paris: Éditions Alexander Lacassagne and Éditions Eska, 1996). These two authors distinguish between missions of consultation and reflection, missions of diffusion, and missions of representation.

158. See table 2E in appendix 2.

159. F. LENOIR, *Le temps de la responsabilité,* (Paris: Fayard, 1991).

160. Mireille DELMAS-MARTY, *Le flou du droit* (Paris: PUF, 1986).

161. Dominique THOUVENIN, "Les comités d'éthique en France." in *Bioéthique et droits de l'Homme,* by F. FURKEL and H. JUNG (Berlin: Carl Hymanns Verlag, K.G., 1993), 32.

162. Dominique THOUVENIN, "Les comités d'éthique en France," in *Bioéthique et droits de l'Homme,* by F. FURKEL and H. JUNG (Berlin: Carl Hymanns Verlag, K.G., 1993), 113.

163. LAW REFORM COMMISSION OF CANADA, "Toward a Canadian Advisory Council on Biomedical Ethics—Study Paper (Ottawa: Law Reform Commission of Canada, 1990).

164. As an example, one could mention France, whose ethics committee has been operating for 13 years. Over these 13 years, techniques have evolved, sometimes quite rapidly. Thus, in regard to the issue of research on embryos, it is enough to compare two opinions of the committee, one from 1986 and the other from 1989. In the same way, it is interesting to look at the two opinions rendered on genetic therapy, or, the 1985 opinion on prenatal diagnosis and that of 1996 on predictive medicine.

165. Ethical reflections on medical research and medically assisted reproduction are the most blatant examples. Medical research in these areas has been going on for many years, but only since the beginning of the 1980s have social and ethical issues been examined in a more general fashion. Techniques like *in vitro* fertilization, embryo donation, and even surrogate motherhood developed and established themselves in the medical landscape without much thought having

been given to them beforehand. Reflection came in *reaction* to these techniques and their development and not in *anticipation* of them, as has been the case with human genetics, AIDS, euthanasia, and the neurosciences.

166. See table 2E in appendix 2.
167. Philippe LAZAR, *L'éthique biomédicale en question* (Paris: Liana Levi, 1995), 40.
168. See table 2F in appendix 2.
169. Canada, Denmark, France, Italy, and the United States; see table 2F in appendix 2.
170. See table 2E, column 5, in appendix 2.
171. See *supra* the comments on personnel and budget.
172. See table 2E in appendix 2.
173. See table 2E in appendix 2.
174. C. NERINCK, ed., *Bioéthique et bio-droit* (Paris: L.G.D.J., 1995); Dominique Thouvenin, "Les comités d'éthique en France," in *Bioéthique et droits de l'Homme*, by F. FURKEL and H. JUNG (Berlin: Carl Hymanns Verlag, K.G., 1993); and Christian BYK and Gérard MÉMETEAU, *Le droit des comités d'éthique*, Collection médecine et droit (Paris: Éditions Alexandre Lacassagne and Éditions Eska, 1996).
175. Philippe LAZAR, *L'éthique biomédicale en question* (Paris: Liana Levi, 1995), 53.
176. Philippe LAZAR, *L'éthique biomédicale en question* (Paris: Liana Levi, 1995), 40. [translation]
177. See table 2E in appendix 2.
178. F. A. ISAMBERT, "Révolution biologique ou réveil éthique," *Science, technologie et société* 11 (1986): 9.
179. J. HAMBURGER, *Monsieur Littré*, (Paris: Flammarion, 1988), 253. [translation]
180. Denmark and Germany; see table 2E in appendix 2.
181. Canada, the Czech Republic, France, Greece, Malta, Norway, and Romania; see table 2E in appendix 2.
182. Greece, the Holy See, Poland, and Romania; see table 2F in appendix 2.
183. Canada, the Czech Republic France, Greece, Italy, Malta, the Netherlands, Poland and Romania; see table 2E in appendix 2.
184. Except for Greece, the Holy See, Poland, and Romania; see table 2F in appendix 2.
185. See table 2F in appendix 2.
186. See, for example, UNIVERSITÉ LAVAL, GROUPE DE RECHERCHE EN ÉTHIQUE MÉDICALE, *Les comités d'éthique au Québec: guide des ressources en centres hospitaliers* (Québec City: Department of Health and Social Services, 1991); John B. DOSSETOR and Janet L. STORCH, "Roles for Ethics Committees in Relation to Guidelines for New Reproductive Technologies: A Research Position Paper," in *New Reproductive Technologies: Ethical Aspects*, vol. 1 of the *Research Studies for the Royal Commission on New Reproductive Technologies* (Ottawa: Supply and Services Canada, 1993).
187. See MEDICAL RESEARCH COUNCIL OF CANADA, *Guidelines on Research Involving Human Subjects, 1987* (Ottawa: Supply and Services Canada, 1987). We wish to emphasize that some university policies refer to the 1978 version of the Medical Research Council of Canada's guidelines; see MEDICAL RESEARCH COUNCIL OF CANADA, *Ethics in Human Experimentation* (Ottawa: Supply and Services Canada, 1978).

188. This was also found in a study carried out by the NATIONAL COUNCIL ON BIOETHICS IN HUMAN RESEARCH, "Protecting and Promoting the Human Research Subject: A Review of the Function of Research Ethics Boards in Canadian Faculties of Medicine," *Communiqué NCBHR* 6 (1): (1995).

189. See table 3A in appendix 3.

190. See table 3A in appendix 3.

191. MEDICAL RESEARCH COUNCIL OF CANADA, *Ethics in Human Experimentation* (Ottawa: Supply and Services Canada, 1978).

192. In its study of hospital ethics committees, the Groupe de recherche en éthique médicale observed that "Between 1970 and 1984, 26 research ethics boards were established in Quebec, whereas during the same period, 5 clinical ethics committees were established. On the other hand, between 1985 and 1989, 25 clinical ethics committees were established, with only 11 new research ethics boards." [translation] See UNIVERSITÉ LAVAL, GROUPE DE RECHERCHE EN ÉTHIQUE MÉDICALE, *Les comités d'éthique au Québec: guide des ressources en centres hospitaliers* (Quebec City: Department of Health and Social Services, 1991), 8.

193. See table 3B in appendix 3.

194. Moreover, the Canadian Hospital Association made a statement of principle, approved by its board of directors on March 17, 1986, supporting the establishment of ethics committees. It also published materials intended to help institutions that wanted to establish a clinical ethics committee. See Heather SHERRARD, *A Planning Proposal for Institutional Ethics Committees* (Ottawa: Canadian Hospital Association, 1986); Brenda MYERS, *Institutional Ethics Committees: Are They Justified?* (Ottawa: Canadian Hospital Association, 1987).

195. Hubert DOUCET, "Ethics Committees: Protection for Patients," *Hospital Trustee* 9 (1985): 27.

196. Specifically, in the section describing management operations and responsibilities, "Acute Care: Large Community and Teaching Hospitals," CCHSA, 1992; Management Services, Standard Area II, Organization and Direction, standard 4.1, p. MGT-7.

197. Jules MARTIN, M.D., Associate Executive Director, Canadian Council on Health Services Accreditation, letter to author, May 30, 1996.

198. For example, the Association des hôpitaux du Québec published *Les comités d'éthique en centre hospitalier: proposition de planification* in June 1987.

199. For example, in British Columbia, the Minister's Advisory Committee on Ethical Issues in Health Care prepared a brochure to help institutions that wish to establish such a committee; see BRITISH COLUMBIA, MINISTER'S ADVISORY COMMITTEE ON ETHICAL ISSUES IN HEALTH CARE, *Institutional Ethics Committees*, 1995. (Victoria: Ministry of Health and Ministry Responsible for Seniors).

200. D. AVARD, G. GRIENER and J. LANGSTAFF, "Hospital Ethics Committees: Survey Reveals Characteristics," *Dimensions in Health Service* 62 (1985): 24. J. STORCH and G. GRIENER, *Final Report of a Pilot Study to Assess the Effectiveness of Institutional Ethics Committees* (Ottawa: Health and Welfare Canada, National Health Research and Development, 1991); UNIVERSITÉ LAVAL, GROUPE DE RECHERCHE EN ÉTHIQUE MÉDICALE, *Les comités d'éthique au Québec: guide des ressources en*

centres hospitaliers (Quebec City: Department of Health and Social Services, 1991); John B. DOSSETOR and Janet L. STORCH, "Roles for Ethics Committees in Relation to Guidelines for New Reproductive Technologies: A Research Position Paper," in *New Reproductive Technologies: Ethical Aspects*, vol. 1 of the *Research Studies for the Royal Commission on New Reproductive Technologies* (Ottawa: Supply and Services Canada, 1993).

201. J. STORCH and G. GRIENER, *Final Report of a Pilot Study to Assess the Effectiveness of Institutional Ethics Committees* (Ottawa: Health and Welfare Canada, National Health Research and Development, 1991), 10.

202. J. L. STORCH, G. G. GRIENER, D. A. MARSHALL and B. A. OLINECK, "Ethics Committees in Canadian Hospitals: Report of the 1989 Survey," *Healthcare Management Forum* 3 (1990): 3 and 4. For example, the authors report the use of terms such as "Ethics and Biomedical Assessment Committee, Ethics Interest Group, Ethics Consultation Committee, Medico-Moral Committee, Patient Rights and Ethics Committee, and Bioethics Committee."

203. UNIVERSITÉ LAVAL, GROUPE DE RECHERCHE EN ÉTHIQUE MÉDICALE, *Les comités d'éthique au Québec: guide des ressources en centres hospitaliers* (Quebec City: Department of Health and Social Services, 1991), 8.

204. UNIVERSITÉ LAVAL, GROUPE DE RECHERCHE EN ÉTHIQUE MÉDICALE, *Les comités d'éthique au Québec: guide des ressources en centres hospitaliers* (Quebec City: Department of Health and Social Services, 1991), 7.

205. For example, BRITISH COLUMBIA, MINISTER'S ADVISORY COMMITTEE ON ETHICAL ISSUES IN HEALTH CARE, *Institutional Ethics Committees* (Victoria: Ministry of health and Ministry Responsible for Seniors, 1995), 2

206. UNIVERSITÉ LAVAL, GROUPE DE RECHERCHE EN ÉTHIQUE MÉDICALE, *Les comités d'éthique au Québec: guide des ressources en centres hospitaliers* (Quebec City: Department of Health and Social Services, 1991), 9.

207. See table 3B in appendix 3, which shows that, in addition to doctors and health professionals such as nurses, social workers and pharmacists, these boards include a law professional and often a community representative as well.

208. UNIVERSITÉ LAVAL, GROUPE DE RECHERCHE EN ÉTHIQUE MÉDICALE, *Les comités d'éthique au Québec: guide des ressources en centres hospitaliers* (Quebec City: Department of Health and Social Services, 1991), 9; J. L. STORCH, G. G. GRIENER, D. A. MARSHALL and B. A. OLINECK, "Ethics Committees in Canadian Hospitals: Report of the 1989 Survey," *Healthcare Management Forum* 3 (1990): 11; ALBERTA HOSPITAL ASSOCIATION, *To Be or Not to Be...Involved: The Role of Hospital Trustees and Management in Bio-ethical Decision Making.* 1983 President's Paper (Edmonton: Alberta Hospital Association, 1983), 50–51. These committees nearly always have doctors as members, and the doctors are usually in the majority, along with nurses and a member of pastoral services; in addition, there are representatives from administration, a social worker, a patients' representative and, increasingly, a legal professional.

209. No doubt, this reflects the standards of the Canadian Council on Health Services Accreditation, which states that the pastoral service is responsible for "the task of watching over the dignity and the rights of the beneficiary and the personnel involved in interpreting and evaluating questions related to morality and ethics

that occur in the paying of health benefits and the making of decisions that touch on bioethics; participation on appropriate committees ..." PAST. –8–.

210. See table 3B in appendix 3.

211. See table 3B in appendix 3.

212. UNIVERSITÉ LAVAL, GROUPE DE RECHERCHE EN ÉTHIQUE MÉDICALE, *Les comités d'éthique au Québec: guide des ressources en centres hospitaliers* (Quebec City: Department of Health and Social Services, 1991), 9; J. L. STORCH, G. G. GRIENER, D. A. MARSHALL and B. A. OLINECK, "Ethics Committees in Canadian Hospitals: Report of the 1989 Survey," *Healthcare Management Forum* 3 (1990): 11.

213. John B. DOSSETOR and Janet L. STORCH, "Roles for Ethics Committees in Relation to Guidelines for New Reproductive Technologies: A Reserch Position Paper," in *New Reproductive Technologies: Ethical Aspects*, vol. 1 of the *Research Studies for the Royal Commission on New Reproductive Technologies* (Ottawa: Supply and Services Canada, 1993).

214. Pierre DESCHAMPS, Patrick VINAY and Sylvia CRUESS, *Rapport sur l'évaluation des mécanismes de contrôle en matière de recherche clinique au Québec.* Submitted to the Quebec Minister of Health and Social Services, 1995, 68–69.

215. See table 3C in appendix 3.

216. See table 3D in appendix 3.

217. J. L. STORCH, G. G. GRIENER, D. A. MARSHALL and B. A. OLINECK, "Ethics Committees in Canadian Hospitals: Report of the 1989 Survey," *Healthcare Management Forum* 3 (1990): 11.

218. P. A. F. MORRIN, "Establishing a Hospital Ethics Committee," *Ontario Medical Review* 62 (1995): 53.

219. UNIVERSITÉ LAVAL, GROUPE DE RECHERCHE EN ÉTHIQUE MÉDICALE, *Les comités d'éthique au Québec: guide des ressources en centres hospitaliers* (Quebec City: Department of Health and Social Services, 1991), 12; J. L. STORCH, G. G. GRIENER, D. A. MARSHALL and B. A. OLINECK, "Ethics Committees in Canadian Hospitals: Report of the 1989 Survey," *Healthcare Management Forum* 3 (1990): 12.

220. See table 3D in appendix 3.

221. Éric GAGNON, "Les comités d'éthique pour la recherche comme entreprise d'interprétation," *Recherches sociographiques* 32 (1991): 221.

222. HEALTH AND WELFARE CANADA, *Drugs Directorate Guidelines, Conduct of Clinical Investigations* (Ottawa: Supply and Services Canada, 1989), 7.

223. See table 3E in appendix 3.

224. See table 3F in appendix 3.

225. See table 3E in appendix 3.

226. *Civil Code of Quebec*, section 21.

227. John B. DOSSETOR and Janet L. STORCH, "Roles for Ethics Committees in Relation to Guidelines for New Reproductive Technologies: A Research Position Paper" in *New Reproductive Technologies: Ethical Aspects*, vol. 1 of the *Research Studies for the Royal Commission on New Reproductive Technologies* (Ottawa: Supply and Services Canada, 1993), 340–341.

228. For example, the *Ontario Medical Review*, published monthly by the Ontario Medical Association, has a column devoted to ethics, entitled "Medical Ethics."

229. For example, at its 1995 annual convention, the theme of which was "L'accessibilité aux médicaments et aux soins pharmaceutiques est-elle possible?" ["Is accessibility to medication and pharmaceutical care possible?"], the Ordre des pharmaciens du Québec presented a lecture covering the ethical dimension of the issues involved.

230. For example, see ALBERTA HOSPITAL ASSOCIATION, *To Be or Not To Be…Involved: The Role of Hospital Trustees and Management in Bio-ethical Decision Making.* 1983 President's Paper (Edmonton, Alberta Hospital Association, 1983); ASSOCIATION DES HÔPITAUX DU QUÉBEC, *Les comités d'éthique en centres hospitaliers: proposition de planification* (Montréal, 1987).

231. See table 4A in appendix 4: List of research centres and groups interested in ethics. This list was disseminated on the Internet in January 1996 by the Canadian Medical Association.

232. See table 4B in appendix 4, for a list of provinces and territories with law reform commissions.

233. For example, see LAW REFORM COMMISSION OF NOVA SCOTIA, "Living Wills in Nova Scotia: A Discussion Paper,"(Halifax: Law Reform Commission of Nova Scotia, 1994); NEWFOUNDLAND LAW REFORM COMMISSION, "Discussion Paper on Advance Health Care Directives and Attorneys for Health Care," (St. John's: Newfoundland Law Reform Commission, 1992); LAW REFORM COMMISSION OF SASKATCHEWAN, *Proposals for an Advance Health Care Directives Act* (Saskatoon: Law Reform Commission of Saskatchewan, 1991); MANITOBA LAW REFORM COMMISSION, *Self-determination in Health Care: Living Wills and Health Care Proxies* (Winnipeg: Manitoba Law Reform Commission, 1991).

234. For example, see ONTARIO LAW REFORM COMMISSION, *Report on Testing for AIDS* (Toronto: Ontario Law Reform Commission, 1992).

235. For example, see LAW REFORM COMMISSION OF NOVA SCOTIA, *Reform of the Laws Dealing with Adult Guardianship and Personal Health Care Decisions—Final Report* (Halifax: Law Reform Commission of Nova Scotia, 1995).

236. There seems to be a correlation between the existence of a faculty of medicine in a province and the establishment of an agency to foster research development in the health sector through a program of grants and scholarships. These agencies are identified in appendix 4.

237. Section 21, which reads as follows:
"A minor or a person of full age who is incapable of giving his consent may be submitted to an experiment only in the absence of serious risk to his health and of objection on his part, provided that he understands the nature and consequences of the act; the consent of the person having parental authority or of the mandatary, tutor or curator is necessary.
An experiment may be carried out on one person alone only if the benefit to the health of that person may be expected, and the authorization of the court is necessary. An experiment on a group of minor persons or incapable persons of full age shall be carried out within the framework of a research project approved by the Minister of Health and Social Services, upon the advice of an ethics committee of the hospital designated by the Minister or of an ethics committee created by him for that purpose; in addition, such an experiment may be carried out only if a benefit to the health of persons of the same age group and having the same illness or handicap as the persons submitted to the experiment may be expected.

Care considered by the ethics committee of the hospital concerned to be innovative care required by the state of health of the person submitted to it is not an experiment."

238. The name and mandate of such committees clearly establishes their role. For example, British Columbia established a "Special Advisory Committee on Ethical Issues in Health Care," and Prince Edward Island established its "Provincial Health Policy Council"; see table 4B in appendix 4: Comprehensive tables by province or territory.

239. For example, Quebec has at least three permanent councils to advise the Minister on health care matters: the Conseil médical du Québec, the Conseil de la santé et du bien-être, and the Conseil d'évaluation des technologies de la santé du Québec; see table 4B in appendix 4: Comprehensive tables by province or territory.

240. See table 4C in appendix 4: Provincial ethics networks.

241. D. ROY, "Demande de subvention pour la formation du réseau d'éthique clinique chez l'humain soumis au FRSQ, programme 26," *Au Chevet* 1 (1994): 2. [translation]

242. On May 24, 1996, at the first general meeting, the names of the board members were announced. See "A Network of Health Ethics Resources: A First for Alberta," *The Bioethics Bulletin* (July 1996): 11–12.

243. See table 4C in appendix 4: Provincial ethics networks.

244. This became clear in the comparison of information collated in table 4B in appendix 4: Comprehensive tables by province or territory and in table 4C in appendix 4: Provincial ethics networks.

245. CANADIAN MEDICAL ASSOCIATION, *Canadian Medical Association—What it is and what it does* (Ottawa: Canadian Medical Association, 1993). Page 2 of this document says that the Canadian Medical Association, which represents approximately 80 percent of medical staff in Canada, has the role of ethical and legal advisor for Canadian doctors as part of its mandate.

246. John R. WILLIAMS, Director, Ethics Department, Canadian Medical Association, personal communication, May 24, 1996.

247. CANADIAN MEDICAL ASSOCIATION, *Code of Ethics* (Ottawa: Canadian Medical Association, 1990).

248. CMA Webspinners, *Canadian Bioethics Report*. Agencies and Organizations, November 14, 1995. Http://www.cma.ca

249. CMA Webspinners, *Canadian Bioethics Report*. Agencies and Organizations, November 14, 1995. Http://www.cma.ca

250. For example, see CANADIAN NURSES ASSOCIATION, *Ethical Guidelines for Nurses in Research Involving Human Participants*, 2nd ed., rev. (Ottawa: Canadian Nurses Association, 1994); CANADIAN NURSES ASSOCIATION, *A Question of Respect: Nurses and End-of-Life Treatment Dilemmas*, (Ottawa: Canadian Nurses Association, 1994).

251. For example, see Heather SHERRARD, *A Planning Proposal for Clinical Ethics Committees* (Ottawa: Canadian Hospital Association, 1986); Brenda MYERS, *Institutional Ethics Committees: Are They Justified?* (Ottawa: Canadian Hospital Association, 1987); CATHOLIC HEALTH ASSOCIATION OF CANADA, *Health Care Ethics Guide* (Ottawa: Catholic Health Association of Canada, 1991).

252. Shirley CASAVANT, "Society Profile," *Canadian Bioethics Society Bulletin* (March 1996): 4.

253. Agencies and Organizations, *Humane Medicine* 10 (1994), p. 18.

254. ROYAL COMMISSION ON NEW REPRODUCTIVE TECHNOLOGIES, *Proceed with Care, Final Report of the Royal Commission on New Reproductive Technologies*, vols. 1 and 2 (Ottawa: Government Services Canada, 1993).

255. FEDERAL CENTRE FOR AIDS WORKING GROUP ON ANONYMOUS UNLINKED HIV SEROPREVALENCE, "Guidelines on Ethical and Legal Considerations in Anonymous Unlinked HIV Seroprevalence Research," *Canadian Medical Association Journal* 143 (1990): 625–627.

256. For example, *Rodriguez v. British Columbia (Attorney General)* (1993) 3 S.C.R. 519, which clearly dealt with the problem of respect for life and death with dignity.

257. SENATE OF CANADA, *Of Life and Death, Report of the Special Senate Committee on Euthanasia and Assisted Suicide* (Ottawa: Supply and Services Canada, 1995).

258. MEDICAL RESEARCH COUNCIL OF CANADA, *Guidelines on Research Involving Human Subjects 1987* (Ottawa: Supply and Services Canada, 1987).

259. See the text cited in note 191.

260. *Guidelines on Research Involving Human Subjects 1987* briefly describes genetics projects; however, developments in this sector led the Medical Research Council of Canada to publish a new guide devoted to this. See MEDICAL RESEARCH COUNCIL OF CANADA, *Guidelines for Research on Somatic Cell Gene Therapy in Humans* (Ottawa: Supply and Services Canada, 1990).

261. MEDICAL RESEARCH COUNCIL OF CANADA, SOCIAL SCIENCES AND HUMANITIES RESEARCH COUNCIL OF CANADA, and NATURAL SCIENCES AND ENGINEERING RESEARCH COUNCIL OF CANADA, *Code of Conduct for Research Involving Humans* (Ottawa, Minister of Supply and Services Canada, March 1996).

262. See table 5A.

263. NATIONAL RESEARCH COUNCIL OF CANADA, *Procedures for Obtaining Ethical Approval to Conduct Research and Development Involving Human Subjects and Supported by NRC-IRAP* (Ottawa, National Research Council of Canada, 1993); NATIONAL RESEARCH COUNCIL OF CANADA, *Procedures for Obtaining Approval to Conduct Experiments Involving Human Subjects* (Ottawa, National Research Council of Canada, 1992).

264. NATIONAL RESEARCH COUNCIL OF CANADA, *Procedures for Obtaining Approval to Conduct Experiments Involving Human Subjects* (Ottawa, National Research Council of Canada, 1992), section 7; Approval by external ethics committees, article 7.4, p. 7.

265. NATIONAL RESEARCH COUNCIL OF CANADA, *Procedures for Obtaining Ethical Approval to Conduct Research and Development Involving Human Subjects and Supported by NRC-IRAP* (Ottawa, National Research Council of Canada, 1993), section 7; Ethics approval procedure, pp. 8–10.

266. MEDICAL RESEARCH COUNCIL OF CANADA, *Ethics in Human Experimentation* (Ottawa: Supply and Services Canada, 1978).

267. MEDICAL RESEARCH COUNCIL OF CANADA, *Guidelines on Research Involving Human Subjects 1987* (Ottawa: Supply and Services Canada, 1987).

268. Ken POLE, "Why is new ethics body so unsure of its stance?" *The Medical Post* (February 7, 1989), p. 10.

269. Ken POLE, "Why is new ethics body so unsure of its stance?" *The Medical Post* (February 7, 1989), p. 10.

270. See the mission statement in the brochure published by the National Council on Bioethics in Human Research to explain the nature of the organization "Agencies and Associations," *Synapse* (1989), p. 4; see also "Mandate of the National Council on Bioethics in Human Research," *NCBHR Communiqué* 6 (1995).

271. For example, the workshop on ethical problems in clinical research related to pharmaceutical products, May 30 and 31, 1990; the workshop on the ethics of clinical trials for committees on ethics in research, May 2 and 3, 1991; the workshop on ethics in research on children, December 1 and 2, 1992; and the more recent workshop on the ethics of experimentation on human subjects, "Reinventing the Research Ethics Board," March 5 and 6, 1995.

272. For example, see NATIONAL COUNCIL ON BIOETHICS IN HUMAN RESEARCH, *Reflections on Research Involving Children* (Ottawa: National Council on Bioethics in Human Research, 1993); NATIONAL COUNCIL ON BIOETHICS IN HUMAN RESEARCH, *Ethical Aspects of Pharmaceutically-based Clinical Investigations* (Ottawa: National Council on Bioethics in Human Research, 1990).

273. NATIONAL COUNCIL ON BIOETHICS IN HUMAN RESEARCH, Annual Report, 1991.

274. NATIONAL COUNCIL ON BIOETHICS IN HUMAN RESEARCH, "Protecting and Promoting the Human Research Subject: A Review of the Function of Research Ethics Boards in Canadian Faculties of Medicine" *NCBHR Communiqué* 6 (1995).

275. See table 5B, which explains the composition of the NCBHR.

276. NATIONAL COUNCIL ON BIOETHICS IN HUMAN RESEARCH, *NCBHR Brochure*, 1st. ed., p. 6.

277. NATIONAL COUNCIL ON BIOETHICS IN HUMAN RESEARCH, *NCBHR Brochure*, 2nd ed., 1992, p. 6.

278. NATIONAL COUNCIL ON BIOETHICS IN HUMAN RESEARCH, *NCBHR Brochure*, 2nd ed., 1992, p. 6.

279. NATIONAL COUNCIL ON BIOETHICS IN HUMAN RESEARCH, "Council News," *NCBHR Communiqué* 6 (1995).

280. NATIONAL COUNCIL ON BIOETHICS IN HUMAN RESEARCH, "Council News," *NCBHR Communiqué* 6 (1995): this committee "is to serve as a forum for discussion and collaboration on institutional research ethics initiatives and as a forum for the provision of financial support and oversight of NCBHR in the discharge of its responsibilities."

281. MEDICAL RESEARCH COUNCIL OF CANADA, SOCIAL SCIENCES AND HUMANITIES RESEARCH COUNCIL OF CANADA, and NATURAL SCIENCES AND ENGINEERING RESEARCH COUNCIL OF CANADA, *Code of Conduct for Research Involving Humans* (Ottawa, Minister of Supply and Services Canada, 1996).

282. NATIONAL COUNCIL ON BIOETHICS IN HUMAN RESEARCH, "Council News," *NCBHR Communiqué* (1995): 6.

283. For comments on this role of the NCBHR, see Judith MILLER, "What to Do Until the Philosopher Kings Come: Bioethics and Public Policy in Canada," *Politics and the Life Sciences* February (1994): 93–95; Judith MILLER, "Research Ethics Boards in Canada—A Time of Review and Renewal," *International Journal of Bioethics* 6 (1995): 246–248.

284. See 30 & 31 Victoria, c. 3 (U.K.)

285. On this topic, see Henri BRUN and Guy TREMBLAY, *Droit constitutionnel,* 2nd ed. (Cowansville: Les Éditions Yvon Blais, 1990), 478–479; Peter W. Hogg, *Constitutional Law of Canada,* 3rd ed. (Toronto: Carswell, 1992), 476–477.

286. See comments by Justice Dickson in *Schneider v. Regina*, [1982] 2 S.C.R. 112, at 137: "This view that the general jurisdiction over health matters is provincial (allowing for a limited federal jurisdiction either ancillary to the express heads of power in S. 91 or the emergency power under peace, order and good government) has prevailed and is now not seriously questioned (see *Rinfret v. Pope* (1886), 12 Q.L.R. 303 (Que. C.A.), *Re Bowack, supra, Labatt Breweries of Canada Ltd. v. Attorney General of Canada*, [1980] 1 S.C.R., 914, *per* Estey J.)."

287. See Justice Estey's analysis in *Schneider v. Regina*, [1982] 2 S.C.R. 112, at 131, as well as the following decisions: *Fawcett v. Attorney General of Ontario*, [1964] S.C.R. 625, *Re Bowack* (1892), 2 B.C.L.R. 216, *Reference re Intoxicated Persons Detention Act*, [1981] 1 W.W.R. 333 (C.A. Manitoba), and *Greene v. Livermore*, [1940] O.R. 381.

288. For more information, consult Henri BRUN and Guy TREMBLAY, *Droit constitutionnel,* 2nd ed. (Cowansville: Les Éditions Yvon Blais, 1990), 484–498; Peter W. Hogg, *Constitutional Law of Canada,* 3rd ed. (Toronto: Carswell, 1992), ch. 17.

289. The opening words of section 91 of the Constitution Act, 1867 stipulates that "It shall be lawful for the Queen, by and with the Advice and Consent of the Senate and House of Commons, to make Laws for the Peace, Order, and good Government of Canada, in relation to all Matters not coming within the Classes of Subjects by this Act assigned exclusively to the Legislatures of the Provinces."

290. Martha JACKMAN, "The Constitution and the Regulation of New Reproductive Technologies," in *Overview of Legal Issues in New Reproductive Technologies,* vol. 3 *Research Studies for the Royal Commission on New Reproductive Technologies* (Ottawa: Supply and Services Canada, 1993).

291. Henry BRUN and Guy TREMBLAY, *Droit Constitutionnel,* 2nd ed. (Cowansville: Les Éditions Yvon Blais, 1990), 488. [translation]

292. First mentioned by Lord Watson in *Ontario A.G. v. Dominion A.G.*, [1896] A.C. 348, at 361; the theory of national dimension was studied in some depth by the Supreme Court of Canada for *R. v. Crown Zellerbach Canada Ltd.*, [1988] 1 S.C.R. 401.

293. Statement by Justice Le Dain in *R. v. Crown Zellerbach Ltd.*, [1988] 1 S.C.R. 401, at 432.

294. See statements by Justice Rand in *Reference re Validity of Section 5(a) of the Dairy Industry Act*, [1949] S.C.R. 1, at 49–50.

295. This federal jurisdiction was on several occasions contested by companies that considered the control implemented to be interfering. In *Standard Sausage Co. v. Lee, Protor v. Standard Co.*, [1933] 4 D.L.R. 501 (C.A. B.C.) Justice Macdonald recognized this jurisdiction. This position is confirmed in *R. v. Westmore et al.*, [1983] 2 S.C.R. 284.

296. R.S.C. (1985), c. F-27.

297. R.S.C. (1985), c. N-1.

298. *RJR-MacDonald Inc v. Canada (AG)*, [1995] 3 S.C.R. 199, at 246 (Justice La Forest).

299. For a brief examination of the relevant case law, see Martha JACKMAN, "The Constitution and the Regulation of New Reproductive Technologies," in *Overview of Legal Issues in New Reproductive Technologies*, vol. 3 of the *Research Studies for the Royal Commission on New Reproductive Technologies* (Ottawa: Supply and Services Canada, 1993).

300. In the form of tax incentives applied to research and development of pharmaceutical substances and NRT- related products and services, as well as in the form of tax credits for individuals using NRT, as suggested in Martha JACKMAN, "The Constitution and the Regulation of New Reproductive Technologies," in *Overview of Legal Issues in New Reproductive Technologies*, vol. 3 of the *Research Studies for the Royal Commission on New Reproductive Technologies* (Ottawa: Supply and Services Canada, 1993), 13.

301. For more information, consult Henri BRUN and Guy TREMBLAY, *Droit constitutionnel*, 2nd ed. (Cowansville: Les Éditions Yvon Blais, 1990), 511–516.

302. P. E. TRUDEAU, *Les subventions fédérales-provinciales et le pouvoir de dépenser du Parlement canadien* (Ottawa: Queen's Printer, 1969), as cited in André TREMBLAY, *Précis de droit constitutionnel* (Montreal: Éditions Thémis, 1982), 153. [translation]

303. For example, health care insurance program, Canada Health Act, R.S.C. c. C-6.

304. Will KYMLICKA, "The Paradox of Liberal Nationalism," *The Literary Review of Canada* (November 1995): 13, which states, "Quebec nationalists have become more and more preoccupied with maintaining and enhancing their provincial jurisdiction, even as they become more and more similar to other Canadians in their basic values."

305. See appendix 7: Summary of Approaches.

306. Guy ROCHER, *Études de sociologie, du droit et de l'éthique* (Montreal: Les Éditions Thémis, 1996), 108. [translation]

APPENDICES

APPENDIX 1

Comprehensive Tables on International Ethics Bodies – 1996

Table 1A

Description of international ethics bodies

Institution	Title of document	Year of document	Name	Scope
Group of Advisers on the Ethical Implications of Biotechnology of the European Commission (GAEB)	Group of Advisers on the Ethical Implications of Biotechnology of the European Commission (GAEB)	1996	Group of Advisers on the Ethical Implications of Biotechnology of the European Commission (GAEB)	– All biotechnology issues, in the broadest sense of the term
HUGO-ETHICS Committee	HUGO-ETHICS Committee Operating Rules and Procedures		HUGO-ETHICS Committee	See role (table 1B).
UNESCO (International Bioethics Committee)	UNESCO International Bioethics Committee (IBC), Proceedings 1995 Vol. 1/United Nations Educational, Scientific and Cultural Organization, International Bioethics Committee, Report of 1st session (1993)/Speaking of ethics, Letter from UNESCO IBC, 1995	1993, 1995	International Bioethics Committee (IBC)	– Define an intellectual platform and guidelines for the development of a declaration on the human genome – Appraise the conditions in which genetic advances may contribute to a more balanced world, and to the battle against injustice, poverty, disabilities, and illness

Table 1B

Functions and activities of international ethics bodies

Institution	Composition	Established by	Parent organization	Role	Mode of reference	Frequency of meetings
GAEB	9 members, including the chair – 2 law professionals – 3 philosophers – 2 geneticists – 1 biologist – 1 doctor For each file, the GAEB brings in a scientific expert and a legal expert Other experts may be consulted Consultation with patients associations or consumer groups	General Secretariat, European Commission	General Secretariat of the European Commission The biotechnology coordination committee (BCC) is responsible for relations between the GAEB and the directorates of the Commission whose functions involve biotechnology Group totally independent (may investigate matters on its own initiative and freely organize its working methods)	Strictly advisory role: opinions not binding Triple mission: – To identify and define the ethical issues raised by biotechnology – To assess, from the ethical viewpoint, the impact of the Community's activities in the field of bio-technology – To advise the Commission, in the exercise of its powers, on the ethical aspects of biotechnology and to ensure that the general public is kept informed	The European Commission may refer to the GAEB any request for an opinion on a specific issue The GAEB may also decide to examine a problem on its own initiative For each opinion, a rapporteur is designated to summarize all the scientific, technical and ethical aspects, and to prepare a draft opinion Approval of all members required for opinion to be final	Average of once every 6 weeks To tighten links with ethics committees that exist in certain countries, and with any other national authorities interested in ethical reflection, an annual meeting is held in a member country To extend dialogue with representatives of various interest groups and current lines of thought, the GAEB periodically organizes meetings-debates

Table 1B (cont.)

Institution	Composition	Established by	Parent organization	Role	Mode of reference	Frequency of meetings
HUGO-ETHICS Committee	14 members at large including the chair and 2 cochair(s) 1 or 2 further members may be nominated and *ad personam* if the HUGO-ETHICS Committee so chooses The president and 3 vice-presidents of HUGO Council ex officio (non-voting) Representatives (non-voting) of funding agencies and international governmental as well as nongovernmental organizations active in ethical, legal, and social issues of the Genome Initiative may be invited by the chair, cochair(s), or secretariat to attend meetings as observers In the interest of drawing advice as widely as possible, no more than 2 voting members will also be members of HUGO Council	Human Genome Organization	HUGO Council	HUGO-ETHICS Committee aims: i) to promote discussion and understanding of social, legal, and ethical issues as they relate to conduct of knowledge derived from the Human Genome Initiative. This includes consideration of research results, and the issues of human diversity, privacy and confidentiality, intellectual property rights, patents and commercialization, disclosure of genetic information to third parties, the non-medical use of information about genetic susceptibilities, and the medical, legal and social aspects of testing, screening, accessibility, banking, and genetic research;		The HUGO-ETHICS Committee and/or its subcommittees will normally meet at least once a year

Table 1B (cont.)

Institution	Composition	Established by	Parent organization	Role	Mode of reference	Frequency of meetings
HUGO-ETHICS Committee (cont.)				ii) to act as an interface between the scientific community, policymakers, educators, and the public; iii) to foster greater appreciation of human variation and complexity; iv) to collaborate with other international bodies in genetics, health, and society with the goal of disseminating information; v) to report annually to HUGO Council		
IBC	Approximately 50 (scientists and others): world specialists in biology, genetics and medicine, law, philosophy, and the humanities	Director general of UNESCO	Director general of UNESCO and Permanent UNESCO Conference	Responsible for identifying statements of principle that could make it possible to meet the main ethical concerns raised by advances in the life sciences Forum for exchange of information and ideas	Not specified	Not specified

Table 1B (cont.)

Institution	Composition	Established by	Parent organization	Role	Mode of reference	Frequency of meetings
IBC (cont.)				Intended to raise and promote the international conscience Platform for proposals to develop an international instrument for the protection of the human genome Education, training, and information: – specialist bioethics training (doctors, scientists, legal experts, philsophers...) and public decision makers to ensure that they speak the same language; – public awareness, in particular aimed at youth in various countries; – improve dialogue with the media; – making people aware of their responsibilities to future generations		

APPENDIX 2

Comparative Comprehensive Tables for National Ethics Bodies

Table 2A

Sources of information
(as of July 15, 1996)

Country	Source
Australia	Australian Health Ethics Committee, National Health and Medical Research Council, GPO Box 9848, Canberra ACT 2601; tel.: (06) 289-6992; fax: (06) 289-7802. Source: Mr. Stuart Cameron (secretary general)
Belgium	Ms. Hennau-Hublet, Faculté de droit, Université Louvain-la-Neuve
Canada	National Council on Bioethics in Human Research (NCBHR), 774 Echo Drive, Ottawa, K1S 5N8; tel.: (613) 730-6225; fax: (613) 730-8251. Source: Dr. Abbyann Lynch (president)
Cyprus	Office of the Attorney General of the Republic, Nicosia. Source: Ms. Frosso Parrisiadou (senior council of the Republic)
Czech Republic	Czech Republic Ministry of Health, Department of International Cooperation, Palackého nam. 4, 128 01 Praha 2; tel.: (44 2) 29-47-66; fax: (42 2) 29-69-83. Source: Ms. Katarina Ciharova (director of the Department of International Cooperation)
Denmark	The Danish Council of Ethics, 2–4 Ravnsborggade, 2200 Copenhagen N; tel.: 45-35-37-58-33. Source: Mr. Lars Nordskov Nielsen (president), Ms. Nina Schultz-Lorentzen (executive director)
Finland	Finish National Research, Prime Minister Office, Aleksan Terinktu 3, SF. Helsinki
France	Comité consultatif national d'éthique pour les sciences de la vie et de la santé, 71 rue Saint Dominique 75007 Paris. Mr. Jean Michaud (vice-president)
Germany	Bundesministerium für Gesundheit, Deutschherrenstr. 87, 5300 Bonn 2; tel.: (02 28) 930-2013; fax: (02 28) 930-2221. Source: Dr. Mathy
Holy See	Permanent Mission of the Holy See to the Council of Europe, 2 rue Le Nôtre, 67000 Strasbourg. Source: Mgr Carlo Maria Vigano
Italy	Comitato nazionale per la bioetica, Via Veneto, 56-00187 Roma; tel.: 4819-944; fax: 4816-1493. Dr. Giovanni Incorvati
Luxemburg	Comité consultatif national d'éthique pour les sciences de la vie et de la santé, 20 montée de la Pétrusse, L-2912 Luxemburg; tel.: (352) 478-6628; fax: (352) 41-887. Source: Mr. Serge Thill (administrative attaché)
Malta	Health Ethics Consultative Committee, c/o Ministry for Social Policy, Paiazzo Ferreria, Vailetta, Malta; tel.: (0356) 243166; fax: (0356) 243017. Source: Dr. J.L. Grech
Mexico	Comisión Nacional de Bioetica, Antiguo Claustro Del Hospital Juarez, Plaza San Pablo, 06090 Mexico, DF; tel.: (525) 542-2195; fax: (525) 542-2006. Source: Mr. Manuel Velasco-Suarez (president)

Table 2A (cont.)

Country	Source
Netherlands	Ministry of Welfare, Health and Cultural Affairs, Postbus 5406, 2280 HK Rijswijk. Source: Ms. Johanna H.W. Kits Nieuwenkamp
Norway	The National Committee for Medical Research Ethics, Gaustadalléen 21, 0371 Oslo 3; tel.: (47 22) 95-87-80, fax: (47 22) 69-84-71. Dr. Kant W. Ruyts
Philippines	Philippine Council for Health Research and Development, Department of Science and Technology, Dost Building, General Santos Avenue, Bicutan, Taguig, Metro Manila Philippines; tel.: (632) 837-29-24; fax: (632) 837-29-42. Ms. Myrna I. Consolación (administrator)
Poland	Polish Medical Council Ethics Committee, Ul. Weadystawa 9, 81-703 Sopot; tel./fax: 0-58-51-43-76. Source: Mr. Jerzy Umiastowski (president)
Portugal	National Ethics Committee for the Life Sciences, Precsdencia do Consleho de Mnistros, Rua Prof. Gomes Teizeira, 1300 Lisbon; tel.: 351-1-397-7001; fax: 351-1-39-84-48. Source: Ms. Sonia Taveira (principal secretary)
Romania	Ministry of Health. Source: Dr. C. Maximilian (member of CAHBI)
Spain	Institut Borja de Bioethica, Llaseres, 30 Sant Cugat del Vallès, 08190 Barcelona, Spain; tel.: (3) 674-47-66; fax: (3) 674-79-80. Source: Dr. Francesc Abel (director)
Sweden	The National Council on Medical Ethics in Sweden, Ministry of Health and Social Affairs, 103 33 Stockholm, Sweden; tel.: 0046/8-405 -33-44; fax: 0046/8-21-34-06. Source: Ms. Wanja Gavelin
Switzerland	– Swiss Academy of Medical Science, Central Ethics Commission. Source: Bernard Courvoisier, Hôpital Beau-Séjour, 1206 Geneva. – Centre for European Legal Studies, Faculty of Law, University of Geneva, 12 Boulevard des Philosophes, 1205 Geneva; tel.: (022) 20-93-33 int. 2170; fax: (022) 20-04-97. Source: Olivier Guillod
Tunisia	Public Health Ministry, National Medical Ethics Committee, Place Pasteur, Belvédère, 1002 Tunis; tel.: (01) 783-828, fax: (01) 791-833. Source: Béchir Hamza (president)
Turkey	Permanent Turkish Representation on the Council of Europe, 23 boulevard de l'Orangerie, 67000 Strasbourg; tel.: 88-36-50-94
United Kingdom	The Nuffield Foundation, 28 Bedford Square, London WC1B 3EG; tel.: 071-6321-0566; fax: 071-323-4877. Source: Mr. David Shapiro
United States	Mr. Daniel Wikler, University of Wisconsin, Madison, Wisconsin

Table 2B

Overview of national ethics committees[1] – 1996

Country	National ethics advisory committee Est'd	National ethics advisory committee Planned	Name	Date	Establishing authority
Australia	No	No	–	–	–
Belgium	Yes	–	National Advisory Bioethics Committee	1993	Government
Canada	No	No	–	–	–
Cyprus	No	Under study	–	–	–
Czech Republic	No	No	–	–	–
Denmark	Yes	–	Danish Council of Ethics	06/1987	Parliament (bill no. 353 dated 3 June 1987)
Finland	Yes	–	Research Ethics Advisory Council	11/1991	Government (Order in Council moved by the Ministry of Education)
France	Yes	–	National Consultative Ethics Committee for Health and Life Sciences	02/1983	President of the Republic (Council of Ministers decree)
Germany	No	No	–	–	–
Greece	Yes	–	National Ethics Board for Health Sciences	1992	Government (Ministry of Health, Welfare and Social Services)
Holy See	No	No	–	–	–
Italy	Yes	–	National Bioethics Committee	03/1990	Government (decree by President of Council of Ministers)

Table 2B (cont.)

Country	National ethics advisory committee Est'd	Planned	Name	Date	Establishing authority
Luxembourg	Yes	–	National Ethics Advisory Committee for the Life and Health Sciences	09/1988	Government (regulation by government in council)
Malta	Yes	–	Health Ethics Advisory Committee	08–1989 (for 3 years)	Government (decree moved by the Ministry of Social Affairs)
Mexico	Yes	–	Comisión Nacional de Bioetica (National Bioethics Committee)	1992	Government (General Health Council of the Republic of Mexico)
Netherlands	Yes	–	Provisional National Ethical Review Board (KEMO)	01/1989	Government (Ministry of Welfare, Health and Cultural Affairs)
Norway	Yes	–	National Biotechnology Advisory Council	1991	Government (Ministry of Health and Social Affairs)
Philippines	No	No	–	–	–
Poland	No	No	–	–	–
Romania	No	–	–	–	–
Spain	No	Yes, draft royal decree	National Bioethics Commission	–	Government (decree of Council of Ministers; moved by Ministry of Health)
Sweden	Yes	–	National Council on Medical Ethics	1985	Government
Switzerland	No	Yes	National Ethics Committee	–	Federal Council
Tunisia	Yes	–	National Medical Ethics Committee	1994	Government (Ministry of Public Health)

Table 2B (cont.)

Country	National ethics advisory committee		Name	Date	Establishing authority
	Est'd	Planned			
Turkey	No	No	–	–	–
United Kingdom	No	No	–	–	–
United States	No[2]	No	–	–	–

1. This table includes only those national ethics committees established in reference to the Comité consultatif national d'éthique (in France) (National Ethics Committee) which was the first of its kind. All other national, regional, or local bodies will be listed in table 2C. The manner in which the committees were established, and the scope of their mandates, were the key criteria in differentiating between national committees and national ethical bodies. Thus we retained the name "national ethics committee" where the body was established under executive or legislative authority, and the mandate included both research ethics and applied ethics. For the others, we have used the more general name of "national ethics body" (or authority).

2. From 1978 to 1980, an advisory ethics committee attached to the Federal Health and Social Services Department became interested in ethical issues relating to in vitro fertilization and to prenatal diagnosis. In addition, from 1979 to 1983, a president's commission was established to study ethical problems in medicine and biomedical and behavioural research (President's Commission for the Study of Ethical Problems in Medicine and Biomedical and Behavioural Research).

Table 2C

National,[1] regional,[2] and local ethics bodies – 1996

Country	Exists	Territorial status			Other ethics bodies		
		National	Regional	Local	Nature		
					Ad hoc	Specialized	
Australia	Yes	Yes National Health and Medical Research Council subdivided into specialized subcommittees – Australian Health Ethics Committee – Medical Research Committee – Public Health Research and Development Committee – National Health Advisory Committee – Strategic Planning and Evaluation Committee	Yes	Yes	?	The specialized subcommittees of the National Health and Medical Research Council are: – animal care – genetic therapy – quality of care etc.	
Belgium	Yes	Yes National Council of the College of Physicians	Yes Unofficial ethics committees approved by the National Council of the College of Physicians	Yes Unofficial ethics committees approved by the National Council of the College of Physicians	Yes Local or regional committees in hospitals, medical and university services	Yes Evaluation of research on humans	

1. The adjective "national" is used in the generic sense of the term to include unitary states, federal states, confederations of states, etc.
2. The adjective "regional" is used in the generic sense of the term to include republics, Länder, provinces, cantons, etc.

Table 2C (cont.)

Country	Exists	Other ethics bodies					
		Territorial status			Nature		
		National	Regional	Local	Ad hoc	Specialized	
Canada	Yes	Yes – National Council on Bioethics in Human Research (1991) – Canadian Bioethics Society – Standing Committee on Ethics and Experimentation of the Canadian Medical Research Council – Biomedical Ethics Committee of the Royal College of Physicians and Surgeons of Canada – Ethics Committee of the Canadian Medical Association	Yes	Yes – Research ethics boards in faculties, hospitals, and research institutes – Hospital ethics committees	–	Yes – Evaluation of research – Guidelines proposals – Assistance to research ethics boards (REB) to resolve contentious and other issues – Promotion of education, communication, and understanding between stakeholders and the public at large – Coordination between various parties with respect to guidelines and statements concerning research ethics	
Cyprus	Yes	Yes – Medical Council – College of Physicians	?	?	?	?	
Czech Republic	Yes	Yes Ministry of Health Central Ethics Committee	Yes For each republic	Yes	Yes	No	

Table 2C (cont.)

Country	Exists	Other ethics bodies					
		Territorial status				Nature	
		National	Regional	Local	Ad hoc	Specialized	
Denmark	Yes	Yes 1 Central Research Ethics Committee	Yes 7 research ethics committees	–	–	Yes Research evaluation	
Finland	Yes	Yes – Finnish Academy Research Ethics Committee – Ethics Advisory Committee of the National Health and Welfare Agency	–	Yes Over 100	–	Yes – Evaluation of research (including Finnish Academy) – Many ethics committees involved in animal research	
France	Yes	Yes Including in the various national colleges of the medical professions	Yes Committees to protect subjects of biological research	Yes Committees in hospitals, universities, and research centres	No	Yes – Cardiology – Geriatrics – Transplants – Resuscitation, etc.	
Germany	Yes	Yes – Central Commission for the Observance of Ethical Principles in the areas of Reproductive Medicine, Human Embryo Research, and Genetic Therapy (1986)	Yes Ethics committees for the regional medical associations (Länder)	Yes University ethics committees	Yes Central Commission for the Observance of Ethical Principles in the areas of Reproductive Medicine, Human Embryo Research, and Genetic Therapy	Yes Research evaluation committee – Clinical trials	

Table 2C (cont.)

Country	Exists	Other ethics bodies				
		Territorial status			Nature	
		National	Regional	Local	Ad hoc	Specialized
Germany (cont.)		– Central Commission for the safeguard of ethical principles in medicine and related fields				
Greece	Yes	No	No	Yes 2 or 3 hospital committees	Yes University of Athens School of Medicine	Yes Society for the study of AIDS and sexually transmitted diseases
Holy See	Yes	Yes – Congregation for the Doctrine of the Faith (1542) – Ethics Committee for the national conferences of bishops	Yes – Ethics committee for the regional councils of bishops	Yes – Ethics committees in most Catholic hospitals	Yes – Explanation of the Catholic position towards certain ethical problems that actually arise in hospitals	–
Italy	Yes	No	Yes	Yes Hospital ethics committees	No	Yes
Luxembourg	No	–	–	–	–	–
Malta	Yes	Yes Medical Council of Malta	No	No	No	No

Table 2C (cont.)

Country	Other ethics bodies					
	Exists	Territorial status			Nature	
		National	Regional	Local	Ad hoc	Specialized
Mexico	Yes	No	Yes The National Bioethics Committee participated in establishing regional ethics committees	Yes – Centro de Estudios e Investigaciones de Bioetica, A.C. – Centro de investigación en Bioetica, Universitad de Guanajuato	No	No
Netherlands	Yes	Yes – The Health Council's Standing Focus Group on Ethics and Law – Central Ethical and Medical Research Committee – Animal Experimentation Advisory Committee – Genetic Modification Committee – Animal Biotechnology Committee	Yes Various regional advisory committees	Yes Many local committees, primarily in hospitals	Yes – The Health Council's Standing Advisory Group on Ethics and Law – Ethics Committee of the Royal Society of Physicians – Netherlands Hospital Council Ethics Committee – Transplant Society Ethics Committee	Yes – Royal Society of Physicians Ethics Committee – Netherlands Hospital Council Ethics Committee – Transplant Society Ethics Committee – Ethics committees of medical faculties and universities – Ethics Committee on Pediatrics and the Mentally Disabled

Table 2C (cont.)

Country	Exists	Other ethics bodies				
		Territorial status			Nature	
		National	Regional	Local	Ad hoc	Specialized
Netherlands (cont.)					– Ethics committees of medical faculties and universities – Ethics Committee for Pediatrics and the Mentally Disabled	
Norway	Yes	Yes – National Committee for Medical Research Ethics (1990) – National Committee for Research Ethics in Science and Technology (1990) – National Committee for Research Ethics in Social Sciences and Humanities (1990)	Yes 1 research ethics committee in each of 5 regions	No	Yes	Yes
Philippines	Yes	National Health Research Ethics Committee (NEC)	Yes Regional ethics committees to advise the regional health research development committees	–	Yes Institutional research ethics committees	–

Table 2C (cont.)

Country	Exists	Other ethics bodies				
		Territorial status			Nature	
		National	Regional	Local	Ad hoc	Specialized
Poland	Yes	Yes National Human Research Monitoring Committee (1982)	Yes	No	Yes National College of Physicians Ethics Committee	Yes Research evaluation
Portugal	Yes	Yes College of Physicians Medical Ethics Committee	No	Yes Hospital ethics committees	Yes	Yes
Romania	Yes	Yes Academy of Medical Science Bioethics Committee (1991)	?	Yes Hospital ethics committees in major cities	–	Yes
Spain	Yes	Yes Ad hoc national commissions of the National Assembly	Yes Bioethics Advisory Committee in the Province of Catalonia	Yes Research ethics committees in all major hospitals have been mandatory since the passage of the Drug Act in December 1990	Yes Commissions of the National Assembly	Yes Future research ethics committees => evaluation of research

Table 2C (cont.)

Country	Exists	Other ethics bodies				
		Territorial status			Nature	
		National	Regional	Local	Ad hoc	Specialized
Sweden	Yes	Yes – National Health Council – College of Physicians	Yes Regional research ethics committees within each medical faculty and university	Yes Hospital ethics committees	No	Yes – Evaluation of medical research – National Health Council Ethics Committee – College of Physicians Committee
Switzerland	Yes	Yes – Central Ethics Committee of the Swiss Academy of Medical Science (1979) – Medical Experimentation Ethics Committee	Yes Committees in the cantons of Tessin and Neuchâtel	Yes Research hospital ethics committees	Yes Canton committees	Yes Research evaluation => hospital committees
Tunisia	?	?	?	?	?	?
Turkey	Yes	Yes – Senior Health Council – Senior Disciplinary Committee of the Turkish Medical Association – Bioethics Section of the Turkish Philosophical Society – Ministry of Health Central Ethics Committee	Yes Ankara Federation of Physicians Ethics Committee	Yes	No	Yes Bioethics Section of the Turkish Philosophical Society

Table 2C (cont.)

Country	Exists	Other ethics bodies					
		Territorial status				Nature	
		National	Regional	Local	Ad hoc	Specialized	
United Kingdom	Yes	Yes – Nuffield Council on Bioethics – Royal College of Physicians – Committees established by government – British Medical Association	Yes Research ethics committees	Yes Hospital research ethics committees	Yes – Warnock Commission => fertilization and human embryology – Polkinghorne Commission => use of foetal tissue – Clothier Commission => genetic therapy	Yes Most Royal Colleges of Medicine => ethics committees by field of specialization	
United States	Yes	Yes – Within the various professional societies and organizations for medicine and research – National Bioethics Advisory Commission	Yes – State task forces (including New York and New Jersey) – Non-government organizations	Yes – Institutional ethics committees (IEC) – Institutional review boards (IRB)	Yes IRBs in universities, hospitals, and medical schools	Yes – The Task Force => Medical ethics – ELSI Committee => Human genetics – IRB: Review of research protocols	

Table 2D

Functions of national ethics bodies[1] – 1996

Country	Mode of reference	Supervisory authority	Composition	Name	Salary	Assignment Amount	Expenses	Personnel	Facilities	Nature	Budget Source	Budget Amount	Purpose
Australia	By the National Health and Medical Research Council	National Health and Medical Research Council	20 members: – one chairperson – members from the health sciences, the humanities (philosophy, theology, law), research, social science, a person representing beneficiaries of the health system, one person representing the disabled	By the Minister	Yes In the form of honoraria	?	Yes	Yes	Yes	?	Government	?	?
Austria	–	–	–	–	–	–	–	–	–	–	–	–	–
Belgium National Advisory Bioethics Committee	– By the presidents of the House of Representatives, the Senate, and of a community council – By 10 senators or community councillors	?	35 members: – 16 members from the university environment (multidisciplinary) – 6 doctors – 2 lawyers – 2 magistrates	Council of Ministers	?	?	?	?	?	?	?	?	?

Table 2D (cont.)

Country	Mode of reference	Supervisory authority	Composition	Name	Salary	Assignment Amount	Expenses	Personnel	Facilities	Budget Nature	Budget Source	Budget Amount	Purpose
Belgium (cont.)			– Other members designated by the French- and German-speaking communities – Representatives from the ministries of justice, public health, and science										
	– By a member of the government – By a scientific agency, health care institution, or higher education institution – By a local ethics committee												
Canada National Council on Bioethics in Human Research	?	– Royal College of Physicians and Surgeons of Canada – Medical Research Council of Canada – Health Canada – Natural Sciences and Engineering Research Council – Sciences Human Research Council	15 members (could eventually reach as high as 20): – 2 from the research committee of the Royal College of Physicians and Surgeons of Canada – 3 from the medical ethics committee of the Royal College of Physicians and Surgeons of Canada	Appointed by the Royal College of Physicians based on nominations by each of the organizations in question	No	–	Yes	– Has its own personnel – Permanent full-time secretariat – Other staff on contract basis for projects – Director a specialist in medical ethics, research, and science policy	– Own facilities – Same building as Royal College	Own budget	Principally Research Council of Canada, Royal College, and Health and Welfare Canada	$375, 000	– Operating expenses – Council activities – Research works – Publications – Symposia

1. The term ethical body is used in this table in the broad sense, and covers both National Ethics Committes as well as the major national ethics bodies, as identified for the various countries (cf. tables 2B and 2C).

Table 2D (cont.)

Country	Mode of reference	Supervisory authority	Composition	Name	Salary	Assignment Amount	Expenses	Personnel	Facilities	Nature	Budget Source	Budget Amount	Purpose
Canada (cont.)		– Councils of other organizations involved in this field	– 1 representative from the Canadian Medical Association										
			– 1 representative from the College of Family Physicians of Canada										
			– 1 representative from the Canadian Nurses Association										
			– 1 representative from the Canadian Society for Clinical Investigation										
			– 1 representative from Health and Welfare Canada										
			– 1 representative from the Medical Research Council										
			– 1 law professional										
			– 1 philosopher										
			– 2 public representatives										

Table 2D (cont.)

Country	Mode of reference	Supervisory authority	Composition	Name	Salary	Assignment Amount	Expenses	Personnel	Facilities	Nature	Budget Source	Budget Amount	Purpose
Cyprus Medical Council	?	Independent	– Director general of the Ministry of Health – Director of Medical Services – Doctors	– Director general and director of Medical Services are ex-officio members – Doctors are elected by local or country-wide medical associations	No	–	No	?	Health Ministry facilities	Health Ministry budget	Health Ministry	?	Current expenses
Czech Republic Central Ethics Committee	– Local ethics committees	Independent	29 members: – 1 chair – 2 secretaries – 4 law professionals – 17 specialist doctors – 1 general practitioner – 1 nurse – 2 theologians – 1 member of the legislature – 2 psychologists – 1 bio-engineer	Appointed by Health Ministry Science Council and approved by the Minister	No	–	?	– Assistance of Ministry of Health	– No facilities of its own	Falls under budget of Ministry of Health	Ministry of Health	U.S.$ 2,000	?

Table 2D (cont.)

Country	Mode of reference	Supervisory authority	Composition	Name	Salary	Assignment Amount	Expenses	Personnel	Facilities	Nature	Budget Source	Budget Amount	Purpose
Denmark Danish Council of Ethics	– Parliament – Ministry of Health – Health authorities – Population	– Parliament – Ministry of Health	17 members: – Multidisciplinary – People with experience and skills in health ethics and the sciences – Equal representation by men and women	– 8 members appointed by the parliamentary committee responsible for the Ethics Council – 9 members appointed by the Ministry of Health	No, except for the president	Very low remuneration for president	Yes	– Seconded from Ministry of Health – 1 permanent secretariat consisting of 5 full-time persons with 3 academic members, including the president and 2 secretaries – Specific skills of academic team	?	Portion of the annual national budget	?	40,000 Danish crowns	– Remuneration of permanent secretariat – Publications – Research works – Symposia and debates – Information and communications
Finland Research Ethics Advisory Council	Not determined	Independent	10 members: – 1 president – 1 vice-president – 8 representatives of various specialties involved in research ethics	Ministry of Science and Education	No	–	Yes Travel and symposium costs based on allowance granted to all members of government committees	– Seconded from Ministry of Science and Education: – 1 secretary general plus 1 permanent secretariat	Ministry of Science and Education	Own budget	Ministry of Science and Education	Not determined	– Secretariat – Symposia – Publications

Table 2D (cont.)

Country	Mode of reference	Supervisory authority	Composition	Name	Salary	Assignment Amount	Expenses	Personnel	Facilities	Nature	Budget Source	Budget Amount	Purpose
France National Consultative Ethics Committee for Health and Life Science	– President of the National Assembly – President of the Senate – Government members – Public institutions or recognized foundations working in the public interest whose main activity is research or technological development – Higher education institutions – Independent	Independent according to statutes. In practice, notices are sent to the Ministry of Social Affairs and the Ministry of Research	40 members: – 1 chair – 5 representatives from principal religious congregations – 18 members with expertise who are involved in ethical thought – 16 persons from the research sector	– 6 members appointed by the President of the Republic – 18 members appointed by ministries, legislative assemblies and senior administrative and legal authorities – 16 members appointed by universities, academies, and national research centres	No	–	Yes Flat-rate travel costs	– No personnel of its own – Secretary General seconded from Ministry of Health – Secretary = personnel from INSERM[2]	– No facilities of its own – INSERM[2] facilities	Own budget	Ministry of Research	?	– Publications – Symposia (annual days) – Honoraria

2. INSERM = Institut national de la santé et de la recherche médicale (National Institute for Health and Medical Research).

Table 2D (cont.)

Country	Mode of reference	Supervisory authority	Composition	Name	Salary	Assignment Amount	Expenses	Personnel	Facilities	Budget Nature	Budget Source	Budget Amount	Purpose
Germany Central Commission for the Observance of Ethical Principles in the areas of Reproductive Medicine, Human Embryo Research, and Genetic Therapy	?	Federal Medical Council	- Minimum 5 members representing specialist organizations - 4 doctors - 1 law professional	Appointed by the director of the Federal Medical Council	?	?	Yes Reimbursement of costs	Assistance from Federal Medical Council	No facilities of its own	Budget headings of Federal Medical Council	Federal Medical Council	?	- Operations - Member costs - Research works
Central Commission for the safeguard of ethical principles in medicine and related fields	?	Federal College of Physicians	12 members: - 5 doctors - 2 philosophers or theologians - 2 scientists - 1 expert in social science - 2 law professionals	Proposed by the government and approved by the Federal College	?	?	?	?	?	?	?	?	?
Greece National Ethics Council for the Health Sciences (Bill)	?	- Probably the Ministry of Health	- Doctors, philosophers, law professionals, theologians, and other ethics consultants	?	?	–	–	?	?	?	- Likely the Ministry of Health	?	?

Table 2D (cont.)

Country	Mode of reference	Supervisory authority	Composition	Name	Salary	Assignment Amount	Expenses	Personnel	Facilities	Budget Nature	Budget Source	Budget Amount	Purpose
Holy See Congregation for the Doctrine of the Faith	– Independent – By the Pope – By the bishops – By the members of the Church	Financial decision by Plenary Assembly of the Congregation after consultation with the Pope	– 21 members for Plenary Assembly (21 cardinals and bishops) – Over 30 consultants selected for their expertise in ethics – 12 permanent officers from different countries	– The members of the Plenary Assembly are chosen by the Pope – Officers and consultants are chosen by the Cardinal Prefect	– Members of the Plenary Assembly are not remunerated – Officers are salaried	–	Consultants expenses are covered	– Own personnel – 12 permanent members selected for their expertise	Own facilities	Own budget	Funded by the Holy See	?	Salaries of permanent staff
Italy National Ethics Committee	Government members	President of Council of Ministers	40 members – Multidisciplinary	Decree by President of Council of Ministers	No	–	Reimbursement of travel costs and per diem expenses for members not living in Rome	– Own facilities – Full-time secretariat – Contract staff (documentation specialists and writers)	Own facilities	Included under the expenditure headings for the President of the Council of Ministers	President of the Council of Ministers	$300,000	– Remuneration of secretariat – Travel costs – Research works – Translation of notices into French and English
Luxembourg National Ethics Advisory Committee for the Life and Health Sciences	– Government members – Independent	Responsible Ministry	15 members: – 1 chair – 1 vice-chair – no less than 5 with medical expertise – no less than 5 with humanities and social sciences expertise	Appointed by the government	Yes Attendance fees	1,000 Flux per session	Yes – Fees – Travel costs – Documentation and training costs	– Seconded from the public service – Coordinator – 1 researcher, executive (half-time) – 1 secretary	Own facilities	Own budget	Government	– Open-ended – 510,000 Flux for 1997	– Operating expenses – Training – Information

Table 2D (cont.)

Country	Mode of reference	Supervisory authority	Composition	Name	Salary	Assignment Amount	Expenses	Personnel	Facilities	Nature	Budget Source	Budget Amount	Purpose
Malta Health Ethics Consultative Committee	– Honorary Secretary – Ministry of Social Affairs	– Ministry of Social Affairs – Government	21 members: – 1 chair – 1 secretary – 19 members	– Appointed by the Ministry of Social Affairs	No	–	?	Assistance with secretariat from Ministry of Social Affairs	Facilities of the Ministry of Social Affairs	Own budget	Ministry of Social Affairs	LM 1,000	Essentially to establish a documentary centre accessible to everyone
Mexico	?	?	– 1 chair – 2 vice-chairs – 1 advisory committee – administrative and technical secretaries – committee members (number not specified) – 1 executive committee	Members are volunteers who are health professionals, scientists, etc.	No	–	No	Own personnel	National Health Ministry	Donations	–	Indeterminate	Operating costs
Netherlands IProvisional National Ethical Review Board (KEMO)	Local ethics committees	– Annual report	10 members: – 1 president, doctor, vice-president of Health Council – 4 ethicists – 2 doctors – 2 law professionals specializing in health – 1 representative of the public	– The president is appointed by the Minister of Welfare, Health and Cultural Affairs – Members are selected by the President of the Council	No Attendance fees	–	Yes Travel costs	No Assistance from Health Council secretariat – 1 person (law professional) from the Occupational Health Council (half time) – 1 person (chemist) from the Health Council works 1 day per week	No – Facilities of National Health Council	National Health Council budget heading	National Health Council, whose annual budget is set by the Minister of Welfare, Health and Cultural Affairs	?	– Remuneration of personnel – Operating expenses – Documentation – Symposium expenses

Table 2D (cont.)

Country	Mode of reference	Supervisory authority	Composition	Name	Salary	Assignment Amount	Expenses	Personnel	Facilities	Nature	Budget Source	Budget Amount	Purpose
Norway National Bio-technology Advisory Council	– Independent – Government agencies – Ministries	Independent	23 members: – 7 reps. from medicine, law, and research – 7 reps. from private organizations – 7 reps. from government ministries and agencies – 2 ethics specialists	Appointed by the Ministry of Social Affairs	Yes	Based on the salary rules established for members of government committees and agencies	–	– Own personnel – Team of 4 full-time staff (2 biologists, 1 information officer, and 1 secretary)	Own facilities	Own budget	Ministry of Health and Social Affairs	NOK 3 million for 1991	– Remuneration of personnel – Remuneration of members – Research works – Information activities
National Committee for Medical Research Ethics	?	Annual report to Ministry of Education and Research	12 members: – 3 medical experts – 3 ethics specialists – 1 person from the humanities – 2 legal specialists – 2 representatives of the public	Appointed by the Ministry of Education and Research on the recommendation of the Norwegian Research Council for the Sciences and Humanities	Yes Attendance fees	–	–	– Own personnel – Director of secretariat + information officer = full time – Secretary = half time – Secretariat director to be a specialist in ethics	– Own facilities – Located at the Medical Ethics Centre of the University of Oslo	Own budget	Norwegian Council for the Sciences and Humanities	NOK 1.5 million	– Committee activities – Secretariat remuneration

Table 2D (cont.)

Country	Mode of reference	Supervisory authority	Composition	Name	Salary	Assignment Amount	Expenses	Personnel	Facilities	Nature	Budget Source	Budget Amount	Purpose
Norway (cont.) National Committee for Research Ethics in Science and Technology	?	Annual report to Ministry of Education and Research	12 members	Ministry of Education and Research on the recommendation of the Norwegian Council for Research in the Sciences and Humanities	Yes Attendance fees	–	–	– Own personnel – Director of secretariat + information officer = full time – Secretary = half time	– Own facilities – Located at the Medical Ethics Centre of the University of Oslo	Own budget	Norwegian Council for the Sciences and Humanities	NOK 0.5 million	– Committee activities – Secretariat remuneration
National Committee for Research Ethics in the Social Sciences and the Humanities	?	Annual report to Ministry of Education and Research	12 members	Ministry of Education and Research upon recommendation by the Norwegian Research Council for the Sciences and Humanities	Yes Attendance fees	–	?	– Own personnel – Director of secretariat and information officer = full time – Secretary = part time	– Own facilities – Rented from University of Oslo Medical Ethics Centre	Own budget	Norwegian Council for the Sciences and Humanities	NOK 0.5 million	– Committee activities – Remuneration of secretariat
Philippines National Health Research Ethics Committee	– Institutional research ethics committee – Other agencies	– Department of Science and Technology	8 members: – Doctors, theologian, environmentalist, sociologist, researchers	Appointed by the secretary of the Department of Science and Technology	Yes	In the form of honoraria for each meeting	–	No	No Facilities for meetings are supplied by the Department of Science and Technology	No budget of its own	Expenses covered by the Department of Science and Technology	?	– Member honoraria – Operating expenses

Table 2D (cont.)

Country	Mode of reference	Supervisory authority	Composition	Name	Salary	Assignment Amount	Expenses	Personnel	Facilities	Nature	Budget Source	Budget Amount	Purpose
Poland National Human Research Monitoring Committee	– Ministry of Public Health – Ministry of Public Health Science Council – Regional commission – Researchers appealing a decision of the regional commission	Ministry of Public Health Science Council	– Medical sciences researchers – Medical specialist representatives from the National Surveillance of medical specialization – Persons with practical experience in the commission's activities – Members representing various ministries, universities, and academies	Appointed by the Ministry of Public Health Designated by their institutions	No	–	?	Personnel assistance from Health Ministry Science Council	No facilities of its own	Expenses covered by Ministry of Health budget	Ministry of Health	?	?
Polish Medical Council Ethics Committee	?	Polish Medical Council	Chairman and 22 members	By the Polish Medical Council	No	–	–	– 1 full-time secretary – 1 part-time secretary	?	?	The Committee is funded by the Polish Medical Council	?	?
Portugal National Council for Life Sciences	– Parliamentary Assembly – Agencies designating Council members	Reports to President of Council of Ministers	20 members: – 1 president – 6 members, political groups	– Appointed by the First Minister – Appointed by Parliament	No	–	Yes Travel expenses	Secretary seconded	– No facilities of its own – Located in facilities of Council of Ministers	Included under budget of President of Council of Ministers	Government	?	– Operating expenses – Information – Symposia

Table 2D (cont.)

Country	Mode of reference	Supervisory authority	Composition	Name	Salary	Assignment Amount	Expenses	Personnel	Facilities	Nature	Budget Source	Budget Amount	Purpose
Portugal (cont.)			– 7 representatives from the humanities and social sciences – 7 members representing the pure sciences and medical sciences	– Designated by Social Affairs ministries and institutions – Designated by scientific and medical ministries and institutions									
Romania Academy of Medical Sciences Bioethics Commission	– Doctor – Patient or family	Independent	Doctors only	Selected by doctors	No	–	No	Seconded by Academy of Medical Sciences	Within facilities of Academy of Medical Sciences	Not yet	Academy of Medical Sciences	?	?
Spain National Bioethics Committee (Bill)	?	Ministry of Health	– Multidisciplinary – Experience and skills in medical ethics and research	By Ministry of Health	No	–	Yes Travel expenses	?	?	?	?	?	?

Table 2D (cont.)

Country	Mode of reference	Supervisory authority	Composition	Name	Salary	Assignment Amount	Expenses	Personnel	Facilities	Nature	Budget Source	Budget Amount	Purpose
Sweden National Council on Medical Ethics	– Independent – By government	Government	20 members: – 1 president – 7 members of political parties – 12 multidisciplinary experts (arts, law, philosophy, theology, National Health Council, College of Physicians, etc.)	Appointed by the government	No	3,000 SKR/year	Yes Per diems for meetings	– Own personnel – 1 full-time person (secretary) – 1 part-time assistant	Own facilities	Own budget	Ministry of Health	SEK 1.5 million	– Personnel salary – Travel expenses – Publications – Conferences
Switzerland National Ethics Commission (Bill)	– Parliament – Federal Council – Cantons	– Federal Council – Reports to federal Department of the Interior	– Multidisciplinary composition – Equal representation by both sexes	Federal Council	?	?	?	?	?	?	?	?	?
Tunisia	– President of the Chamber of Deputies – President of constitutional council – President of economic and social council – Member of government – Higher education or research institute – Health sciences association	Ministry of Public Health	14 members: – 1 president – other members appointed from the categories stipulated in the decree	Members are designated by their respective ministries or institutions	?	?	?	Seconded by hospitals under the Ministry of Public Health	?	?	?	?	?

Table 2D (cont.)

Country	Mode of reference	Supervisory authority	Composition	Name	Salary	Assignment Amount	Expenses	Personnel	Facilities	Nature	Budget Source	Budget Amount	Purpose
Turkey Senior Health Council	Through the Ministry of Health	In principle, independent	9 members	Appointed by Minister of Health	Yes Honoraria for residents of Ankara	?	Yes Travel expenses and per diems for others	Assistance from Ministry of Health personnel	No facilities of its own	Ministry of Health budget	Ministry of Health	?	Operating expenses
United Kingdom Nuffield Council on Bioethics	Not yet determined	Independent	15 members: – 4 health professionals – 3 scientists – 2 administrators – 2 law professionals – 1 philosopher – 1 theologian – 1 educator – 1 journalist	Appointed by the Nuffield Foundation Administration Committee	No	–	Yes Travel expenses	– Has its own personnel – 3 full-time members – Qualifications in science and humanities	Own facilities	Own budget	– Medical Research Council – Wellcome Trust	£150,000	– Remuneration of personnel – Operating expenses – Contracting out of work

Table 2D (cont.)

Country	Mode of reference	Supervisory authority	Composition	Name	Salary	Assignment Amount	Expenses	Personnel	Facilities	Budget Nature	Budget Source	Budget Amount	Purpose
United States National Bioethics Advisory Commission	– Independently – Federal agencies – Congress – Public	President's National Science and Technology Council (NSTC)	– No more than 15 members, including the chairman – Multidisciplinary: bioethics/theology, social sciences, law, health sciences, and biomedical research. Three members from the public at large with expertise in areas other than the above – Search for a balance between scientists and nonscientists	By the president	No	–	Yes	– Personnel provided by the Department of Health and Human Services and other agencies of the National Science and Technology Council – 6 full-time employees	Supplied by other agencies of the National Science and Technology Council	Own budget	Government	$2 million	– Operating expenses – Full-time personnel ($500,000) – Compensation and travel costs of members

Table 2E

Activities of national ethics bodies[1] – 1996

Country	Field of activity	Specific activities					Action priorities		Obstacles
		Opinions and recommendations	Education and training	Information, communication, and advice	Scientific evaluation and research ethics	Other	Nature	Priority setting	
Australia Australian Health Ethics Committee	Studies and advice on ethical, legal, and social issues as they concern public health, medical practice, and human research	Yes – To board – On research involving human subjects – On compliance with Privacy Act	Yes – Promote debate on health ethics issues	Yes – Coordinate the work of research ethics committees – Monitor international activities in health ethics	?	?	– Human research – Protection of privacy – In addition, working groups on: 1) transplant ethics 2) legal problems 3) reproductive technologies 4) women and clinical trials	– Under the Act itself and where the Minister deems it appropriate	
Belgium National Advisory Bioethics Committee	Give an opinion on problems raised by research and applications in biology, health, and medicine	Yes	?	Yes	?	?	?	?	–

1. The term "ethics body" is used in its broadest sense to include national committees and the principal national ethics bodies as identified for the various countries (cf. tables 2B and 2C).

Table 2E (cont.)

Country	Field of activity	Specific activities					Action priorities		Obstacles
		Opinions and recommendations	Education and training	Information, communication, and advice	Scientific evaluation and research ethics	Other	Nature	Priority setting	
Canada National Council on Bioethics in Human Research	The ethics of research on human subjects in the humanities and health sciences	Yes – Opinions on the formulation of guidelines with respect to evaluation mechanisms of research ethics boards and the research ethics review process	Yes – The promotion of education, communications and understanding within the scientific and medical community with respect to ethical principles and practices that must provide a framework for research involving human subjects – Public awareness	Yes – To clinical research ethics committees – To government agencies – To the scientific and medical communities (universities, hospitals, etc.)	Yes – Opinions on the implementation of decision-making principles and criteria developed by the Medical Research Council to guide local research committees – Establishment of an ongoing evaluation mechanism for research ethics board functions	–	Yes The application and interpretation of research ethics standards in biomedicine and the health sciences, that involve human subjects	Priorities set by the Council itself pursuant to its mandate, generally in consultation and in response to the needs of research ethics boards	Yes Scope of mandate in view of limited resources
Cyprus Medical Council	Establishment of a code of ethics	Yes	No	Yes	–	–	?	?	?

Table 2E (cont.)

Country	Field of activity	Specific activities					Action priorities		Obstacles
		Opinions and recommendations	Education and training	Information, communication, and advice	Scientific evaluation and research ethics	Other	Nature	Priority setting	
Czech Republic Central Ethics Committee	Statement of ethical principles concerning practices at health institutions and research centres in compliance with the Helsinki Declaration and other international declarations	Yes	Yes – To the scientific and medical community – To the public – To regional and local ethics bodies	Yes – To the government – To elected representatives – To the scientific community – To regional and local ethics authorities	Yes	No	Yes – Development of codes – Participation in preparation of legal standards	?	No
Denmark Danish Council of Ethics	Ethical implications of biomedical research involving human subjects	Yes Opinions and recommendations to Parliament	Yes – Preparation of pedagogical materials for health personnel with respect to patient information – Development of educational materials on bioethical issues for secondary schools and colleges	Yes Organization of debates on bioethics issues	?	Yes – Film presentations – Television programs – Organization of public hearings – Debates surrounding Council publications	Yes – Ethical, social, and legal impact of Human Genome Project – Ethical evaluation of issues surrounding the recording, keeping, and use of genetic information – Ethical components of priorities to be determined in health services	Priorities set on the basis of the Council's mandate and public debates	?

Table 2E (cont.)

Country	Field of activity	Specific activities					Action priorities		Obstacles
		Opinions and recommendations	Education and training	Information, communication, and advice	Scientific evaluation and research ethics	Other	Nature	Priority setting	
Finland Research Ethics Advisory Council	– Research ethics	Yes Advise government authorities on possible legislation and other research ethics issues	Yes Advice on specific research ethics problems	Yes – Promotion of debate and meetings in the area of research ethics – Provide information on research ethics issues	No Specific evaluation agency exists	Yes Understanding and participation in international development in this area of activity	?	?	No
France National Consultative Ethics Committee [for Health and Life Sciences	– Advisory body – Ethical evaluation in biological, medical, and health research	Yes	Yes – To the scientific and medical community – To the public – To local and regional ethics bodies	Yes – To government – To elected representatives – To the scientific and medical community – To regional or local authorities	Yes	–	Yes – Responds to questions asked – Studies fundamental problems	By the Committee	Yes – Legislative gaps – Defining the boundaries between research ethics and professional ethics

Table 2E (cont.)

Country	Field of activity	Specific activities					Action priorities		Obstacles
		Opinions and recommendations	Education and training	Information, communication, and advice	Scientific evaluation and research ethics	Other	Nature	Priority setting	
Germany Central Commission for the Observance of Ethical Principles in the Areas of Reproductive Medicine, Human Embryo Research, and Genetic Therapy	Promote compliance with appropriate guidelines	Yes − To government − To elected representatives − To board of trustees of Federal Medical Council	Yes Development of consistent standards of practice	Yes − To government − To elected representatives − To regional and local committees − To institutions involved in human embryo research − To the board of trustees of the Federal Medical Council	?	Yes Advise the Science Committee of the Federal Medical Council on certain specific subjects	No	–	?
Central Commission for the Safeguard of Ethical Principles in Medicine and Related Fields	Develop a standpoint on sensitive societal issues such as medically assisted death, transplants, assisted reproduction, abortion, genetic engineering	?	?	?	?	?	Yes Labelling of food undergoing genetic engineering processes	By the Committee itself	–

Table 2E (cont.)

Country	Field of activity	Specific activities					Action priorities		Obstacles
		Opinions and recommendations	Education and training	Information, communication, and advice	Scientific evaluation and research ethics	Other	Nature	Priority setting	
Greece National Health Sciences Ethics Council	Participates in formulating policy for the Department of Health with respect to biomedical matters	Yes – Gives opinions on medical ethics issues – Gives opinions on issues pertaining to future institutional ethics committees	Yes – To the scientific and medical community – To the public – To regional or local ethics bodies	Yes – To government – To elected representatives – To the scientific and medical community – To regional and local ethics authorities	Yes Only at the second level	–	– Develops directives for dealing with problems such as: – ethical conflicts in medical practice – moral dilemmas in hospital medicine – clinical experimentation – biomedical research on human subjects – conflicts between various hospital ethics committees	Not specified	– Limited medical expertise, therefore "imports" from other European models – Lack of ethics education for health professionals, who are not all that interested in such committees
Italy National Bioethics Committee	– Government advisory body – Formulates opinions to government authorities and provides information to the public	Yes	No	Yes – To chair of Committee – To government – To Parliament – To the public	Yes On request	–	Yes Questions relating to the safeguarding of life	Assembly of Council	No

Table 2E (cont.)

Country	Field of activity	Specific activities					Action priorities		Obstacles
		Opinions and recommendations	Education and training	Information, communication, and advice	Scientific evaluation and research ethics	Other	Nature	Priority setting	
Luxembourg National Ethics Advisory Committee for the Life and Health Sciences	– Advisory body – Ethical evaluation of possible solutions to modern problems related to life and health	Yes To government	No But plans to publish opinions and to have greater contact with the public and provide training to the public	Yes – To government – To elected representatives	–	–	No	By supervising ministry	Difficult to reach quorum required at plenary assemblies to be able to take decisions (votes on opinions, etc.)
Malta Health Ethics Consultative Committee	– Government advisory body – Ethical evaluation of problems posed by biomedical progress	Yes To government	Yes – To students of medicine and pharmacology – To the public	Yes – Essentially to the government – To elected representatives on request – To the scientific community on request	Yes	Yes Advice to Department of Health on specific issues	Yes	As a function of the specific problems that arise in Malta	Yes – Committee slow to gain recognition – Limits on scope of its opinions as the Committee's voice has no binding power – No recognized status => credibility problem

Table 2E (cont.)

Country	Field of activity	Specific activities					Action priorities		Obstacles
		Opinions and recommendations	Education and training	Information, communication, and advice	Scientific evaluation and research ethics	Other	Nature	Priority setting	
Mexico	Research and review of subjects related to life, health, welfare, and social security	Yes	?	Yes	Yes	–	Study and recommendations in professional ethics, biomedical activities related to life, health, and ecology	?	?
Netherlands Provisional National Ethical Review Board (KEMO)	– Advisory body for local hospital committees – Advice and support for complex or interesting issues to the country as a whole	Yes – To the scientific community – To regional and local committees	No	Yes – To government – To elected representatives – To the scientific community	Yes This is the specific activity of the council	No	No Not at this time	–	Yes Has trouble obtaining an overview of all aspects of research projects, both in terms of researchers, local committees, and funding agencies

Table 2E (cont.)

Country	Field of activity	Specific activities					Action priorities		Obstacles
		Opinions and recommendations	Education and training	Information, communication, and advice	Scientific evaluation and research ethics	Other	Nature	Priority setting	
Norway National Biotechnology Advisory Council	– Advisory body – Ethical evaluation of research and practical applications of biotechnology as they relate to humans, animals, plants, and microorganisms	Yes – To government authorities with respect to the safety and evaluation of biotechnological risks	Yes – To the public	Yes – To government – To elected representatives – To the scientific and medical community – To local and regional ethics bodies – To the public	No	–	Yes – Ethical issues relating to biotechnology	– By the Council itself	?
National Committee for Medical Research Ethics National Committee for Research Ethics in Science and Technology National Committee for Research Ethics in the Social Sciences and Humanities	Deliberation on research ethics in those areas assigned to them by statute	Yes	Yes – To the scientific and medical community – To the public – To local and regional ethics committees	Yes – To government – To local and regional committees	Yes Coordination and assistance to regional research ethics committees	–	Yes – Advisory and coordination role with respect to professional committees under their jurisdiction – Inform researchers, administrators, and the public on issues raised in their areas of jurisdiction	The committees set their own priorities	Yes The committee for medical research ethics of the Norwegian Council for the Sciences and Humanities spent 11 years acquiring formal national status and became the current National Committee for Research Ethics in the Social Sciences and the Humanities

Table 2E (cont.)

Country	Field of activity	Specific activities					Action priorities		Obstacles
		Opinions and recommen- dations	Education and training	Information, communication, and advice	Scientific evaluation and research ethics	Other	Nature	Priority setting	
Philippines National Health Research Ethics Committee	– Formulate directives for the ethical evaluation of research pro- jects in the health field and for the establishment of institutional ethics commit- tees and the accreditation of these committees – Carry out studies proposed by various agencies	Yes	Yes Seminars and training on how to organize an institutional ethics committee	Yes Organize seminars on specific topics (e.g., research involving children, the mentally ill, status of the foetus, etc.)	Yes Restructuring of research protocols	–	Yes Evaluation of research	?	– Cultural differences between people – Budgetary limitations

Table 2E (cont.)

Country	Field of activity	Specific activities					Action priorities		Obstacles
		Opinions and recommendations	Education and training	Information, communication, and advice	Scientific evaluation and research ethics	Other	Nature	Priority setting	
Poland National Human Research Monitoring Commission	Appraisal of the eligibility of human medical experimentation in view of ethical and practical principles	Yes	No	Yes – To the Minister of Health – To the scientific community – To regional and local ethics bodies	Yes	Yes – Preparation of draft regulations – Periodic control of the activities of regional and local committees	No	–	Yes – Inadequate autonomy in terms of finance, day-to-day operations, and organization – No regulatory power – Criteria for the establishment of the Commission are much too imprecise
Polish Medical Council Ethics Committee	– Bioethics, medical ethics – Establishment and interpretation of medical ethics code	Yes	Yes – For the scientific and medical community – For regional and local ethics bodies	Yes – To the government – To elected representatives – To the scientific community – To regional and local ethics bodies	No	–	Yes The teaching of bioethics in medical faculties	–	Poor understanding of the Polish Medical Code of Ethics by the media

Table 2E (cont.)

Country	Field of activity	Specific activities					Action priorities		Obstacles
		Opinions and recommendations	Education and training	Information, communication, and advice	Scientific evaluation and research ethics	Other	Nature	Priority setting	
Portugal National Ethics Council for the Life Sciences	– Advisory body – Evaluation of ethical issues in the life sciences	Yes – To government – To elected representatives	Yes	Yes – To government – To elected representatives	?	?	No	–	– Limited budget – Limited secretariat – Lack of documentation services
Romania Academy of Medical Science Bioethics Committee	?	Yes	Yes – To the scientific community – To regional and local ethics bodies – To the public	Yes – To the scientific community – To regional and local ethics authorities	Yes	–	– Life-prolonging medical treatment – Human experimentation – Animal experimentation – Passive euthanasia	By the Committee itself	– Limited financial resources – Lack of international contacts
Spain National Bioethics Committee (Bill)	?	Yes – To government – To the scientific community – To ethics bodies – To Parliament – To the public	Yes – Of the scientific community – Of the public	Yes – Government – Local and regional ethics bodies – Public	No There are specific committees	–	Not yet determined	By the Commission itself	Yes Some members of colleges of physicians are reluctant concerning the establishment of such a commission

Table 2E (cont.)

Country	Field of activity	Specific activities					Action priorities		Obstacles
		Opinions and recommendations	Education and training	Information, communication, and advice	Scientific evaluation and research ethics	Other	Nature	Priority setting	
Sweden National Council on Medical Ethics	– Advisory body – Approaches to medical ethics issues from a societal standpoint – Intermediary role between scientists, politicians, and citizens	Yes To the government	Yes Indirectly through its publications	Yes – To the government – To elected representatives, indirectly – Very little to the scientific community and to local and regional committees	No	No	Yes	At the request of government, but the Committee may also take its own initiatives	No
Switzerland National Ethics Committee (Bill)	– Advisory body – Monitors developments in reproduction and genetics engineering or any other questions chosen by the Federal Council	Yes Directives to complement legislation	?	Yes on request: – To Parliament – To the Federal Council – To the cantons	No	No	?	?	–

Table 2E (cont.)

Country	Field of activity	Specific activities					Action priorities		Obstacles
		Opinions and recommendations	Education and training	Information, communication, and advice	Scientific evaluation and research ethics	Other	Nature	Priority setting	
Switzerland (cont.) Central Ethics Committee of the Swiss Academy of Medical Science	– Advisory body – Deliberation on contemporary medical ethics problems	Yes – To the Confederation, to the cantons – To the Federation of Physicians	Yes Coordination among hospital and institutional ethics committees	Yes on request: – To the government – To elected representatives – To the scientific and medical community – To regional and local ethics bodies	No	Yes – Investigates the scope of rules of conduct proposed for practitioners – Exchanges with international, national, and regional agencies involved in medical ethics	Yes Formulation of directives and opinions	By the Committee and its president	Yes Business interests
Tunisia	– Opinions on moral problems raised by research – Formulation of major principles to reconcile technological progress with ethical and legal standards	Yes	?	?	?	?	?	?	?

Table 2E (cont.)

Country	Field of activity	Specific activities					Action priorities		Obstacles
		Opinions and recommen-dations	Education and training	Information, communication, and advice	Scientific evaluation and research ethics	Other	Nature	Priority setting	
Turkey Senior Health Council	– Review of health and social issues – Participates in deliberation on medical practice	Yes	No	Information and advice to government	No	Review of draft regulations	No	–	Yes Wide variety of functions
United Kingdom Nuffield Council on Bioethics	– Advisory body – Identify and define ethical issues raised by recent progress in medical and biological research	Yes To appropriate institutions	?	Yes – To the government – To the public – To organiza-tions on request	No	– Organizes symposia – Encourages the public to speak out on biomedical issues	– Foetal surgery – Over-the-counter test kits	By the Foundation itself	–

Table 2E (cont.)

Country	Field of activity	Specific activities					Action priorities		Obstacles
		Opinions and recommendations	Education and training	Information, communication, and advice	Scientific evaluation and research ethics	Other	Nature	Priority setting	
United States National Bioethics Advisory Commission	Bioethical implications of biomedical research and its applications	Yes To National Science and Technology Council and other concerned parties, as well as to the public	?	?	?	No	– Issues surrounding the management and utilization of genetic information – Protection of research subjects' rights and welfare	– 4 criteria used to establish priorities: 1) urgency of public policy or public health 2) relationship between bioethical issues and federal objectives in terms of investment in science and technology 3) unavailability of jurisdiction of another body to deliberate the issue 4) interest in the issue throughout government (i.e., not only one department or agency)	?

Table 2F

Communications, publications, and recommendations – 1996

Country	Public perception		Publication		National ethics bodies reporting structure/Other regional and local bodies		Opinions and recommendations	
	Yes/no	Means	Yes/no	Means	Yes/no	Means	Topics covered	Topics being considered
Australia Australian Health Ethics Committee	?	?	Yes	Through the National Health and Medical Research Council	Yes	The AHEC closely monitors and gives advice to the various institutional ethics committees	Through the working groups: – Privacy – Transplants – Reproductive technologies – Women and clinical trials	?
Belgium National Advisory Bioethics Committee	No	–	?	?	–	–	?	Problems raised by research and its application in biology, medicine and health, whether these problems affect humans, social groups, or all of society
Canada National Council on Bioethics in Human Research	Yes	– Public participation in Council workshop – Public representation on Council and in its expert groups	Yes	– Publication of a bulletin: *Communiqué* – Proceedings of workshops – Discussion papers	No	– Cooperation – No subordination – Coordination committee functions as a forum for discussion and cooperation for institutional initiatives in research ethics	– The ethics of clinical trials – Preparation of a national data bank on ethics evaluation in Canada – The ethics of research using children – Pedagogical requirements of institutions establishing research ethics boards and persons appointed to these boards – Preparation of a procedures manual for research ethics boards – Research ethics into somatic genetic therapy in compliance with the guidelines of the Medical Research Council	– Research on the mentally disabled – The introduction of changes acceptable for ethics assessment at the local level – Research on embryos and the foetus – Other areas of ethics involving research using human subjects in the health sciences

Table 2F (cont.)

Country	Public perception		Publication		National ethics bodies reporting structure/Other regional and local bodies		Opinions and recommendations	
	Yes/no	Means	Yes/no	Means	Yes/no	Means	Topics covered	Topics being considered
Cyprus Medical Council	Yes	– Symposia – Round tables	No	–	?	?	?	?
Czech Republic Central Ethics Committee	Yes	– Annual meeting with a representative of each ethics committee in the Czech Republic – Round tables	No	Published through the press	No	–	– Euthanasia – Medically assisted reproduction – Embryo research – Transplants – Grafts – Neonatology – Abortion – Cessation of treatment – International adoption	– Status of the embryo – Patient information and diagnosis of incurable diseases – The concept of death with dignity – Protection of information – Genetic studies
Denmark Danish Council of Ethics	Yes	– Field visits – Conferences – Round tables – Public hearings – Surveys – Press inserts	Yes	– Publicity through press conferences – Extensive distribution of certain documents and reports free of charge – Bookstore sales	No	– Cooperation with various ethics and scientific committees – No reporting structure	– Criteria and definition for death – Protection of gametes, fertilized eggs, embryos, and foetuses – Informed patient consent – Genetics – Health services – Genetic screening – The use of genetic tests for insurance – Premature birth	?

Table 2F (cont.)

Country	Public perception		Publication		National ethics bodies reporting structure/Other regional and local bodies		Opinions and recommendations	
	Yes/no	Means	Yes/no	Means	Yes/no	Means	Topics covered	Topics being considered
Finland Research Ethics Advisory Committee	Too early	–	Too early	–	No	–	–	– The use of genetic therapy – Use of genetically modified organisms – Research on embryos and foetuses – Human research – Protection of personal data collected for research purposes – The use of animals in research – Reliability of scientific research – Independence of scientific research – Value judgments and the role of the researcher
France National Consultative Ethics Committee for Health and Life Sciences	Yes	– Yearly ethics days – Public lectures	Yes	– Publicity through press releases – Publication of annual reports – Publication of working groups reports	No	Council only	– 41 opinions given on various aspects of life and health Principal topics: – The use of embryonic tissues – Medically assisted impregnation – Prenatal diagnosis – AIDS – Marketing the body – The use of human cells and derivatives – Donating gametes and embryos	– Ethics and money – Ethics and the environment – Eugenics – Gestational and other forms of maternity

Table 2F (cont.)

Country	Public perception		Publication		National ethics bodies reporting structure/Other regional and local bodies		Opinions and recommendations	
	Yes/no	Means	Yes/no	Means	Yes/no	Means	Topics covered	Topics being considered
France (cont.)							– Preimplantation genetic diagnosis – Embryo experimentation – Genetic therapy – Blood transfusions – DNA identification – The grafting of nerve cells – Assistance to the dying – Epidemiological registries and studies – Ethics and neuroscience – Predictive medicine, etc.	
Germany Central Commission for the Observance of Ethical Principles in the Areas of Reproductive Medicine, Human Embryo Research, and Genetic Therapy	No	–	Yes	– Annual report Medicine-Ethics – Reports published in the German practitioners' Gazette	No	Cooperation	– Embryo disposal – Genetic therapy – Research using fertilized eggs – Evaluation of research applications – Registration of research activities – Methods and purposes of reproductive medicine centres	Research on foetal tissues, including ethical problems involved in abortion
Central Commission for the Safeguard of Ethical Principles in Medicine and Related Fields	?	?	?	?	?	?	?	?

Table 2F (cont.)

Country	Public perception			Publication			National ethics bodies reporting structure/Other regional and local bodies		Opinions and recommendations	
	Yes/no	Means		Yes/no	Means		Yes/no	Means	Topics covered	Topics being considered
Greece National Health Sciences Ethics Council	?	–		?	–		Yes	In the event of disputes, referral to the Committee	–	– Euthanasia – AIDS – Medically assisted reproduction – Truth and information to patients
Italy National Bioethics Committee	Yes	Public hearings		Yes	Publication of opinions by the Council Information and Publication Department		No	–	– Genetic therapy – Definition of and criteria for death – Assistance to terminally ill patients – Processing of seminal fluid for diagnostic purposes – Biotechnology security – Organ transplants in children – Drug experimentation – Patentability of living organisms – Informed consent – Operation of ethics committees – Antenatal diagnosis	– Bioethics training – Genetic tests for medico-legal purposes – Assistance to terminally ill patients – Organ donations for therapeutic grafting – Ethical guidelines for medically assisted reproduction

Table 2F (cont.)

Country	Public perception		Publication		National ethics bodies reporting structure/Other regional and local bodies		Opinions and recommendations	
	Yes/no	Means	Yes/no	Means	Yes/no	Means	Topics covered	Topics being considered
Luxembourg National Ethics Advisory Commission for the Life and Health Sciences	Not organized	The Commission aims at increased contact with the public, through publication of its notices and press conferences, and other avenues	Yes	Opinions to be sent to government and Parliament	No	–	– Haemoglobin irregularities during prenuptial examination – The dissemination of genetically modified organisms – Youth protection – Patentability of biotechnological inventions – Mandatory HIV screening tests – Prolongation of life by medical means	– Medically assisted reproduction – Euthanasia – Hospital ethics committees – Anonymous delivery – Systematic review of stereotypes in children up for adoption
Malta Health Ethics Consultative Committee	Yes	– Public debate – Lectures	No	–	No	–	– Patient consent for treatment, surgery, and medical experimentation – Medically assisted reproduction (in progress)	– Dialysis – Organ and tissue transplants – The use of genetic tests for medical, civil, and criminal purposes
Mexico	Yes	The Commission receives and regularly provides opinions on the country's medical practice	Yes	– Publication of work through the *Bulletin* – Briefs on activities and events – Proceedings of First International Congress on Bioethics	No	–	Establishment of moral principles for the respect of all forms of life	– Genetics – Human rights – Reproduction – Biomedical research and experimentation – Ethical aspects of organ transplants – Legal aspects of bioethics

Table 2F (cont.)

Country	Public perception		Publication		National ethics bodies reporting structure/Other regional and local bodies		Opinions and recommendations	
	Yes/no	Means	Yes/no	Means	Yes/no	Means	Topics covered	Topics being considered
Norway National Biotechnology Advisory Council	Yes	?	Yes	Publicizing all opinions and decisions rendered	?	?	Opinions on the forthcoming Genetic Engineering Act	– Biotechnological safety and risk assessment – Dissemination and use of genetically modified organisms – Research ethics and practical applications of biotechnology
National Committee for Medical Research Ethics	Yes	– Annual days – Organization of debates	Yes	Publication by the Norwegian Council for Science and the Humanities (essentially the National Committee for Medical Research Ethics)	No	Coordination and advice	– Medical ethics – Informed consent – Child research – In vitro fertilization and in vitro fertilization services – Processing of sensitive personal data – Foetal research	– Ethical issues surrounding the recording of genetic abnormalities – Setting of medical ethics priorities – Relationship between ethics and law with respect to the research structure
National Committee for Research Ethics in Science and Technology National Committee for Research Ethics in the Social Sciences and the Humanities	Yes	– Annual days – Organization of debates	Yes	Publication by the Norwegian Council for Science and the Humanities (essentially the National Committee for Medical Research Ethics)	No	Coordination and advice	?	– Risk assessments – Environmental ethics – Computer science

Table 2F (cont.)

Country	Public perception		Publication		National ethics bodies reporting structure/Other regional and local bodies		Opinions and recommendations	
	Yes/no	Means	Yes/no	Means	Yes/no	Means	Topics covered	Topics being considered
Netherlands Provisional National Ethical Review Board (KEMO)	Yes	– Submission of final report on television – Activities of public members	Yes	Publication of an annual report	No officially Yes in practice based on expertise of council members	?	– Embryo research (including preimplantation diagnosis) – Human genetic therapy – The use of foetal tissue – Research projects involving legally incapable persons – The use of human tissues	– In-depth studies of the consequences of the use of foetal tissues – Embryo research (including preimplantation diagnosis) – Human genetic therapy – Research projects involving legally incapable persons
Philippines National Health Research Ethics Committee	Yes	?	Yes	Philippine Council for health research and development is responsible for its publications	Yes	The National Ethics Committee acts as an arbiter when differences between regional and institutional bodies cannot be settled	– Issues concerning HIV/AIDS – Organ transplants – The genetics industry – Medically assisted reproduction	– The development of new technologies (such as organ transplants) – The prolongation of life (quality of life issues)
Poland National Human Research Monitoring Commission	No	–	No	–	Yes	?	– Monitoring of regional committee activities – Safety of research and respect for patient	Application of prenatal diagnoses
Polish Medical Council Ethics Committee	Yes	?	Yes	In the medical press	Yes	Representatives of regional committees attend committee meetings	– Formulation of Polish Medical Ethics Code	?

579

Table 2F (cont.)

Country	Public perception			Publication			National ethics bodies reporting structure/Other regional and local bodies			Opinions and recommendations	
	Yes/no	Means		Yes/no	Means		Yes/no	Means		Topics covered	Topics being considered
Portugal National Ethics Council for the Life Sciences	No	–		No	–		?	–		– Organ donation – Medically assisted reproduction	– Informed consent – Status of the embryo – Definition and criteria of death
Romania Academy of Medical Science Bioethics Committee	Yes	– Use of media – Organization of conferences and lectures for doctors and the public at large		Yes	Articles in the Romanian Academy Journal *Academica*		Yes	The Commission recommends positions to be adopted to local and regional committees		– The terminal phases of life – Active and passive euthanasia – The ethics of medical emergencies – Eugenics – Death as viewed by children	– Medically assisted reproduction – Abortion – Allocation of resources in a poor country – The status of disabled children – AIDS – The treatment of the chronically ill – Contemporary medicine in a developing country
Spain National Bioethics Commission (Bill)	?	?		?	?		No	–		–	Pursuant to s. 2 of the bill: – Experimentation – Clinical trials – Therapy and diagnostic research – Medically assisted impregnation – Genetic manipulations – Contraception – Abortion – Use of human blood, organs, and tissues – Confidentiality and information – Consent

Table 2F (cont.)

Country	Public perception		Publication		National ethics bodies reporting structure/Other regional and local bodies		Opinions and recommendations	
	Yes/no	Means	Yes/no	Means	Yes/no	Means	Topics covered	Topics being considered
Switzerland Central Ethics Committee of the Swiss Academy of Medical Science	Yes	– Symposia – Lectures – Televised programs	Yes	– Annual bulletin of the Swiss Assembly of Medical Sciences – Bulletin of the Swiss Physicians Federation	?	?	– Medically assisted reproduction – Human research – Animal research – Organ transplants – Euthanasia – The use of foetal tissue – Human genetic screening	Prenatal and postnatal diagnosis
National Ethics Committee (Bill)	?	?	?	–	?	?	–	Medically assisted reproduction
Tunisia	?	?	?	?	?	?	?	?
Turkey Senior Health Council	No	–	No	–	?	?	– Problems with social and health services – Medical practice	– Problems with social and health services – Medical practice
United Kingdom Nuffield Council on Bioethics	Yes	– Promotion of public understanding and discussion – Publication of reports	Yes	– Publication of an annual report – Publication of research reports	No	–	– Genetic screening – The use of human tissue – Xenotransplantation	– Foetal testing kits – Over-the-counter test kits
United States National Bioethics Advisory Commission	Yes	– Possibility of reference by the public – Meetings of the Commission are public	Yes	– Annual report – Publication of reports on specific issues	No	–	?	?

APPENDIX 3

Canada – University Research Ethics Boards

Table 3A

Identification of board – 1996

Institutions	Title of references	Year of publication	Board name
University of Alberta	*University Standards for the Protection of Human Research Participants*	1991	Ethics Review Committee
University of British Columbia	*Policy and Procedure Handbook, Policy #87*	1992	Screening committees
University of Calgary	*Research Policy – Ethics of Human Studies, Structure, Procedure and Guidelines for Ethical Review of All Research Proposals and Projects Involving Human Subjects*	1986 and 1992	Conjoint Medical Ethics Committee
Dalhousie University	*Form I-A and I-B, Summary of Ethical Guidelines and Approval Form and Form II, Information Sheet for Faculty Requesting Ethical Review of Research Proposal and Form III, Request for Ethical Evaluation Form*	1992	Ethics Committee
Université Laval	*Comité provisoire chargé de coordonner l'étude des aspects déon-tologiques de la recherche à l'Université Laval (Rapport final)*	1980	Comité de déontologie de la recherche/Comités d'évaluation déontologique
University of Manitoba	*General Guidelines for Human Research*	1976	Faculty Committee on the Use of Human Subjects in Research
McGill University	*Ethical and Legal Aspects of Research Involving Human Subjects Conducted in the Faculty of Medicine and Affiliated Hospitals Policies and Procedures*	1993	Research Ethics Committee of the Faculty (RECF) and Research Ethics Boards (REBs)
McMaster University	*Research Bulletin (09-09-88)*	1988 and 1989	President's Committee on the Ethics of Research on Human Subjects

Table 3A (cont.)

Institutions	Title references	Year of publication	Board name
Memorial University	Letter from Dr. Verna M. Skanes, Ph.D., assistant dean, Research and Graduate Studies (Medicine)	27 May 1996	
Université de Montréal	*Politique relative à l'utilisation des êtres humains en recherche: Comité de la recherche*	1993	Comités d'éthique pour la recherche portant sur les êtres humains
University of Ottawa	*Ethics, School of Graduate Studies and Research*	1993–1994	University Human Research Ethics Committee
Queen's University	*Queen's University Health Sciences and Affiliated Teaching Hospitals Human Research Ethics Board, Procedural Guidelines*	1994	Research Ethics Board
University of Saskatchewan	*Policies Related to Ethical and Safety Considerations; Conflict of Interest; Ethics in Research (1990)/Ethics in Human Experimentation*	1990	University Advisory Committee on Ethics in Human Experimentation (Health Sciences) and University Advisory Committee on Ethics in Human Experimentation (Behavioural Sciences)
Université de Sherbrooke	*Guide et critères d'évaluation, Projets de recherche clinique*	1991	Comité de déontologie de la recherche chez l'humain
University of Toronto	*Guidelines on the Use of Human Subjects* (1979) *Regulations of Research Activities as appended to the University Hospital Affiliation Agreement, appendix E, Arrangements with Respect to Research (October 1986)	1979, 1986	Human Subjects Review Committee of the Research Board/Review Committee on the Use of Human Subjects
University of Western Ontario	Not received		

Table 3B

Structure of board – 1996

Institutions	Composition		Establishment	Reporting authority
	Science community	Nonscience community		
University of Alberta	At least 4 local faculty members 1 or more members from another unit	Additional members at the discretion of the ERC chair, including lay representation	Not specified	Policy Committee for Human Research Ethics, a standing committee of the Vice-President (Research) comprised of 7 members
University of British Columbia	4 must be chosen with a view to having representatives familiar with the general field of the projects being submitted by investigators	1 must be from the Faculty of Law 1 must be from a faculty other than those presenting applications	With the advice of the deans of the faculties concerned, committees are to be appointed by the president	Not specified
University of Calgary	The chair Faculty member(s) not engaged in clinical practice, engaged in clinical practice and clinical and/or bench research/or not in clinical investigation Assistant dean (medical bioethics), associate dean (research), dean—all of them ex officio	The lay community A practicing or academic lawyer Representative(s) with graduate training and research background in social sciences Representative(s) with graduate or postgraduate training in bioethics	Not specified	Minutes submitted to the dean, associate dean (research), assistant dean (medical bioethics), the chair of the General Faculties Council Standing Committee on the Ethics of Human Studies, chair of the Research Committees of the Faculty and Affiliated Institutions

Table 3B (cont.)

Institutions	Composition		Establishment	Reporting authority
	Science community	Nonscience community		
University of Calgary (cont.)	Representatives from selected hospitals, health dciences, medical student, medical sciences (graduate) student, postgraduate (resident)	*Quorum: Dean or delegate plus 7 members		
Dalhousie University	Not specified	Not specified	Not specified	Dean
Université Laval	*Comité de déontologie:* 5 university professors *Comité d'évaluation déontologique:* Normally 3 persons, at least 2 of whom are appointed from the list established by the Comité de déontologie, and where required, 1 or more persons from outside the university (the Comité de déontologie is responsible for ensuring that appointees have no decision authority over the researcher's career)	*Comité de déontologie:* 1 person from outside (for example, a representative of the Human Rights Office)	*Comité de déontologie de la recherche:* Members appointed by the Conseil de l'Université upon the recommendation of the Vice-Rector Academic and Research *Comité d'évaluation déontologique:* Established for specific projects by the Comité de déontologie	*Comité de déontologie de la recherche:* Annual report to the Conseil de l'Université
University of Manitoba	Not specified	Not specified	Not specified	Not specified

Table 3B (cont.)

Institutions	Composition		Establishment	Reporting authority
	Science community	Nonscience community		
McGill University	*Research Ethics Committee of the Faculty* (RECF): Not specified REB (minimum total of 5): 1 physician or scientist who is not in the employ of the university or hospital to which the REB reports Sufficient membership to address the need for scientific assessment in the areas of investigation most frequently submitted	RECF: Not specified REB: 1 or more community volunteer(s) 1 bioethicist, lawyer (preferably not the Institution's Counsel), or theologian 1 patient advocate *Quorum: Majority and must include at least 1 physician with a clinical appointment and at least 1 member whose primary responsibility is neither clinical nor scientific	RECF: Dean and approval of the directors of Professional Services REB: Not specified	RECF: Not specified REB: Principal of the university if research conducted on campus (Faculty of Medicine, dean and he may delegate to associate dean [research])/board of directors of the hospital for research conducted in a hospital (may be delegated to Research Institute directors or director of Professional Services)
McMaster University	The makeup and specialities needed are first discussed and agreed upon with the chairman of Medical Advisory Committee (hospital), associate dean of research, committee chairperson, and members before any changes		President's Council	The Medical Advisory Committee, the Deanery, the president of the university through the chairman of the President's Ethics Committee

Table 3B (cont.)

Institutions	Composition		Establishment	Reporting authority
	Science community	Nonscience community		
Université de Montréal	*Comité universitaire:* 1 representative of the vice-rector (research); 1 representative of the dean of the Faculty of Graduate Studies; chairs of the 4 sectoral committees; chair of the Research Committee; 1 master's or doctoral student representative *Comités facultaires dits sectoriels:* E.g., Medicine. No less than: 1 representative of the dean of the Faculty of Medicine; 3 professors or researchers conducting research on the main university campus; 1 professor or clinical researcher working in a hospital or affiliated institute; 1 master's or doctoral student	*Comité universitaire:* 1 professor or researcher specializing in law 1 professor or researcher specializing in ethics 1 outside person without any links to the university	Not specified	Vice-rector (research)

Table 3B (cont.)

Institutions	Composition		Establishment	Reporting authority
	Science community	Nonscience community		
Université de Montréal (cont.)	*Comité d'évaluation:* No less than 3 professors or researchers, including 1 member of the appropriate sectoral committee. At least 1 member shall come from the same unit as the person in charge of the project and no less than 2 from different units. Two experts may be added to the committee			
University of Ottawa	*University Human Research Ethics Committee (UHREC):* 4 voting members shall hold academic appointments with the U and be members of the School of Graduate Studies and Research; 2 members shall be elected by the Commission of Graduate Studies in the Humanities and 2 shall be elected by the Commission of Graduate Studies in the Sciences. The faculty members normally shall not be concurrently chairpersons of their respective Ethics Subcommittees	*University Human Research Ethics Committee:* 1 voting member shall be a member of the legal profession (either a faculty member or a member of the community at large) appointed by the dean of the School of Graduate Studies and Research in consultation with the chairperson of the Committee and the director of Research Services; 1 voting member shall be from the community at large and appointed by the dean of the School of Graduate Studies and Research	Not specified	School of Graduate Studies and Research/Senate of the University of Ottawa

Table 3B (cont.)

Institutions	Composition		Establishment	Reporting authority
	Science community	Nonscience community		
University of Ottawa (cont.)	The dean of the School of Graduate Studies and Research and the director of the Office of Research Services shall be ex-officio, nonvoting members			
	The chairperson of the Committee shall be appointed by the dean of the School of Graduate Studies and Research from among the members of the Committee			
	The chairperson of the Ethics Subcommittees (or delegate) may attend UHREC meetings as nonvoting members			
	Subcommittees in the faculties of Administration, Arts, Education, Health Sciences, Medicine, Social Sciences, School of Psychology	*Subcommittees:* At least 1 member must be a member of the community at large		
	Membership of these subcommittees will be determined by the academic units concerned but must include at least 2 persons who are not members of the unit			

Table 3B (cont.)

Institutions	Composition		Establishment	Reporting authority
	Science community	Nonscience community		
Queen's University	10 members, including at least: 2 active researchers in biomedical research, at least one of whom shall be a physician 1 nurse involved in research 1 scientist with expertise in research design	1 community representative 1 clinical psychologist or other mental health expert 1 lawyer 1 bioethicist, philosopher, or theologian	Principal, with appropriate consultation and interactions with the hospitals through the Joint Committee Executive	Principal
University of Saskatchewan	The University Committee on Ethics in Human Experimentation (health sciences) shall be broadly based and include qualified persons from within and without the university and from within and without the health science disciplines 4 persons nominated by the dean of the College of Medicine 2 persons nominated by the president of the university hospital The assistant dean (research), College of Medicine, ex officio The director of Research Services, College of Graduate Studies and Research, ex officio	Up to 3 persons selected from the nonmedical research community A person competent in the law	University Advisory Committee on Ethics in Human Experimentation (health sciences): President on the advice of the associate vice-president (research) University Advisory Committee on Ethics in Human Experimentation (behavioural sc.): Associate vice-president (res.)	Not specified

Table 3B (cont.)

Institutions	Composition		Establishment	Reporting authority
	Science community	Nonscience community		
Université de Sherbrooke	Not specified	Not specified	Not specified	Not specified
University of Toronto	Monitoring of research proposal is undertaken by the *Human Subjects Review Committee of the Research Board*. It exercises its responsibility through the Review Committee on the use of human subjects, which is a select committee struck for each research proposal which requires review *Review Committee on Human Subjects*: 2 specialists in the investigator's area who are not themselves involved in the proposed research 1 member of the staff of the Office of Research Administration who has experience in working with research involving the use of human subjects Additional persons may be nominated if their special expertise can contribute to the review	*Human Subjects Review Committee of the Research Board*: Not specified *Review Committee*: Members are drawn from the administration of the university, the Faculty of Law and, not infrequently, the departments of philosophy or theology 1 person experienced in ethical and legal aspects of research (often a professor of law)	*Human Subjects Review Committee of the Research Board*: Not specified *Review Committee*: Members are nominated by the head of the academic department or division in which the research is to be conducted. The investigator may advise the head of department of appropriate nominees Office of Research Administration will nominate the specialist in ethics and law	Not specified

Table 3C

Mandate of board – 1996

Institutions	Statement of scope
University of Alberta	All persons who intend to conduct research involving human participants must have their plans reviewed and approved by an ethics review committee (ERC) prior to commencement of the research. Human participation in research includes the direct or indirect involvement of persons who are the focus of a researcher's inquiry, the use of extant documents and other records and materials (e.g., blood and tissue samples) containing information about persons when the collection and the use of such information could deprive them of their dignity or jeopardize their physical or mental well-being. Persons studied on the basis of information contained in newspaper and journal articles, or other public materials, are not deemed to be research participants for the purposes of this policy. The standards apply to members of the U who are all faculty, staff, sessional instructors, administrators, students, visiting or adjunct scholars, fellows and chairs, paid and unpaid research associates and assistants, and any other person in a like position, whether they are principal investigators or junior collaborators.
University of British Columbia	Any project carried out by a person connected with the U which involves human subjects must conform with the U Policy on Research and Other Studies Involving Human Subjects and must have the approval of the appropriate university screening committee. The policy of the U is that no research or other study involving human subjects may be undertaken by anyone associated with the U, nor may U facilities or services be used, nor may funds for such purposes be accepted, nor accounts opened by Financial Services unless the following requirements have been met and the appropriate certificate of approval for procedures in research and other studies involving human subjects has been completed.
University of Calgary	Examining any research proposal or project submitted or otherwise referred to it to ensure that it meets acceptable ethical standards in relation to human subjects. Each local review committee shall review those proposals or projects that originate within the faculty in question.
Dalhousie University	Review any research proposal (funded or nonfunded) involving human subjects from faculty members of health professions with the following exceptions: a. A proposal may be reviewed by any other Dalhousie University ethics committee (e.g., graduate studies, medicine). For legal reasons, reviews by ethics committees from other institutions (e.g., hospitals) may not be substituted for reviews by Dalhousie University committees. Collaborative research with faculty members from other universities should also be reviewed by a Dalhousie University committee if subjects are to be tested here b. Proposals which represent partial fulfilment of requirements for graduate degrees should be reviewed by the Ethics Committee of Graduate Studies. If a faculty member continues a research project subsequent to the graduation of the student, a proposal needs to be submitted in the faculty member's name to one of the university ethics committees c. Proposals which represent partial fulfilment of requirements for undergraduate degrees and courses should be reviewed by the ethics committee of the school/college d. No ethical review is necessary for students participating as subjects in laboratories for specific courses
Université Laval	It has been recommended that compliance with ethical standards be applied throughout the university to all projects, no matter what their source of funding, that fall within their purview.

Table 3C (cont.)

Institutions	Statement of scope
University of Manitoba	Approval of the appropriate ethics review subcommittee must be acquired before research involving human subjects can proceed.
McGill University	The REB has responsibility to review research performed within the boundaries of its institution including research performed by nonaffiliated or non-employed members from another institution. The REB has the responsibility to review a staff member's research that the institution administers even if such research is carried out in a different geographical location. The extent to which an REB serves a part-time physician who carries out research in a private setting should be left to the discretion of the board of directors of the hospital.
	The REB shall review all research involving human subjects (irrespective of source of funding) during the course of which an investigator obtains data through intervention or interaction with the individual or obtains identifiable private information, for the purpose of developing or contributing to generalizable knowledge (Code of Federal Regulations 46.102, appendix E).
	Review and approval of certain types of research may be carried out by responsible individuals in the faculty or hospital: Research conducted in established or commonly accepted educational settings, involving normal educational practices, such as (i) research on regular and special education instructional strategies, or (ii) any disclosure of the human subjects' responses outside the research could reasonably place the subjects at risk of criminal or civil liability or be damaging to the subjects' financial standing, employability, or reputation; research, involving the collection or study of existing data, documents, records, pathological specimens, or diagnostic specimens, if these sources are generally available or if the information is recorded by the investigator in such a manner that subjects cannot be identified, directly or through identifiers linked to the subjects.
	Any faculty members with the rank of assistant professor or above including part-time or GFT-H appointees may submit protocols and act as principal applicants. Hospital employees, including attending staff and other professionals, may also submit protocols to the REB of their employing organization.
McMaster University	It must be emphasized that all research involving human subjects (even if only interviews or questionnaires are used) falls within the jurisdiction of the ethics committee, irrespective of the source of financial support (if any) and of the location of the project (McMaster or elsewhere), so long as the investigator represents the work as McMaster research.
	Graduate student research: M.A. and Ph.D. research should undergo ethics review, unless the work has been fully described in an approved proposal by the student's supervisor.
	Undergraduate student research: In courses that require students to carry out projects or that have a laboratory involving human subjects, the instructor is responsible for review of the student's activities, with McMaster's ethical principles in mind.
Université de Montréal	Ensure that professors and researchers, as well as master's- and Ph.D.-level students in the university, follow the general ethics rules in their human research.
University of Ottawa	The University of Ottawa has adopted procedures for the ethical review of all research involving human subjects (including thesis research and research undertaken as part of graduate or undergraduate course requirements) conducted under its jurisdiction and involving its professors and students as either investigators or experimental subjects.
	The mandate of the University Human Research Ethics Committee is to examine and sanction the ethical aspects of all human research projects prior to their inception.
Queen's University	All research protocols involving human subjects for the Faculty of Medicine and the three teaching hospitals, School of Nursing, and Kingston Psychiatric Hospital. All applications and experimental protocols of health sciences U faculty are required to go through the board review process.

Table 3C (cont.)

Institutions	Statement of scope
University of Saskatchewan	It is the policy of the U that research or other studies involving human subjects not be undertaken by anyone associated with the U, or any U facilities or services used, or funds for such purposes accepted, or accounts established unless the following requirements have been met and the appropriate certificates of approval issued. All research projects involving human subjects shall be reviewed by a competent group of peers to ensure compliance with the highest standards of ethical conduct.
Université de Sherbrooke	The basic mandate of the Comité de déontologie de la recherche chez l'humain is to evaluate the ethical implications of all projects directly or indirectly involved in human research. Any research projects to be carried out on human patients or unidentifiable human tissue at the university hospital shall be submitted for the approval of the Clinical Research Centre.
University of Toronto	The policy of the U on the use of human subjects will apply to proposed research if, in the course of investigation, an investigator: (a) will administer a drug, take a blood sample, do a test, or perform any procedure, clinical, therapeutic or otherwise, upon the investigator himself or someone else, for research rather than treatment; (b) will ask people questions whether by telephone, letter, survey, questionnaire, or interview; (c) will be using nonpublic records (e.g., not the telephone book) which contain identifying information about anyone; or (d) will be observing anyone's responses to behaviour, either directly or indirectly.

Table 3D

Functions – 1996

Institutions	Evaluation of protocols	Evaluation of courses	Training	Regulation	Other
University of Alberta	Y	Y	Responsibility of principal investigator	Y	
University of British Columbia	Y	N	N	Y (Exec. Comm. for Research)	
University of Calgary	Y	Y	N	Y	Participate in research in biomedical ethics Constructing appropriate protocols by which committee members themselves will engage in such research
Dalhousie University	Y	N	N	N	
Université Laval	Y	Y	Y	Y	*Comité de déontologie de la recherche:* Receives all complaints with respect to a presumed failure to observe research ethics principles, investigates and submits a substantiated opinion to the vice-rector (academic and research)
University of Manitoba	Y	N	N	N	
McGill University	Y	N	Y	Y	RECF: Act as a central Policy and Procedures Committee for REBs and assist in the establishment of local REB (campus and affiliated hospitals)

(Y: yes, N: not specified)

Table 3D (cont.)

Institutions	Evaluation of protocols	Evaluation of courses	Training	Regulation	Other
McMaster University	Y	Y	Y	Y	To make the U community aware of its existence, of its interest in matters of ethical concerns, and of its availability for consultation on such matters To maintain a current file on matters related to such research
Université de Montréal	Y	Y	N	Y	*Comité universitaire:* Coordination of sectoral committees/Checks that affiliated hospital research centres and research institutes enforce the general ethics rules/Liaises with NCBHR and funding agencies/Evaluates the structure and operations of ethics committees and recommends changes to the Vice-rector (research) *Comités sectoriels:* Make suggestions to the Comité universitaire concerning evaluation criteria, ethics, and other rules/Review and submit opinions to the Comité universitaire concerning the annual reports of the hospital and research institute committees affiliated to the university by contract

Table 3D (cont.)

Institutions	Evaluation of protocols	Evaluation of courses	Training	Regulation	Other
University of Ottawa	Y	N	Y	Y	To set the policies of the U in matters relating to ethical approval of research conducted on human subjects
					To approve the terms of reference of sub-committees, to ensure that similar standards are used by all subcommittees, and to make subcommittees aware of pertinent ethical standards in other disciplines
					To review policies and procedures at timely intervals.
					To monitor the review process carried out by the subcommittees
					To be available for consultation by ethics sub-committees, individual researchers, and interested groups within the university community
					To direct research projects to the appropriate subcommittee for review when appropriate
					To examine research proposals referred by sub-committees for adjucation and to issue ethics clearance to projects meeting ethical standards
					To review cases in which the decision of the subcommittee is being appealed and to confirm or modify the subcommittee's decision, after con-sultation with the subcommittee
					To advise the dean of the School of Graduate Studies and Research, and the director of Research Services to suspend work on any project involving human subjects that is deemed not to meet the ethical standards

Table 3D (cont.)

Institutions	Evaluation of protocols	Evaluation of courses	Training	Regulation	Other
Queen's University	Y	Y	N	Y	Dealing with other matters concerned with human-based research including those referred to the Board Preparing an annual report for submission to the hospital boards and the U
University of Saskatchewan	Y	N	N	Y	To be the U's resource and authority in the ethics of human experimentation in health research To establish and periodically review policies, practices, and procedures at the U relating to the ethical review of research activities in the health sciences involving human subjects To familiarize itself with competent authorities in this field of human behaviour; to remain informed upon the evolving body of though, in the area of the Committee's concern To advise the President of the U and/or the President of the U hospital on such matters coming to its attention, within its general terms of reference, as it may deem appropriate To undertake such other related tasks which may be referred to it by the President of the U and/or the President of the U hospital. To advise the President of the U and/or the President of the U hospital on such matters coming to its attention, within its general terms of reference, as it may deem appropriate To undertake such other related tasks which may be referred to it by the President of the U and/or the President of the U hospital

Table 3D (cont.)

Institutions	Evaluation of protocols	Evaluation of courses	Training	Regulation	Other
Université de Sherbrooke	Y	N	Y	N	
University of Toronto	Y	N	N	N	

Table 3E

Evaluation activity – 1996

Institutions	Possible decisions	Review if modifications	Renewal	Follow-up	Appeal
University of Alberta	Approval/disapproval/cooperation with researcher for modification	Y	Y	Y	Y
University of British Columbia	Approval/disapproval	Y	Y	Y	Y
University of Calgary	Approval/disapproval	Y	Y	N	Y
Dalhousie University	Approval/substantiated disapproval with rationale	N	N	N	N
Université Laval	Approval/substantiated disapproval with rationale/cooperation with researcher for modifications if negative	N	N	Y	Final decision at the level of the Comité de déontologie de la recherche
University of Manitoba	Not specified	Y	N	Y	N
McGill University	Approve/require modification/disapprove Suspend/terminate	Y	Y	Y	Y
McMaster University	Approval/modifications/disapproval	N	N	Y	Y

(Y: yes, N: not specified)

Table 3E (cont.)

Institutions	Possible decisions	Review if modifications	Renewal	Follow-up	Appeal
Université de Montréal	*Comité d'évaluation:* Unconditional approval of project/approval under conditions specified/ rejection of project/declare inability to reach decision and refer to appropriate sectoral committee	N	N	Y	Y
University of Ottawa	Unconditional approval Approval for initial stage only Some concerns must be addressed before approval is given Decision deferred pending receipt of supplementary information or documentation as specified by UHREC Not approved. The reasons will be provided	N	Y	Y	Y
Queen's University	Approved Some concerns must be addressed before approval is given. The Board endorses protocol with some changes and mandates the chair to grant approval when the concerns have been satisfactorily addressed Decision deferred pending receipt of supplementary information or documentation as specified by the REB. The Board will rereview the material Not approved. The reasons will be provided	Y	Y	Y	Y
University of Saskatchewan	Approbation/further review of a research proposal's scientific merit is warranted/substantiated disapproval	Y	Y	N	N

Table 3E (cont.)

Institutions	Possible decisions	Review if modifications	Renewal	Follow-up	Appeal
Université de Sherbrooke	Not specified	N	N	Y	N
University of Toronto	Approval/disapproval/modifications	N	N	N	Y

Table 3F

Evaluation procedures – 1996

Institutions	Contact method	Decision process	Frequency of meetings
University of Alberta	P or M	Consensus If consensus not reached: Majority vote	Not specified
University of British Columbia	Not specified	Majority	Not specified
University of Calgary	Preevaluation by chairperson If consensus deemed to be reached: M If lack of consensus possible: P Expedite review if possible	Consensus If protocol has been studied by at least 3 persons from different disciplines, and if the chairperson believes that there is consensus between them, approval	At least 11 times per year
Dalhousie University	Not specified	Not specified	Not specified
Université Laval	Not specified	*Comité d'évaluation déontologique:* Forwards unanimous or majority recommendation to Comité de déontologie *Comité de déontologie:* Forwards positive decisions to appropriate authorities with identification of members of Comité d'évaluation	Not specified
University of Manitoba	Not specified	Not specified	Once per month except in July, August, and December
McGill University	Not specified	Consensus	Minimum: Once per month

(P: in person, M: by mail)

Table 3F (cont.)

Institutions	Contact method	Decision process	Frequency of meetings
McMaster University	P	Not specified	Monthly
Université de Montréal	Not specified	Not specified	The Comité universitaire as the comités sectoriels meet at least twice a year
University of Ottawa	Not specified	*Subcommittees:* Unanimity Otherwise referred to UHREC	Not specified
Queen's University	• Distribution by M of protocol to all members 7 days prior to meeting with 2 members designated primary reviewers • Meeting with report of primary reviewers: P	Not specified	At least monthly
University of Saskatchewan	Submitted to director of Research Services, College of Graduate Studies and Research, who refers the matter to the appropriate committee	2/3 of the votes of those members present and voting at the meeting at which it is considered *Quorum: 60% of the appointed and ex-officio members	U Committee on Ethics in Human Experimentation: Normally once per month
Université de Sherbrooke	Not specified	Not specified	Not specified
University of Toronto	M or P depending on the Office of Research Administration's decision (subject to the advice of the members of the Review Committee)	If contact by M: Unanimity	Not specified

APPENDIX 4

Canada – Provincial or Territorial Bodies (1996)

Table 4A

List of Research Centres and Groups Interested in Ethics*

Clinical Research Institute of
Montreal
Centre for Bioethics
David J. Roy, Director
110 Pine Avenue West
Montreal, Quebec
H2W 1R7
Tel.: (514) 987-5615
Fax: (514) 987-5695
E-mail: royd@ircm.umontreal.ca

McGill University
Centre for Medicine, Ethics and Law
Margaret Somerville, Director
3690 Peel Street
Montreal, Quebec
H3A 1W9
Tel.: (514) 398-7400
Fax: (514) 398-4668
E-mail: somerv m@falaw.lan.mcgill.ca

Dalhousie University
Office of Bioethics Education and
Research
Nuala Kenny, Director
Room C5CRC - 5849 University
Avenue
Halifax, Nova Scotia
B3H 4H7
Tel.: (902) 494-3801
E-mail: skenny@adm.da.ca

St. Joseph's College
St. Joseph's College Ethics Centre
University of Alberta
Edmonton, Alberta
T6G 2J5
Tel.: (403) 492-7681
Fax: (403) 492-8145

Groupe de recherche en génétique et
éthique du Québec
Marcel J. Melançon, Directeur
Collège de Chicoutimi
534, Jacques-Cartier Est
Chicoutimi, Québec
G7H 1Z6
Tel.: (418) 549-9520
Fax: (418) 549-1315

St. Paul University
Centre for Techno-Ethics
Jean-Marc Larouche, Director
223 Main Street
Ottawa, Ontario
K1S 1C4
Tel.: (613) 236-1393
Fax: (613) 782-3001
E-mail: techno-ethics@spu.st.paul.
uottawa.ca

The Hospital for Sick Children
Department of Bioethics
Christine Harrison, Acting Director
555 University Avenue
Toronto, Ontario
M5G 1X8
Tel.: (416) 813-5000
Fax: (416) 813-4967
E-mail: christine.harrison@mailhub.
sickkids.on.ca

The Salvation Army Ethics Centre
Dr. James E. Read, Executive Director
447 Webb Place
Winnipeg, Manitoba
R3B 2P2
Tel.: (204) 957-2412
Fax: (204) 957-2418
E-mail: saethics@mbnet.mb.ca

Sunnybrook Health Science Centre
Clinical Ethics Unit
Eric Meslin, Director
Room G326, 2075 Bayview Avenue
North York, Ontario
M4N 3M5
Tel.: (416) 480-4818
Fax: (416) 480-6191
E-mail: clinical=ethics%common%
smc@smc.sunnybrook.utoronto.ca

University of Alberta
Bioethics Centre
John B. Dossetor, Director
ANR 222, 8220 - 114th St.
Edmonton, Alberta
T6G 2J3
Tel.: (403) 492-6676
Fax: (403) 492-0673
E-mail: jdosseto@grp.srv.ualberta.ca
World Wide Web site: www.gpu.srv.
ualberta.ca/ethics.bethics.htm

Université de Montréal
Centre de recherche en droit public
Jacques Frémont, Directeur
Faculté de droit
C.P. 6128, Succursale centre-ville
Montréal, Québec
H3C 3J7
Tel.: (514) 343-7210
Fax: (514) 343-7508
E-mail: frémontj@droit.umontréal.ca

University of British Columbia
Centre for Applied Ethics
Michael McDonald, Director
227 – 6356 Agricultural Road
Vancouver, British Columbia
V6T 1Z2
Tel.: (604) 822-5139
Fax: (604) 822-8627
E-mail: mcdonald@ethics.ubc.ca
World Wide Web site: www.ethics.
ubc.ca

Université du Québec à Rimouski
Groupe de recherche ETHOS
Pierre Fortin, Directeur
300, avenue des Ursulines
Rimouski, Québec
G5L 3A1
Tel.: (418) 724-1784
Fax: (418) 724-1525
E-mail: pierre fortin@uqar.uquebec.ca

University of British Columbia
Office of the Co-ordinator of Health
Sciences
Division of Health Care Ethics
Alister Browne, Director
#400 - 2194 Health Sciences Hall
Vancouver, British Columbia
V6E 1Z3
Tel.: (604) 822-3028
Fax: (604) 822-2495

Université Laval
Groupe de recherche en éthique
médicale de l'Université Laval
Marie-Hélène Parizeau, Directrice
Faculté de philosophie
Québec, Québec
G1K 7P4
Tel.: (418) 656-2244
Fax: (418) 656-7267
E-mail: cz53@musica.McGill.ca

University of Calgary
Medical Ethics Research Program
Douglas Kinsella, Director
Faculty of Medicine
3330 Hospital Drive N.W.
Calgary, Alberta
T2N 4N1
Tel.: (403) 220-7990
Fax: (403) 220-4740
E-mail: dkinsell@acs.ucalgary.ca

University of Manitoba
Centre for Professional and Applied
Ethics
Arthur Schafer, Director
University College
500 Dysard Rd.
Winnipeg, Manitoba
R3T 2M8
Tel.: (204) 474-9107
Fax: (204) 261-0021
E-mail: schafer@cc.umanitoba.ca

University of Toronto
Joint Centre for Bioethics
Peter Singer, Director
88 College Street
Toronto, Ontario
M5G 1L4
Tel.: (416) 978-2709
Fax: (416) 978-1911
E-mail: rhonda.martin@utoronto.ca

**Westminster Institute for Ethics and
Human Values**
Barry Hoffmaster, Director
361 Windermere Road
London, Ontario
N6G 2K3
Tel.: (519) 673-0046
Fax: (519) 673-5016
E-mail: medcem@uwoadmin.uwo.ca

York University
Centre for Practical Ethics
Don MacNiven, Director
102 McLaughlin College
4700 Keele Street
North York, Ontario
M3J 1PE
Tel.: (416) 736-5128, ext. 30446
Fax: (416) 736-5436
E-mail: praceth@nexus.yorku.ca

---

* This list was posted on the Internet in January 1996 by the Canadian Medical
Association. CMA address: http://www.jwc.ca:8400/homw-f.htm

Table 4B

Comprehensive Tables by Province or Territory (1996) – ALBERTA

| Identification | | | Mandate and achievements | |
Agencies	Year established	Composition	Roles	Publications
Alberta Law Reform Institute	1968		It has been established by the Government of Alberta, the University of Alberta and the Law Society of Alberta for the purposes, among others, of conducting legal research and recommending reforms in the law	*Advance Directives and Substitute Decision Making in Personal Health Care, Report for Discussion* (1992)*
Alberta Public Health Advisory and Appeal Board	July 1985	8 members with varied professional backgrounds who represent all parts of the province	PHAAB is (a) to advise the Minister of Health on matters pertaining to the public health; (b) to make investigations or inquiries into, to collect information relating to, or to conduct research into, any matter relating to public health and make its report in the manner and at the time specified by the Minister of Health; (c) on the request of the lieutenant-governor-in-council, to hold public hearings for the purpose of receiving submissions on matters pertaining to public health and make its report to the Minister of Health; and (d) to hear appeals, pursuant to section 4 of the Public Health Act	*Annual Report 93–94**
Alberta Provincial Health Ethics Network	December 1995	12 individuals: – 4 of whom will be elected by the membership – 4 of whom will be elected by the Council of Chairs of the Regional Health Authorities – 4 by the Board itself	Facilitate examination, discussion, and decision making with respect to ethical issues in health and health care in the Province of Alberta	No
Alberta Heritage Foundation for Medical Research		Scientific Advisory Council Program Advisory Council Health Advisory Committee	Support a community of researchers who generate knowledge that improves the health and quality of life for Albertans and people throughout the world. A long-term commitment to fund basic, patient, and health research based on international standards of excellence and carried out by new and established investigators and researchers in training (funding agency)	*Annual Report 1994–1995**

* Documents consulted.

Table 4B

Comprehensive Tables by Province or Territory (1996) – BRITISH COLOMBIA

Identification			Mandate and achievements	
Agencies	Year established	Composition	Roles	Publications
Law Reform Commission of British Columbia				No relevant works
Special Advisory Committee on Ethical Issues in Health Care	June 1987	12 members selected for their background and expertise and not for the organization they represent. They have backgrounds in philosophy, medical ethics, religion, human rights, law, medicine, and nursing. Regional and cultural diversity will be taken into consideration in the selection process	To identify and clarify ethical issues in the field of health care To review the range of standards and solutions extant in other health jurisdictions To seek and develop areas of consensus in British Columbia with respect to such issues To advise the Ministry of Health and develop practical guidelines for handling of such issues by health field in British Columbia To facilitate education of the public, health care providers, and the Health Ministry about ethical issues The Minister of Health will request the Committee to review issues referred by ministry of health officials. The Committee may also undertake to review issues of wide concern including those referred to it by health provider groups, and could act as a resource to regional health boards	*Advisory Committee on Ethical Issues in Health Care, British Columbia Ministry of Health and Ministry Responsible for Seniors (1986)** *Reports by the Ministry of Health Advisory Committee on Ethical Issues in Health Care:* – *Guidelines to Develop Advance Directives and Do Not Resuscitate Orders, 1996* – *HIV Testing for Pregnant Women* – *Institutional Ethics Committees, 1995* – *Mandatory vs. Recommended Prophylaxis Ophthalmia Neonatorum, 1994* – *Ethical Allocation of Health Resources, 1994* – *Euthanasia and Physician-Assisted Suicide, 1994**

BRITISH COLUMBIA (cont.)

Identification			Mandate and achievements		Publications
Agencies	Year established	Composition	Roles		
Special Advisory Committee on Ethical Issues (cont.)					– Ethical Considerations Touching Medical Requirements for Immigrants – Anencephalic Newborns as Organ Donors, 1991 – Responsibilities of Health Care Workers Reporting on HIV, 1991* – Death and Dying and the Living Will, 1989 – Retrieval of Human Gametes, 1988 – Position Paper on Abortion, 1988
British Columbia Health Research Foundation	1991		The objects of the Foundation are to assist and collaborate with organizations conducting research in the field of health, including policy, promotion, and care in the Province of B.C.; to cooperate with community facilities of organizations concerned with the general health of communities in the province; and to accept and receive grants, donations, and other funds for use in carrying out its objects. It awards grants for operating funds to conduct health research projects, to purchase equipment, to develop research proposals, to facilitate research activities, and to fund scholarships for new researchers starting their professional careers and studentships for students pursuing graduate degrees (funding agency)		Annual Report 1994–95

* Documents consulted.

Table 4B

Comprehensive Tables by Province or Territory (1996) – MANITOBA

Identification			Mandate and achievements	
Agencies	Year established	Composition	Roles	Publications
Manitoba Law Reform Commission	1970	5 to 7 commissioners including at least, 1 judge from the Court of Queen's Bench, at least, 1 full-time member of the University of Manitoba Faculty of Law, at least, 1 lawyer entitled to practice in the province but who is not working full time for the Government of Manitoba or one of its agencies, and at least person who is not a lawyer	The duties of the Commission are to inquire and consider any matter relating to law in Manitoba with a view to making recommendations for the improvement, modernization and reform of the law, including, without limiting the generality of the foregoing (a) the removal of provisions of the law that are outdated or inconsistent; (b) the maintenance and improvement of the administration of justice; (c) the review of judicial and quasi-judicial procedures under any act; (d) the development of new approaches to, and new concepts of, law in keeping with and responsive to the changing needs of society and individual members of society; and (e) any subject referred to it by the Minister	– *Report on a Statutory Definition of Death* (1974)* – *Report on Emergency Apprehension, Admissions and Rights of Patients under the Mental Health Act* (1979)* – *Report on Medical Privilege* (1983) * – *Self-Determination in Health Care: Living Wills and Health Care Proxies* (1991) – *Report on Sterilization and Legal Incompetence* (1992)
Manitoba Health Research Council	June 1982		Promote and assist basic, clinical, and applied research in the health sciences in Manitoba and advise the Minister on health research matters referred to Council (funding agency)	*Annual Report 1994–1995**

* Documents consulted.

Table 4B

Comprehensive Tables by Province or Territory (1996) – NEW BRUNSWICK

Identification			Mandate and achievements	
Agencies	Year established	Composition	Roles	Publications
Premier's Council on Health Strategy	1990		Provide independent advice to the government on possible future policy directions that would appropriately address the health status of our citizens. Strategy: 1. Advise the government on strategies that will impact positively on the health of New Brunswickers 2. Recommend broad policy options for improving the health status of N.B. The recommended policies will be cost effective, measurable, and include policies which are beyond the traditional jurisdiction of the health sector 3. Recommend innovative approaches to health services which are sensitive to the needs of the province, foster personal responsibility for health, foster the appropriate use of resources by individuals and health professions, enhance linkages between health and related human services, emphasize health promotion and disease prevention 4. Involve the public and provider groups in identifying strategies that will impact positively on the health of N.B. 5. Appoint such committees as it deems necessary to the attainment of its mandate 6. Make periodic reports to the Government of N.B.	*Summary Report, An Ounce of Prevention... A Prevention Paper on Health Promotion and Prevention Issues* (1992)

Table 4B

Comprehensive Tables by Province or Territory (1996) – NEWFOUNDLAND

Identification			Mandate and achievements	
Agencies	Year established	Composition	Roles	Publications
Newfoundland Law Reform Commission	1971		It is the function of the Commission to inquire into and consider a matter relating to (a) reform of the law having regard to the statute law, the common law, and judicial decisions; (b) judicial and quasi-judicial procedures under the Act; (c) a subject referred to it by the Minister. The Commission may institute and direct legal research for the purpose of carrying out its functions. The Commission shall report to the Minister at the times that the progress of its work makes it advisable, and it shall report to the Minister when requested by him in regard to a matter then under its deliberation	*Working Paper on Powers of Attorney* (1987) *Discussion Paper on Advance Health Care Directives and Attorneys for Health Care* (1992)
Newfoundland Health Industry Sector Development Strategy Working Group, Newfoundland Economic Recovery Commission	1994	Health industry participants, members of the academic and research community and government officials	To investigate the economic development potential within the health industry. Research was directed toward the following sectors within the health industry: Medical devices, biotechnology, toxicology, technical services, health services research, clinical trials, basic science research, education and training, and information and communications. The objectives of the research initiative were to assess the potential of the health industries sector to contribute to economic development within the province and to help both established and nonestablished industry participants identify new commercial opportunities	*Health Industry Sector Development Strategy* (1995)

Table 4B

Comprehensive Tables by Province or Territory (1996) – NOVA SCOTIA

Identification			Mandate and achievements		
Agencies	Year established	Composition	Roles		Publications
Law Reform Commission of Nova Scotia	1969	Not fewer than 10 members nor more than 15 members of whom at least two-thirds shall be persons who are appointed from those who are active or retired judges of the Supreme Court, judges of the Country Court, judges of the Provincial Court, or barristers of the Supreme Court	It shall be the function of the Commission and the Commission shall have power to (a) review at the request of the attorney general any enactment and recommend the repeal, revision, or amendment of an enactment or any part thereof so reviewed; (b) consider at the request of the attorney general any matter that might be the subject of an enactment and, if an enactment is deemed desirable, recommend draft legislation for enactment (research/assistance/inquiries)		*The Legal Status of the Child Born outside of Marriage in Nova Scotia – Final Report* (1995) *Reform of the Laws Dealing with Adult Guardianship and Personal Health Care Decision – Final Report* (1995) *Living Wills in Nova Scotia: A Discussion Paper* (1994) *Adult Guardianship in Nova Scotia: Suggestions for Reform of the Incompetent Persons Act: A Discussion Paper* (1993)
Nova Scotia Task Force on Primary Health Care	April 1992	The Task Force is made up of representatives of a broad range of community and professional groups	To identify primary health care needs in Nova Scotia and to promote a primary health care approach to the delivery of health care services Identify methods of assessing primary health care needs; identify barriers to primary health care; identify specific changes that need to be made in the way health care services are planned, funded, accessed, delivered, and evaluated; consider and recommend for funding, projects and initiatives designed to meet primary health care needs in Nova Scotia's communities		*Toward Primary Health Care in Nova Scotia* (1992)

Nova Scotia (cont.)

| Identification | | | Mandate and achievements | |
Agencies	Year established	Composition	Roles	Publications
Nova Scotia Provincial Health Council	1990 (further to the report of the Nova Scotia Royal Commission on Health Care)	12 volunteer Nova Scotians	Advise the Government on health issues; Monitor the government's public policy decisions to ensure they support health and are consistent with Nova Scotia's health goals; Help Nova Scotians take part in planning how health care is delivered; Suggest ways to make health care delivery more effective, efficient, and affordable; Provide information about health and the health care system to Nova Scotians	*Annual Report 1993–1994* 1991–1992* Nova Scotia's Health Goals: How They Were Developed and What They Mean (1992)*
Cancer Treatment and Research Foundation of Nova Scotia				*Annual Report 1989–1991**

* Documents consulted.

Table 4B

Comprehensive Tables by Province or Territory (1996) – ONTARIO

Identification		Mandate and achievements		
Agencies	Year established	Composition	Roles	Publications
Ontario Law Reform Commission			In November 1982, the Ontario Law Reform Commission received from the Attorney General for Ontario the following letter of reference: I wish to request that the Commission inquire into and consider the legal issues relating to the practice of human artificial insemination, including "surrogate mothering" and transplantation of fertilized ova to a third party. I would be pleased to have the Commission report on the range of alternatives for resolution of any legal issues that may be identified. Considerations to be included: The legal status and legal rights of the child and the safeguards for protecting the best interests of the child/the legal rights and legal duties of each biological parent/the legal rights and legal duties of the spouse, if any, of each biological parent/the nature and enforceability of agreements relating to artificial insemination and related practices/the nature and enforceability of agreements respecting custody of the child/the legal rights and liabilities of medical and other personnel involved in performing artificial insemination and other related practices/the legal procedures for establishing and recognizing the biological parentage of children born as a result of these practices/the applicability of present custody and adoption laws in such cases/the availability of information to identify the child and the parties involved/such medical and related evidence as may have a bearing on the legal issues raised in these cases.	*Report on Human Artificial Reproduction and Related Matters* (vols. 1 and 2, 1985)* *Report on Drug and Alcohol Testing in the Workplace* (1992) *Report on Testing for AIDS* (1992)

ONTARIO (cont.)

Identification		Mandate and achievements		
Agencies	Year established	Composition	Roles	Publications
Ontario Premier's Council on Health, Well-Being and Social Justice	1992–1994	Chaired by the Premier Council members include leaders from the health, education, community and business sectors, as well as government ministers	Working to develop medium- and long-term strategies for social change that will lead to enhanced well-being for Ontario residents The Council identifies strategic issues and assesses the need for change. It proposes and helps launch initiatives to inform policy directions for health and social justice. Created from the merger of the Ontario Premier's Council on Health, Well-Being and Social Justice and the Premier's Council on Economic Renewal. The new Council includes the Premier's Council Projects Committee and the Premier's Council Advisory Committee	*Devolution and Decentralization of Health Care Systems: A Review of Models* (1993) *Decentralization of Health Care and Social Services in Ontario: Refocusing the Debate* (1994)
Ontario Premier's Council	June 1994	Created from the merger of the Ontario Premier's Council on Health, Well-Being and Social Justice and the Premier's Council on Economic Renewal. The new Council includes the Premier's Council Projects Committee and the Premier's Council Advisory Committee	Premier's Council Projects Committee: Directs projects and contracts research Premier's Council Advisory Committee: Gives the Premier essential advice with respect to policy and serves as a forum to review issues of interest	
Health Research and Development Grants, Ministry of Health	1960s			*Health Research and Development Grants, 1993–1994, Program Overview* (1994)*

* Documents consulted.

Table 4B

Comprehensive Tables by Province or Territory (1996) – PRINCE EDWARD ISLAND

| Identification | | Mandate and achievements | | |
Agencies	Year established	Composition	Roles	Publications
Hospital and Health Services Commission of Prince Edward Island				*Prehospital and Emergency Services Study (1990)* *Nutrition and Dietetic Needs Study (1990)* *The Report of the Panel on the Hospitals' Role in the Health Community (1991)*
Provincial Health Policy Council		10–12 members Representation: 5–6 public members 5–6 service providers, representing the broad health system	Its role is to make recommendations to the Minister on issues that affect the health of the general population of P.E.I. in the following areas: (1) the vision and mission of the health system, using health promotion philosophy and principles of primary health care; (2) provincial policy, based on provincial health needs, as identified through regional community needs assessment; (3) the indicators for measuring health status of the general population (e.g., rate of smoking, % of low-birthweight babies, etc.); (4) health status indicator results; (5) the development, monitoring and evaluation of the achievement of provincial health goals and objectives; (6) opportunities for input and discussion of health issues by health service providers, individuals, and communities; *this includes establishment of forums for discussion of ethical issues that may impact on the health of the general population of P.E.I.;* identification and assessment of policy issues that impact on the health of the general population of P.E.I.; publicly stating the views of the Council (authors' emphasis)	

Table 4B

Comprehensive Tables by Province or Territory (1996) – QUEBEC

Identification			Mandate and achievements	
Agencies	Year established	Composition	Roles	Publications
Conseil médical du Québec	December 1991 An Act respecting the Conseil médical du Québec, R.S.Q. C-59.000	15 voting members, at least 8 of whom must be doctors: - 2 general practitioners - 2 specialists - 1 physician chosen from a list of 3 physicians recommended by the Ordre professionnel des médecins du Québec - 1 physician chosen from a list of 3 physicians recommended by the body grouping the councils of physicians, dentists and pharmacists of institutions within the meaning of the Act respecting health services and social services (chapter S-4.2) or within the meaning of the Act respecting health services and social services for Cree Native persons (chapter S-5)	Advisory agency to the Department of Health and Social Services To advise the Minister on any matter relating to medical services, taking into account the needs of the population and the evolving costs of, and ability of the population to pay for, medical services. Matters on which the council may advise the Minister include (1) the orientation of medical services in relation to the priorities of the health care system, especially the evolution, organization and distribution of services and the manner in which medical services dispensed by institutions within the meaning of the Act respecting health services and social services (chapter S-4.2) or within the meaning of the Act respecting health services and social services for Cree Native persons (chapter S-5) may be harmonized with those dispensed in private medical facilities; (2) medical staffing needs in general practice and specialties, viewed as a whole or by specialty, and staff distribution between the regions or territories of Québec in light of the characteristics of the population and the available budgetary resources; (3) the evolution and adaptation of medical practice with regard to emerging needs, new realities and standards of quality; (4) the different types of medical practice having regard to the needs of the population that are to receive priority; (5) draft regulations concerning the coverage of insured medical services within the meaning of the Health Insurance Act (chapter A-29); (6) the most appropriate methods of remuneration of physicians; (7) policies or programs addressing the rationalization of, or priority to be given to, the dispensation of a medical service.	Conseil médical du Québec, *Rapport d'activités 1994–1995** *Avis sur le modèle de projection: Offre et demande de services médicaux*, June 1994 *Avis sur le projet politique triennale des inscriptions dans les programmes de formation doctoral et postdoctorale en médecine de 1995–1996 à 1996–1998*, December 1994 *Avis sur les études de pertinence dans la dispensation des procédures diagnostiques et thérapeutiques*, December 1994 *Avis sur l'intégration professionnelle des diplômés d'écoles de médecine situées hors du Canada et des États-Unis*, March 1995

QUEBEC (cont.)

Identification		Mandate and achievements		
Agencies	Year established	Composition	Roles	Publications
Conseil médical du Québec (cont.)		– 4 persons appointed after consultation with the Rectors of Québec universities having a faculty of medicine and the Deans of such faculties, a body responsible for evaluating health care technology, the Fonds de la recherche en santé du Québec and the Conseil consultatif de pharmacologie – 3 persons appointed after consultation with the health care and social services community – 1 medical resident chosen from a list of 3 residents recommended by the body representing medical residents – 1 doctoral student in medicine chosen from a list of three persons recommended by the body representing doctoral students in medicine	The Minister shall consult the council and obtain its advice on the following matters: (1) draft regulations relating to the clinical organization of medical services dispensed by institutions; (2) policies relating to the medical work force, including policies governing enrollment in programs of medical training at the doctoral and post-doctoral level; (3) the reference framework for medical staff distribution, and in particular the expansion or reduction objectives to be established for each region of Québec. The council shall give its advice on these matters within the time prescribed by the Minister. The council must give its advice to the Minister within the period of time prescribed by the latter on any other matter submitted by the Minister. In the pursuit of its objects, the council may, in addition, (1) initiate consultation, seek advice, accept and hear requests and suggestions from persons, bodies or associations and submit to the Minister any recommendation it considers appropriate; (2) set up committees; (3) conduct or commission a study or survey in accordance with an authorization from the Minister.	*Rapport du Président du comité de réflexion sur les coûts socioéconomiques des deuils non résolus et de l'acharnement thérapeutique,* January 1995

QUEBEC (cont.)

Identification		Mandate and achievements	
Conseil de la santé et du bien-être	May 1992 An Act respecting the Conseil de la santé et du bien-être, R.S.Q. C-56.3	On the recommendation of the Minister of Health and Social Services and following consultation with the representative bodies in the health and social services community which are concerned in each case, the voting members of the council are appointed by the Government in the following manner: – 1 chairman – 3 persons chosen from among the users of health services and social services or their representatives – 3 persons from community organizations involved in the defense of users' rights, the dispensation of services or volunteer work – 6 persons chosen from among practitionners research workers or administrators of whom 3 shall be from the health sector and 3 from the social services sector.	The function of the council is to advise the Minister on the most appropriate ways of improving the health and well-being of the population. Matters on which the council may advise the Minister include the evolution of problems of health or well-being in the population, the causes related to such problems and the most vulnerable groups. The council shall advise the Minister on the objectives of health and social services policies developed by the Minister and on appropriate means for achieving those objectives, taking into account the capacity of the community to mobilize the necessary resources. The council shall advise the Minister on any other matter he submits to it. In pursuing its objectives, the council may in addition (1) initiate consultation, seek advice, accept and hear requests and suggestions from persons, bodies or associations and submit to the Minister any recommendation it considers relevant; (2) set up committees; (3) inform the public. The council may make public any advice, opinion or recommendation it formulates pursuant to sections 16 to 20, 60 days after forwarding it to the Minister.	Conseil de la santé et du bien-être, *Rapport annuel 1994–1995** *Un juste prix pour les services de santé* (1995) *L'évolution macroéconomique et la question budgétaire au Québec* (1994)

QUEBEC (cont.)

Identification		Mandate and achievements		
Agencies	**Year established**	**Composition**	**Roles**	**Publications**
Conseil de la santé et du bien-être (cont.)		– 6 persons from any of the sectors concerned by health and social services policies, such as the municipal, education, economics, labour, income security, environment and justice sectors. The appointments shall, as far as possible, reflect the socio-cultural, ethno-cultural, linguistic and demographic composition of the population as a whole and shall represent women and men and the regions of Québec in the fairest possible way. Nonvoting members: 1 selected from employees of the Department of Health and Social Services, 1 from a regional board mentioned in the Act respecting health services and social services, and 2 others from the departments concerned by health and welfare policy		

QUEBEC (cont.)

Identification		Mandate and achievements		
Agencies	Year established	Composition	Roles	Publications
Conseil d'évaluation des technologies de la santé du Québec			Twofold mandate: 1. Open to all health system stakeholders (population as recipients of care, caregivers, or health services managers): Promote and support the evaluation of health technologies by disseminating results and encouraging the use of these results in decision making by all those involved in the spread of these technologies 2. Advise the Minister on issues concerning the introduction, distribution and use of health technologies, and, accordingly, give opinions based on an evaluation of their effectiveness, safety, cost, and impact on the health system, as well as their economic, ethical, and social implications	*Rapport d'activités 1993–1994**
Fonds de recherche en santé du Québec (FRSQ)	1964		The FRSQ, under the responsibility of the Minister of Health and Social Services, is responsible for promoting and providing financial assistance to research, training, and the development of researchers in the health care field	*Recherche en Santé* (periodical)

* Documents consulted.

Table 4B

Comprehensive Tables by Province or Territory (1996) – SASKATCHEWAN

| Identification | | | Mandate and achievements | |
Agencies	Year established	Composition	Roles	Publications
Law Reform Commission of Saskatchewan	(Since 1992, the Health Services Utilization and Research Commission took on the mandate of the Saskatchewan Health Research Board, which had been established in 1979.)	The Law Reform Commission Act provides that the Minister of Justice shall appoint a chair and not less than two other members of the Commission	The Commission shall take and keep under review all the law of the province, including statute law, common law and judicial decisions, with a view to its systematic development and reform, including the codification, elimination of anomalies, repeal of obsolete and unnecessary enactments, reduction in the number of separate enactments, and generally simplification and modernization of the law (art. 6, the Law Reform Commission Act) Topics for the Commission's research program are brought before meetings of the Commission for consideration. These topics may originate from a recommendation of the Minister of Justice, from the Commission and its staff, from the judiciary, from the legal profession, from other professional organizations, or from the public generally	*Tentative Proposals for a Consent of Minors to Health Care Act (1978)** *Proposals for a Consent of Minors to Health Care Act (1980)** *Proposals for a Human Artificial Insemination Act (1987)** *Proposals for an Advance Health Care Directives Act (1991)*
Saskatchewan Provincial Health Council		16 members from diverse backgrounds	Recommends healthy public policies to the Minister of Health It is responsible for: Investigating the economic, educational, cultural, spiritual, and environmental factors that affect health; consulting widely on health related issues; recommending practical and affordable public policies that can improve health; encouraging the adoption of such policies; and assessing progress in meeting Saskatchewan's health goals	*Population Health Goals for Saskatchewan (1994)**

SASKATCHEWAN (cont.)

| Identification | | Mandate and achievements | | |
Agencies	Year established	Composition	Roles	Publications
Saskatchewan Health Services Utilization and Research Commission	(Since 1992, the Health Services Utilization and Research Commission assumes the mandate of the Saskatchewan Health Research Board established in 1979.)		The mission of the Health Services Utilization and Research Commission is to promote the wellness of the people of Saskatchewan by fostering the efficient and effective utilization of health services and by stimulating, funding, and promoting research in the healing arts and health sciences (funding agency)	*The PSA Test in Early Detection of Prostate Cancer: Guidelines* (1995): Guidelines, Summary Reports, Final Report *Where We've Been and Where We're Going: A Survey of Utilization Management in Saskatchewan* (1995) *Barriers to Community Care: Final Report* (1994) *Technical Report of the Surgery Working Group on Presurgical Admissions and Rates of Day Surgery in Saskatchewan's Twenty Largest Hospitals* (1993) *Annual Report 1993–1994** *Health Services Utilization and Research Commission and Saskatchewan Health Research Board, Annual Report, Period Ending March 31, 1992**

* Documents consulted.

Table 4B

Comprehensive Tables by Province or Territory (1996) – YUKON

Identification		Mandate and achievements		
Agencies	Year established	Composition	Roles	Publications
Yukon Health Social Services Council	1990	14 members with experience in the areas that are the Council's concern Ministers of justice and health and social services sit as exofficio members	Advise the Yukon government on matters related to health and social policy Evaluating programs and services at the request of Cabinet, initiating studies of issues related to health, justice, and social services, and consulting individuals, groups, and the public about health, social, and justice issues with a view to recommending how the government should handle such issues. Suggest new visions for health and social services	*Annual Report 1991–1992**

* Documents consulted.

TABLE 4C

Provincial Ethics Networks – 1996

Identification			Mandate and achievements	
Organizations	Establishment	Composition	Roles	Operations
Provincial Health Ethics Network (Alberta)	Department of Health (1995)	The Network, as a society, is operated by a board of 12 individuals, 4 of whom will be elected by the membership, 4 by the Council of Chairs of the Regional Health Authorities, and 4 by the Board itself. Membership is open to all, including health care professionals and providers, policymakers, administrators, related personnel and their institutions, and interested members of the general public	To provide health care professionals, policymakers, and the general public easy access and connection to each other and to ethics resources in order to discuss, reflect, and deliberate about ethical issues in health and health care. To coordinate and to communicate about ethics activity in the province as would be helpful to those organizing or engaged in these activities, including serving as a centre for housing ethical guidelines, ethical policies, and other documents developed by various clinical ethics committees. To educate and assist in ethics educational endeavours for the public, for health professionals, and for other health care providers as well as agencies/institutions, and their boards. This will include the development of the skills of interested public and health providers to facilitate ethical reflection and decision making. To stimulate public dialogue on health ethics to promote informed and reasoned debate and development of consensus on difficult ethical dilemmas of health and health care. To provide access to ethics consultation to facilitate ethical discussion, while enhancing capabilities for ethical decision making of those involved in the situation	The Network is established as a society in Alberta. The Network has 3 employees: 2 persons are responsible for coordination among the regions and for providing assistance and advice, and 1 person handles the secretarial functions

Table 4C (cont.)

Identification		Mandate and achievements		
Organizations	Establishment	Composition	Roles	Operations
Réseau d'éthique clinique chez l'humain (Quebec)	Fonds de recherche en santé du Québec (1994)	1 coordination centre 6 topical units: Foundations of clinical ethics/clinical ethics in medicine and surgery/pediatrics/psychiatry/oncology and palliative care/clinical ethics and genetics, membership ranging from 2 to 36 1 advisory committee Multidisciplinary (clinicians from various specialties, philosophers and theologians, sociologists, law professionals, and ethicists)	The Réseau's objective is to help practitioners and researchers work in close cooperation with humanities and social sciences professionals. The scope of activity for the Réseau d'éthique clinique chez l'humain extends to research into clinical ethics, health care, and quality of life. It functions only in Quebec The purpose of the Réseau is to promote respect for human integrity, informed freedom of choice, quality of life, and human dignity in Quebec health services. The missions of the Réseau are essentially consultative and educational, in addition to a coordination function	The secretariat coordinates the activities of the 6 units 2 general meetings each year for all members of the Réseau; 4 meetings for directors and codirectors; 4 to 6 meetings for each unit; frequent meetings between coordinator and directors and codirectors

APPENDIX 5

Canada – Canada-Wide Bodies

Table 5A

Federal agencies

Identification			Mandate and achievements		
Organizations	Establishment	Composition	Roles		Operations
Medical Research Council of Canada (MRC)[1]	Parliament (1969)	1 full-time president and chief executive officer 21 volunteer members who represent the scientific and lay community, appointed by the governor-in-council 3 associate members represent the other 2 federal research granting agencies (NSERC and SSHRC) and Health Canada 4 standing committees: Ethics'/business development/ science and research/policy and planning 40 committees charged with evaluating the scientific merit of applications for funds 350 of Canada's leading researchers provide unpaid input into the activities of these committees *Standing Committee on Ethics*:[1] Established in March 1984 Multidisciplinary (consists of scientists, health professionals, law professionals, lay representatives, etc.)	The Medical Research Council of Canada is the major federal agency responsible for funding biomedical research in Canada. Its role is to promote, assist, and undertake basic, applied, and clinical research in Canada in the health sciences. It also has a major role in supporting research training of health scientists and acts as an advisor on health research to the federal Minister of Health. The research it supports is carried out by scientists in universities, hospitals, and research institutes across the country. It also promotes cooperation between university researchers and industry. The Council administers the health sciences portion of the Networks of Centres of Excellence program and is responsible for and administers the Canadian Genome Analysis and Technology program (CGAT) To keep the MRC abreast of developments, the Committee meets regularly to review recent discoveries and problems that ought to be mentioned in the next guidelines		Applications by researchers are carefully considered by scientific review committees made up of experts in many health fields: Applications are assessed for their potential in revealing new knowledge and insights into the functioning of the human body in sickness and in health Ethical aspects are considered by the research ethics committee at the local level

1. Information extracted from Medical Research Council of Canada, http:/www.hc-sc.gc.ca/main/mrc/web/whatis/foldeng.html

Table 5A (cont.)

Identification			Mandate and achievements		
Organizations	Establishment	Composition	Roles		Operations
National Research Council of Canada (NRC)[2]	Federal government (1916)		A leader in the drive to create an innovative, knowledge-based Canadian economy. Its goal has been to improve life for Canadians by performing and supporting relevant research and development		
			Carries out research in 4 strategic technology areas: Biotechnology/construction/information and tele-communications/manufacturing		
		National Research Council of Canada (NRC) Ethics Committee for Research on Human Subjects (ECRHS): Specialists from the fields of medicine and science	The ECRHS, which was established by NRC's Management Committee, is responsible for formulating recommendations to the NRC Management Committee, through the secretary general of the organization on ethical aspects and practices in research and development which use human subjects		NRC research which would involve the participation of human subjects shall not be undertaken without the approval of the NRC Management Committee as to its ethical acceptability. Such approval will be given or withheld taking into consideration the recommendations of the HSREC.
		Law specialists	Areas for ECRHS intervention:		
		Ethicists from institutions other than NRC	There are five main ways in which the NRC Human Subjects Research Ethics Committee may be involved in NRC projects that involve research and development on human subjects:		
			(a) by assessing the scientific and ethical acceptability of selected projects in which NRC is involved, including through IRAP, which are brought to its attention or which it decides to review; (b) by overseeing a process to assess the ethical acceptability of projects which involve the participation of NRC laboratories or facilities; (c) by overseeing a process whereby the ethical acceptability of projects which receive support from the NRC Industrial Research Assistance Program is assessed; (d) by assessing the ethical acceptability of projects that receive support from IRAP where no ethics committee from a Canadian university or a Canadian		All proposed IRAP-supported research and development projects which would involve the participation of human subjects must be approved as scientifically sound and ethical by IRAP.

Table 5A (cont.)

| Identification | | | Mandate and achievements | | |
Organizations	Establishment	Composition	Roles		Operations
National Research Council of Canada (NRC) (cont.)			university teaching hospital is available to conduct this assessment; (e) by reviewing the terms of reference and conditions of NRC contributions (other than from IRAP) or contracts to external research organizations to ensure that any research and development involving human subjects and supported by these contributions or contracts receives adequate ethical and scientific review prior to its commencement.		The basis for such approval will be compliance with the guidelines developed by the NRC Human Subjects Research Ethics Committee (HSREC) and adopted by the NRC Management Committee. As a basis for approving such projects, IRAP Management would normally rely on the evaluation, recommendations, and conclusions of an appropriate external mechanism such as a local ethics committee in a Canadian university or an approved and accredited Canadian university teaching hospital, which the firm would use for the assessment of the scientific and ethical acceptability of a proposed project.

2.Information taken from National Research Council, How to obtain approval to conduct experiments on human subjects, November 1992, and How to obtain approval to conduct research and development on human subjects in projects funded by NRC's IRAP, March 1993, and National Research Council of Canada, http://www.corpserv.nrc.ca/corpserv/m_list_e.html

Table 5B

National Council on Bioethics in Human Research (NCBHR)

History	Composition	Roles	Publications
1989 Established by the Medical Research Council/Health and Welfare Canada/Royal College of Physicians and Surgeons of Canada	The Royal College of Physicians and Surgeons of Canada appoints 2 members from its Research Committee and 3 members from its Biomedical Ethics Committee to the Council. The National Council also includes one representative each from: the Canadian Medical Association, the Association of Canadian Medical Colleges, the College of Family Physicians of Canada, the Canadian Nurses Association, the Canadian Society for Clinical Investigation and Health and Welfare Canada. Renewals or new appointments are made on a staggered basis through nominations from the organization on the Royal College. The public is represented by 4 members, including a philosopher/theologian, a lawyer and 2 community members. The President of the MRC (or his delegate) is an ex officio member of the Council.	The mission of the National Council on Bioethics in Human Research is to encourage compliance with strict ethical standards in biomedical research and health sciences research using human subjects in Canada The National Council will: Interpret and promote existing ethical guidelines for biomedical and health-related research involving human subjects Advise and consult university, hospital and other Research Ethics Boards to establish guidelines and procedures for the evaluationof such boards and of the institutional processes of ethics review of research with human subjects. These may include site visits by invitation or at request Advise and consult on other relevant ethical matters with bodies funding research with human subjects Assist institutional Research Ethics Boards to resolve contentious issues involving biomedical and health-related research with human subjects Foster education and dialogue with health professionnals and the public on ethical aspects of biomedical and health-related research involving human subjects	*NCBHR Communiqué CNBR* *Legal Aspects of Research and Clinical Practice with Children*, 1992 *Legal Aspects of Research and Clinical Practice with Human Beings*, 1992 *Selected Bibliography: Bioethics of Research with Human Subjects in the Health Sciences*, 1995 Protecting and promoting the human research subject: A review of the function of Research Ethics Boards in Canadian Faculties of Medicine, *NCBHR Communiqué CNBR*, 6(1), 1995 *Reflections on Research Involving Children*, 1993 Ethics of clinical trials for Research Ethics Boards: Proceedings of a National Workshop, *NCBHR Communiqué CNBRH*, 2(2), 1991 *Ethical Aspects of Pharmaceutically-Based Clinical Investigations*, 1990 *Ethics Review in Canada: Highlights from a National Workshop*, NCBHR Working Document, 1989

Table 5B (cont.)

History	Composition	Roles	Publications
1995 Revised structure	*CNBRH/NCBHR*: Interdisciplinary group of 15–20 experts in human research ethics. The composition of Council shall be sensitive to the age, gender, ethnicity, language, geographical, cultural, and like characteristics of the Canadian public *Coordinating Committee*: Deputy Minister of Health Canada, the presidents of the MRC, NCBHR, Natural Sciences and Engineering Research Council of Canada, Royal College of Physicians and Surgeons of Canada, Social Sciences and Humanities Research Council, or their delegates	*CNBRH/NCBHR*: The NCBHR mandate now extends beyond biomedical research to include human research ethics in the humanities and health sciences An update of the NCBHR mandate, which includes slight changes, has been made *Coordinating Committee (CC)*: Serves as a forum for discussion and collaboration of institutional research ethics initiatives amongst its membership, particularly as regards NCBHR. It is the intention of members of the CC to provide financial and intellectual support to NCBHR, so as to facilitate the discharge of its important responsibilities and the fulfilment of its mission. Even while offering such support, it is also the clear intention of all founding members that NCBHR discharge its responsibilities on an arm's-length basis from other members of the CC. As such, it is understood that certain tasks shall be delegated to NCBHR by other members of the CC, which are also referred to as the sponsoring organizations. In the performance of these tasks, NCBHR is responsible both to the sponsoring organizations and to the people of Canada Advise NCBHR on nominations for the NCBHR Council: The CC may offer any advice, suggestions, or commentary on the nominees to NCBHR. NCBHR shall then exercise its responsibility for making Council appointments Receive annual reports from NCBHR concerning its activities Promote effective communication and collaboration between NCBHR and its sponsoring organizations Receive reports from the members regarding research ethics initiatives and the implementation of the NCBHR terms of reference Coordinate consultation regarding changes in membership or changes in the terms of reference of the CC	*NCBHR Communiqué CNBRH*

APPENDIX 6

Canada – List of information Providers

A. Provincial and Territorial Ministries of Health

B. Academic Institutions

C. Other Organizations

A. Provincial and Territorial Ministries of Health

Alberta

Alberta Department of Health
Halvar C. Jonson, Minister of Health
228 Legislature Building
Edmonton, Alberta
T5K 2B6

British Columbia

Ministry of Health and Ministry
Responsible for Seniors
Lilian Bayne, Executive Director
Policy, Planning and Economics
5th Floor, 1515 Blanshard Street
Victoria, British Columbia
V8W 3C8

Manitoba

Province of Manitoba, Department of
Health
The Honorable James Collus McCrae,
Minister of Health
Room 302, Legislative Building
Winnipeg, Manitoba
R3C 0V8

New Brunswick

Department of Health and
Community Services
The Honorable Russell Hugh Tennant
King, Minister of Health and
Community Services
P.O. Box 5100
Fredericton, New Brunswick
E3B 5G8

Newfoundland and Labrador

Department of Health
The Honorable Lloyd Matthews,
Minister of Health
P.O. Box 8700
West Block, Confederation Building
St. John's, Newfoundland
A1B 4J6

Northwest Territories

Health and Social Services
David Ramsden, Deputy Minister
Government of the Northwest
Territories
P.O. Box 1320
Yellowknife, Northwest Territories
X1A 2L9

Nova Scotia

Department of Health
The Honorable Ronald D. Stewart,
Minister of Health and Registrar
General
Office of the Minister
P.O. Box 488
Halifax, Nova Scotia
B3J 2R8

Prince Edward Island

Department of Health and Social
Services
The Honorable Walter McEwen,
Minister of Health and Social Services
P.O. Box 2000
Charlottetown, Prince Edward Island
C1A 7N8

Quebec

Ministère de la Santé et des Services
Sociaux
André Jean
15e étage, Édifice Catherine-de-Longpré
1075, chemin Sainte-Foy
Québec (Québec)
G1S 2M1

Saskatchewan

Department of Health
The Honorable Eric Cline, Minister of
Health
Legislative Building
Regina, Saskatchewan
S4S 0B3

Yukon

Department of Health and Social
Services
The Honorable Mickey Fisher,
Minister of Health and Social Services
Box 2703
Whitehorse, Yukon
Y1A 2C6

B. Academic Institutions

University of Alberta

The Bioethics Centre
John B. Dossetor, Director
222 ANR, University of Alberta
8220 - 114 Street
Edmonton, Alberta
T6G 2J3

University of British Columbia

Division of Health Care Ethics,
Office of the Coordinator of Health
Sciences
Alister Browne, Director
#400 - 2194 Health Sciences Mall
Vancouver, British Columbia
V6T 1Z3

University of Calgary

Janet Storch, Dean
Faculty of Nursing
47 Coleridge Cres. N.W.
Calgary, Alberta

Université Laval

Guy Pelletier, Président du Comité
institutionnel
C.H.U.L.
2705 boul. Laurier
Ste-Foy, Québec
G1V 4G2

Memorial University

Dr. Verna Skanes, Assistant Dean
Research and Graduate Studies
(Medicine)
Faculty of Medicine
The Health Sciences Centre
St. John's, Newfoundland
A1B 3V6

University of Ottawa

George P. Biro, Associate Dean
Medical Research and Medical Studies
451 Smyth Rd.
Ottawa, Ontario
K1H 8M5

Queen's University

Dr. Duncan G. Sinclair
Vice-Principal (Health Sciences)
Dean, Faculty of Medicine
Room 234 Botterell Hall, Stuart Street
Kingston, Ontario
K7L 3N6

University of Saskatchewan

Dr. David Popkin, Dean
Room B103, Health Science Building
107 Wiggins Road
Saskatoon, Saskatchewan
S7N 5E5

Université de Sherbrooke

Francyn Lemire, Secrétaire du Centre de recherche clinique et secrétaire du Comité de déontologie de la recherche sur l'humain
Centre universitaire de santé de l'Estrie, Centre de recherche clinique
Site Fleurimont
3001, 12e avenue Nord, pièce 2500
Fleurimont (Québec)
J1H 5N4

University of Toronto

Rosalind Waxman, Coordinator
Research Administration
Faculty of Medecine, Office of the Dean
Room 112–116, 150 College Street
Toronto, Ontario
M5S 3E2

C. Other Organizations

Canadian Healthcare Association
Michelle Albagli, Director
Policy and Communications
17 York St.
Ottawa, Ontario
K1N 9J6

Catholic Health Association of Canada
Maryse Blouin for Richard M. Haughian, President
1247, Kilborn Place
Ottawa, Ontario
K1H 6K9

Association of Canadian Medical Colleges
Dr. D. Hawkins, President
774 Echo Drive
Ottawa, Ontario
K1S 5P2

Canadian Medical Association
John R. Williams, Director
Department of Ethics
1867 Alta Vista Drive
Ottawa, Ontario
K1G 3Y6

British Columbia Health Association
Mary Collins, President and CEO
1333 W. Broadway, Ste. 600
Vancouver, British Columbia
V6H 4C7

The Canadian Institute of Law and Medicine
Gilbert Sharpe, President
P.O. Box 552
Aurora, Ontario
L4G 3L6

The Royal College of Physicians and Surgeons of Canada
Hugh M. Scott, Director General
774 Echo Drive
Ottawa, Ontario
K1S 5N8

Canada Council on Health Services Accreditation
Jules Martin, Associate Director General
1730 St. Laurent Blvd., Suite 430
Ottawa, Ontario
K1G 5L1

Le Conseil de la santé et du bien-être
Norbert Rodrigue, Président
1126, chemin St-Louis
Sillery, Québec
G1S 1E5
Tel.: (418) 643-3040

Canadian Council on Animal Care
Gilles Demers, Directeur associé des
évaluations
1000 - 151 Slater St.
Ottawa, Ontario
K1P 5N3

Le Conseil médical du Québec
Diane Verret pour J.R. Iglesias,
Président
1126, chemin St-Louis, 6e étage
Sillery, Québec
G1S 1E5

**National Council on Bioethics in
Human Research**
Derek J. Jones, Director
774 Echo Drive
Ottawa, Ontario
K1S 5N8

**Law Reform Commission of Nova
Scotia**
Dr. Moira L. McConnell, Executive
Director
1484 Carlton Street, 2nd Floor
Halifax, Nova Scotia
B3H 3B7

Manitoba Law Reform Commission
Jeffrey A. Schnoor, Executive Director
12th Floor of the Woodsworth
Building
405 Broadway
Winnipeg, Manitoba
R3C 3L6

**New Brunswick Health Care
Association**
Michel J. Poirier, Executive Director
861 Woodstock Road
Fredericton, New Brunswick
E3B 4X4

**Newfoundland and Labrador Health
Care Association**
John F. Peddle, Executive Director
Beclin Building
1118 Topsail Road
P.O. Box 8234
St. John's, Newfoundland
A1B 3N4

**Northwest Territories Health Care
Association**
P. Kovich, Executive Director
P.O. Box 1709
3rd Floor, 4920 - 47th Street
Yellowknife, Northwest Territories
X1A 2P3

Ontario Hospital Association
Hilary Short, Vice-President
Public Affairs
200 Front Street West
Suite 2800
Toronto, Ontario
M5V 3L1

APPENDIX 7

Summary of Approaches

Table 7

Advantages/Disadvantages

Approach adopted	Advantages	Disadvantages
Statu quo	– Pluralism – Flexibility – Ethical thinking close to reality => practical ethics rather than principle-based ethics	– Complexity of system – Lack of consistency – Lack of coordination – Poor dissemination of information – Sectoral approach to ethics – Reactive, rarely forward looking
National Ethics Committee	– Stability => continuity in thinking – Approach is forward looking rather than reactive – Independence – Greater legitimacy because institutionalized – High profile; international recognition – Long-term educational role much more effective – Referral body acts as buffer between political level, judiciary, and public opinion – Able to take broader approach to positions adopted – Over time, group dynamics and work become increasingly effective and efficient provided that a membership renewal process is in place to prevent sclerosis or control by a clique * if objective = examining ethics issues raised by research or publicly funded sectors => such a committee an advantage	– Centralization – Can fall out of touch with local reality; discussion theoretical – Difficulty functioning within federal system – Perceived as hegemony – Risk of infiltration and control by clique of ethical thinking – Difficult to implement opinions, especially when impact on medical practice can be anticipated – risk of self-justification to perpetuate itself; these types of organizations do everything possible to take on missions that are not necessarily within their terms of reference – Danger of becoming transformed into an empty shell without adequate resources

Table 7 (cont.)

Approach adopted	Advantages	Disadvantages
National Ethics Body	– More flexible structure – Implementation based on needs – Effectiveness – Specificity (when *ratione materiae*) => plus in-depth deliberation on specific topics * If objective = review of general issues requiring quick assessment => this type of structure useful	– Sectoral approach to ethics – Lack of continuity – Follow-up on work = often leads nowhere – Over time, scope and content of conclusions lose force, especially when not followed by official statements of position – Danger of inconsistency between opinions stated by concomitant bodies – Often inexperienced in implementing and organizing this type of structure – Significant expenses and time required each time committee undergoes renewal
Standing Conference of Ethics Bodies	– Flexible structure – Appropriate to federal legal system – Encourages dissemination of information and dialogue – A gathering place	– Difficult to identify members – Organizationally difficult to operate; requires permanent office – Uncertainty about follow-up to discussions – Publicity for meetings and work often depends on chance circumstances

Series
Canada Health Action: Building on the Legacy
Papers Commissioned by the National Forum on Health

Volume 1
Determinants of Health
Children and Youth

Jane Bertrand
Enriching the Preschool Experiences of Children

Paul D. Steinhauer
Developing Resiliency in Children from Disadvantaged Populations

David A. Wolfe
Prevention of Child Abuse and Neglect

Christopher Bagley and Wilfreda E. Thurston
Decreasing Child Sexual Abuse

Barbara A. Morrongiello
Preventing Unintentional Injuries among Children

Benjamin H. Gottlieb
Strategies to Promote the Optimal Development of Canada's Youth

Paul Anisef
Making the Transition from School to Employment

Pamela C. Fralick and Brian Hyndman
Youth, Substance Abuse and the Determinants of Health

Gaston Godin and Francine Michaud
STD and AIDS Prevention among Young People

Tullio Caputo and Katharine Kelly
Improving the Health of Street/Homeless Youth

Series
Canada Health Action: Building on the Legacy
Papers Commissioned by the National Forum on Health

Volume 2

Determinants of Health

Adults and Seniors

William R. Avison
The Health Consequences of Unemployment

Mary J. Breen
Promoting Literacy, Improving Health

Neena L. Chappell
Maintaining and Enhancing Independence and Well-Being in Old Age

Sandra O'Brien Cousins
Promoting Active Living and Healthy Eating among Older Canadians

Victor W. Marshall and Philippa J. Clarke
Facilitating the Transition from Employment to Retirement

Dr. Robyn Tamblyn and Dr. Robert Perreault
Encouraging the Wise Use of Prescription Medication by Older Adults

Daphne Nahmiash
*Preventing, Reducing and Stopping the Abuse and Neglect of Older Canadian
Adults in Canadian Communities*

Series
Canada Health Action: Building on the Legacy
Papers Commissioned by the National Forum on Health

Volume 3
Determinants of Health
Settings and Issues

Susan A. McDaniel
Toward Healthy Families

Kathryn J. Bennett and David R. Offord
Schools, Mental Health and Life Quality

Michael F. D. Polanyi, Joan Eakin, John W. Frank, Harry S. Shannon and Terrence Sullivan
Creating Healthier Work Environments: A Critical Review of the Health Impacts of Workplace Change

Kimberly A. Scott
Balance as a Method to Promote Healthy Indigenous Communities

Pierre Hamel
Community Solidarity and Local Development: A New Perspective for Building Sociopolitical Compromise

Joseph Zayed and Luc Lefebvre
Environmental Health: From Concept to Reality

Marlies Sudermann and Peter G. Jaffe
Preventing Violence: School- and Community-Based Strategies

Ronald J. Dyck, Brian L. Mishara and Jennifer White
Suicide in Children, Adolescents and Seniors: Key Findings and Policy Implications

John Lord and Peggy Hutchison
Living with a Disability in Canada: Toward Autonomy and Integration

Benjamin H. Gottlieb
Protecting and Promoting the Well-Being of Family Caregivers

Peter A. Singer and Douglas K. Martin
Improving Dying in Canada

Terrence Sullivan, Okuri Uneke, John Lavis, Doug Hyatt and John O'Grady
Labour Adjustment Policy and Health: Considerations for a Changing World

Lars Osberg
Economic Policy Variables and Population Health

Series
Canada Health Action: Building on the Legacy
Papers Commissioned by the National Forum on Health

Volume 4
Striking a Balance
Health Care Systems in Canada and Elsewhere

Geoffroy Scott
International Comparison of the Hospital Sector

Astrid Brousselle
Controlling Health Expenditures: What Matters

Wendy Kennedy
Managing Pharmaceutical Expenditures: How Canada Compares

Centre for International Statistics
Health Spending and Health Status: An International Comparison

Damien Contandriopoulos
How Canada's Health Care System Compares with that of Other Countries: An Overview

Delphine Arweiler
International Comparisons of Health Expenditures

Marc-André Fournier
The Impact of Health Care Infrastructures and Human Resources on Health Expenditures

Ellen Leibovich, Howard Bergman and François Béland
Health Care Expenditures and the Aging Population in Canada

Raisa Deber and Bill Swan
Puzzling Issues in Health Care Financing

Terrence Sullivan
Commentary on Health Care Expenditures, Social Spending and Health Status

Allan M. Maslove
National Goals and the Federal Role in Health Care

Raiser Deber, Lutchmie Narine, Pat Baranek et al.
The Public-Private Mix in Health Care

John Marriott and Ann L. Mable
Integrated Models: International Trends and Implications for Canada

Steven G. Morgan
Issues for Canadian Pharmaceutical Policy

Series
Canada Health Action: Building on the Legacy
Papers Commissioned by the National Forum on Health

Volume 5
Making Decisions
Evidence and Information

Joan E. Tranmer, Susan Squires, Kevin Brazil, Jacquelyn Gerlach,
John Johnson, Dianne Muisiner, Bill Swan, Dr. Ruth Wilson
Factors That Influence Evidence-Based Decision Making

Paul Fisher, Marcus J. Hollander, Thomas MacKenzie, Peter Kleinstiver,
Irina Sladecek, Gail Peterson
Decision Support Tools in Health Care

Charlyn Black
Building a National Health Information Network

Robert B. Butcher
Foundations for Evidence-Based Decision Making

Carol Kushner and Michael Rachlis
*Civic Lessons: Strategies to Increase Consumer Involvement in
Health Policy Development*

Frank L. Graves and Patrick Beauchamp (EKOS Research Associates Inc.);
David Herle (Earnscliffe Research and Communications)
Research on Canadian Values in Relation to Health and the Health Care System

Thérèse Leroux, Sonia Le Bris, Bartha Maria Knoppers, with
the collaboration of Louis-Nicolas Fortin and Julie Montreuil
*The Feasibility of a National Canadian Advisory Committee on Ethics:
Points to Consider*

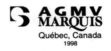

AGMV
MARQUIS
Québec, Canada
1998